health

for life 2

HEALTH EDUCATION IN THE PRIMARY SCHOOL

A TEACHER'S GUIDE TO THREE KEY TOPICS:

The World of Drugs

Keeping Myself Safe

Me and My Relationships

Project team:

Trefor Williams

Noreen Wetton

Alysoun Moon

HEALTH EDUCATION AUTHORITY

THE HEALTH EDUCATION AUTHORITY'S PRIMARY SCHOOL PROJECT

Nelson

Thomas Nelson and Sons Ltd
Nelson House   Mayfield Road
Walton-on-Thames   Surrey
KT12 5PL   UK

51 York Place
Edinburgh
EH1 3JD   UK

Thomas Nelson (Hong Kong) Ltd
Toppan Building 10/F
22A Westlands Road
Quarry Bay   Hong Kong

Distributed in Australia by

Thomas Nelson Australia
102 Dodds Street
South Melbourne   Victoria 3205

and in Sydney, Brisbane, Adelaide and Perth

Nelson Canada
1120 Birchmount Road
Scarborough Ontario
M1K 5G4   Canada

© Health Education Authority 1989
First published by Thomas Nelson and Sons Ltd 1989

ISBN 0-17-423113-X

NPN 9 8 7 6 5 4

Printed and bound in Hong Kong

Contents

How To Use This Guide

This book accompanies *Health for Life 1: A teacher's planning guide to health education in the primary school.*

Health for Life 1 provides you with a lifestyles approach to health education. It enables you to plan the content and sequence of your own programme(s) in a way that will meet the particular needs of your pupils, their families and communities. *Health for Life 1* covers all the key health education topics in a holistic way which will enable you to develop children's awareness of their own and other people's healthy lifestyles. It provides opportunities for you to focus on areas such as growing, growing up, keeping safe, family relationships, healthy eating, healthy environments and the world of drugs.

Health for Life 2 provides a more detailed approach to the three key topics which most often cause parental and public concern:

- **The World of Drugs**
- **Keeping Myself Safe**
- **Me and My Relationships**

Health for Life 2 provides you with a wide range of classroom strategies and activities on these topics. As sensitive issues may arise naturally from these sessions with the children, suggestions are given to help you tackle them in ways appropriate to your class. The strategies are designed both to extend children's understanding and knowledge and enhance their sense of personal responsibility.

Ideally the two books should be used together. *Health for Life 1* will help you plan your broad health education programme and integrate it into the curriculum. *Health for Life 2* will help you to focus on the three key topics.

Health for Life 2 provides an individual programme for each of the three topics consisting of planning materials as well as activities. However, this structure has been designed only to be a guide, and it is to be hoped that each school will adapt the programme to its individual needs and the cultural background of its pupils, make its own decision about when and how to introduce sensitive aspects of the three topics, and choose the materials (which are themselves often subject to contention) which it feels are appropriate.

Many areas of health education which are concerned with issues which some people (not necessarily the children) find sensitive are not always well understood. There is often anxiety among parents, teachers, health professionals and others that children are being introduced to topics too soon, that this will encourage them to experiment, that it will frighten them, or that they will ask questions which adults prefer not to, or feel unable to answer. Some adults plead for schools to preserve childhood innocence for as long as possible, or will deny that young children are daily acquiring 'knowledge' of these issues and making their own sense of them. However, it is erroneous to believe that we can keep children totally innocent in a world dominated by the media. Also, children do have perceptions, misconceptions, and their own unique explanations, of life, death, family life and relationships, sexuality, danger, ways of keeping safe and the world of drugs and the authors take the attitude that it is wise not to ignore these.

The framework of *Health for Life 2* like *Health for Life 1* draws on the results of the Health Education Authority's Primary School Project. The original accounts of the investigations which form the basis of **The World of Drugs, Keeping Myself Safe** and **Me and my Relationships** are published in *The Way in – Five Key Areas of Health Education* by D T Williams, N M Wetton and A M H Moon (Health Education Authority, 1989). The Project investigated children's perceptions of many different aspects of health and health related activities. It sought to identify the changing patterns and trends in these perceptions and to chart some of the underlying explanations. A range of Draw and Write Investigation Techniques, were developed for this purpose which you might like to use. (A guide to their administration and analysis is given in Appendix 1, see page 410.) The analysis of the original investigation results revealed:

- the amount of knowledge the children already had, which comprised health messages, misconceptions, and stereotyped views.

- how they had manipulated newly-acquired information to fit what they already knew.

- how they used language to explain what they knew.

Ideally, you should use the technique with a group of children before you finally decide on your programmes. This will enable you to start from the perceptions, attitudes and information the children bring to their own learning, and to build on this. You can also use the technique again, at the end of a programme, as one way of evaluating the impact of the work you have done with the children.

This book is divided into three sections, one for each topic. Each section contains:

– A photocopiable Scope and Sequence Chart;

– Classroom Strategies and Activities;

– four photocopiable Action Planners, one for each age range;

– and a set of photocopiable Family Worksheet Masters.

The Scope and Sequence Charts are non-prescriptive frameworks which will help you plan programmes for each topic which will suit the needs of your school. You can use the charts in a number of different ways for both short- and long-term planning. For example, they can be used:

– as a guide to help you record what has been taught in order to avoid non-productive repetition, and ensure the continuity of the spiral curriculum.

– as a starting point for consultation with teachers, parents and health professionals.

– as a basis for discussion with feeder schools and schools to which the children will eventually go.

There are three main strands in the chart which run across the whole primary age range (4–11):

1 Children's changing perceptions.
2 Suggested programme content.
3 Suggested skills and strategies.

Each of these strands is an essential component of a successful health education programme. Although the first strand of the Scope and Sequence Chart is based on the results of the Project investigations, you may feel that they are not matched by the perceptions of the children you teach. To remedy any inconsistencies you may find, it is recommended that you investigate the perceptions of your class using the technique mentioned above.

The second strand provides a range of starting points for activities with each age range. This incorporates a number of themes which are developed step-by-step in the programme as the child moves up the school, so all new learning is based upon previous work.

The third strand summarises some of the skills which will enable children to explore their own perceptions and apply the new health information they have learnt.

There are four Action Planners for each topic, one for each age range: 4 and 5, 6 and 7, 8 and 9, and 10 and 11. Each one consists of a series of content boxes which, like the Scope and Sequence Chart, provide starting points for activities, but in more detail. Each content box is composed of a series of questions a child might ask on a specific theme.

The Classroom Strategies and Activities for each age range usually start with the kinds of answers children are likely to give to these questions and then build on what they know. The classroom activities include spoken and written language work and role-play and highlight cross-curricular links, and opportunities for family involvement. You can either use the classroom strategies or activites as they stand, modify them according to your needs, or even create your own using the Scope and Sequence Chart, Key Message lists and Action Planners for guidance.

The Key Messages lists precede the Classroom Strategies and Activities, and provide an easy-to-check guide to the health education 'targets' which they tackle. These targets are sub-divided into skills, or aspects of health, which the children need either to *learn*, or to *practise* or to *understand*.

Finally there is a set of photocopiable worksheets for each topic. These vary in difficulty to cater for all abilities but they are not age-labelled because of the variations in ability within each age range. The worksheets were written so children could explore health education with their families. They can be used with teachers, or by the children alone; but their use creates an effective and valuable channel for school-parent communication.

Health for Life 2 reiterates the major themes of *Health for Life 1*:

- health education is most likely to be effective in a school which sees itself, and is seen as, a community actively seeking to promote health.

- health education is achieved when it is taught as an on-going progressive programme, integrated into the main curriculum in which health topics are visited and revisited in increasingly complex and demanding ways as the child matures, and in which new information always builds on previous experience and understanding.

- children bring to their own health education a wealth of skills, knowledge and 'health messages'. It is from their contribution that any relevant programme must start.

Part One
The World of Drugs

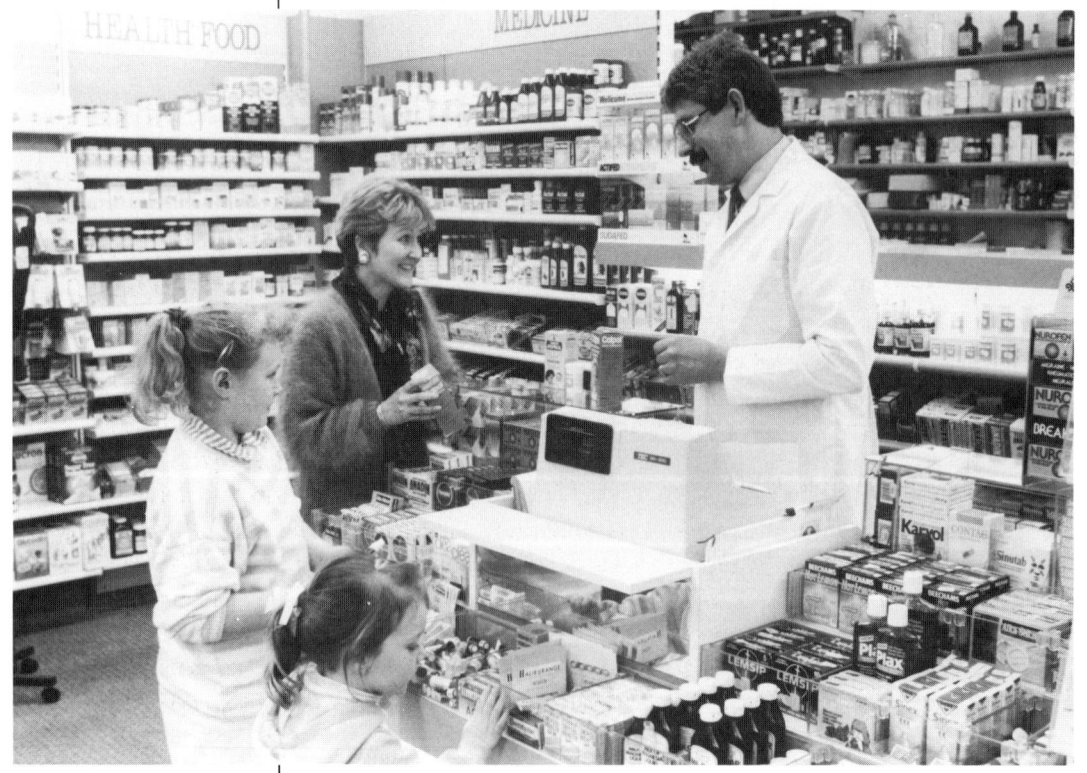

Introduction

● *Why we need drug education*

The **World of Drugs** has been written to help you plan and implement a drug education programme in your school. The reaction of most primary school teachers to the prospect of attempting such work is, understandably, cautious yet positive. Most are aware of the need to do 'something' and realise the need for a sensitive yet unambiguous approach at a time when drug misuse and abuse is increasing.

There remains, however, a tiny minority of people who resist the introduction of even a sensitive drug education programme, basing their judgement upon their own feelings and beliefs rather than upon fact. Often, such opposition to 'drug education' finds expression in comments such as:

- 'We don't need drug education in our school.'
- 'Teaching children about drugs encourages experimentation.'
- 'Our children are far too young to deal with this topic.'
- 'It will frighten them.'
- 'Let's preserve their innocence a little longer.'
- 'We haven't got a drug problem in our community.'
- 'Parents and families don't want drug education.'
- 'Many parents smoke and drink – teaching children about drugs will cause problems.'

These comments fail to recognise that children live in a world where drugs have become commonplace and are used legally and illegally, in both a social context, for example, tobacco, alcohol, tea and coffee, and in a medical context as prescribed and non-prescribed drugs.

Even young children have already begun to build up a store of knowledge, attitudes and experiences related to the world of drugs. Our own extensive research amongst children aged 4–11 has shown that they do have their own perceptions of drugs which are frequently erroneous and focused on their misuse. The analysis of the responses of approximately 2000 children aged four to eleven (known as *Jugs and Herrings*, the results of the drugs investigation of the Health Education Authority's Primary School Project) provides a fascinating insight into children's perceptions of the world of drugs, and provides the basis of the Scope and Sequence Chart, Action Planners and Classroom Strategies and Activities which follow.

These results show that by the age of 6, children formed the view that the world of drugs is bad and dangerous. This gradually replaces their earlier view of drugs as medicines. From this age onwards, the children steadily acquired knowledge of illegal, abused and misused drugs.

The children were beginning to develop a stereotyped view of illegal drug users and drug sellers sometimes as early as 6 years old. This remained until the age of 11, widening at around the age of 9 to include depressed, unhappy people. The stereotype is usually an older, easily identifiable male who intends both to take drugs and to persuade others to use and buy them.

At about the age of nine, some children worried that friends might try to persuade them to take drugs. The notions of the long-term effects of drug abuse and addiction to drugs developed more slowly, although the words 'addict' and 'hooked' were used around the age of 8–9.

The children's understanding of the role of drugs as medicines which can alleviate or cure illnesses was slow to develop and was difficult for them to accept if they had previously equated the word 'drugs' with illegal drug abuse. The ability to see the two sides of the issue was slow to emerge.

Children seemed to be aware of cigarettes and alcohol from about the age of 6, although these were not necessarily seen as drugs in themselves. At around the age of 8 or 9, children did not mention them much which was surprising considering their increasing awareness of illegal drugs. This may have been because they were starting to experiment with them, or that they are aware of their use by adults who do not fit their stereotyped view of drug users.

It was clear that the children made their own sense out of what they heard, saw or experienced in connection with drugs. There appeared to be little difference in the response of children from different social, ethnic or geographical groups.

Our investigations into parents' views revealed a widely-held desire that schools help children understand the drugs issue. Indeed, it is now widely accepted that schools have a responsibility to provide children with a sound understanding of the skills they need to cope with the pressures of everyday life.

The word 'drugs', as it is popularly used, refers to dangerous and harmful substances, rather than to the substances which doctors and nurses refer to as 'drugs'. In the **World of Drugs**, we take a broad view and present drug education as something which should enable children to choose a healthy and happy lifestyle in a world where drugs are used for many good purposes, but are also being misused and abused.

We have concluded from our research findings that a successful drug education programme for children must have four vital characteristics:
- the focus of the programme should be upon the children themselves, and their knowledge, feelings, attitudes and decision-making capabilities, rather than on facts about drugs.

- the programme should be supported by the whole school, including staff and health professionals.

— the programme should be supported by and involve parents at every step, to ensure that drug education provided at school is reinforced by the home.

— the programme should have the support of the wider community.

This type of drug education programme is, therefore, holistic in its approach. It is less concerned with teaching children *about* drugs, than with helping them, as growing and developing individuals, to understand how they can make responsible *decisions* about the increasing range of drugs that are already available to them.

Investigating children's perceptions of drugs in the classroom

Whether you or your colleagues are deciding on the content of your drug education programme (*Health for Life 1* will help you do this) or you are using the Scope and Sequence Chart provided in this book, it is up to the individual teacher to assume the role of mediator and decide what information is appropriate for his or her group, and how to provide learning experiences which will communicate it.

The best way to do this is to discover what the children already know, or think they know, about drugs, and start from there. The investigation method adopted by the Project Team for research into children's perceptions of drugs was a Draw and Write Technique. This is easy for the teacher to organise in the classroom and will reveal the children's knowledge of specific topics, and will provide a rich source of background knowledge from which starting points for the work will emerge. By using this technique before and after teaching the children, it is possible to chart the children's progress.

The analysis of the children's work can either be done quickly and simply to provide a quick overview of the children's perceptions, or, extensively, to provide a detailed picture of their thoughts and ideas. Full details of the technique and suggestions for its administration and analysis are given in Appendix 1 on page 410.

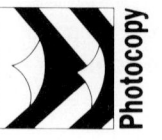

Photocopy

The World of Drugs
Scope and Sequence Chart

Age	Children's changing perceptions of drugs	Suggested programme content	Suggested skills and strategies
4 & 5	The word 'drugs' doesn't mean much to us. We think drugs are the medicines which grown-ups use, especially doctors and nurses.	What goes onto and into my body? When should I say 'No'? When should I ask for help? Who can I trust? What are medicines, pills and injections? Where do we find unsafe substances? Which everyday substances can be harmful? For example, tobacco, sprays, liquids How can I get to know my feelings?	*Language skills:* Talking Listening Reading Writing Describing Vocabulary Categorising Illustration and presentation *General skills:* Empathy Decision making Observing Classroom play
6 & 7	We still think of drugs as medicines, but the world of drugs is already becoming a bad and frightening place for us. Some of us even mention cocaine and heroin. Some of us think cigarettes are part of the 'drug scene' which we associate with 'baddies', teenagers and criminals.	What goes onto and into my body? What happens to the substances which enter my body? When should I say 'No'? When should I ask for help? Where do we find medicines and drugs? Which drugs are contained in cigarettes and certain drinks?	*Language skills:* Talking Listening Reading Writing Vocabulary Categorising Illustration and presentation *General Skills:*

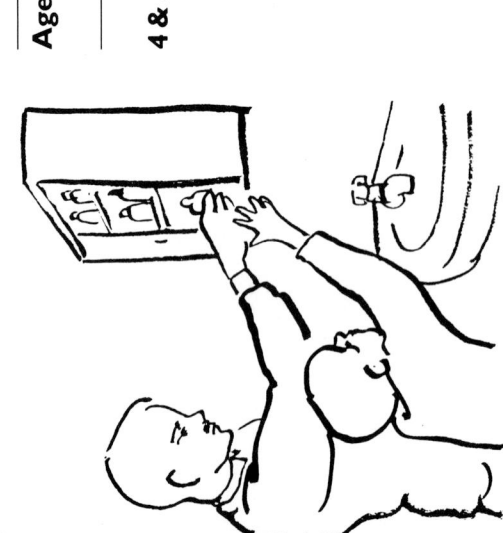

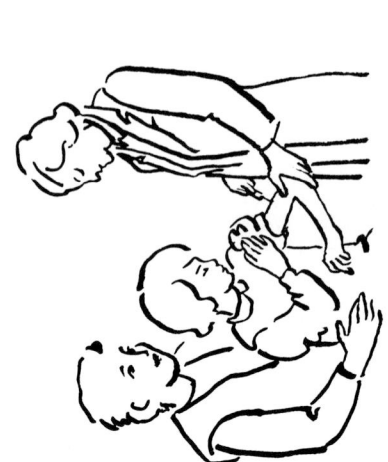

Classroom Strategies and Activities for Ages 4 – 11

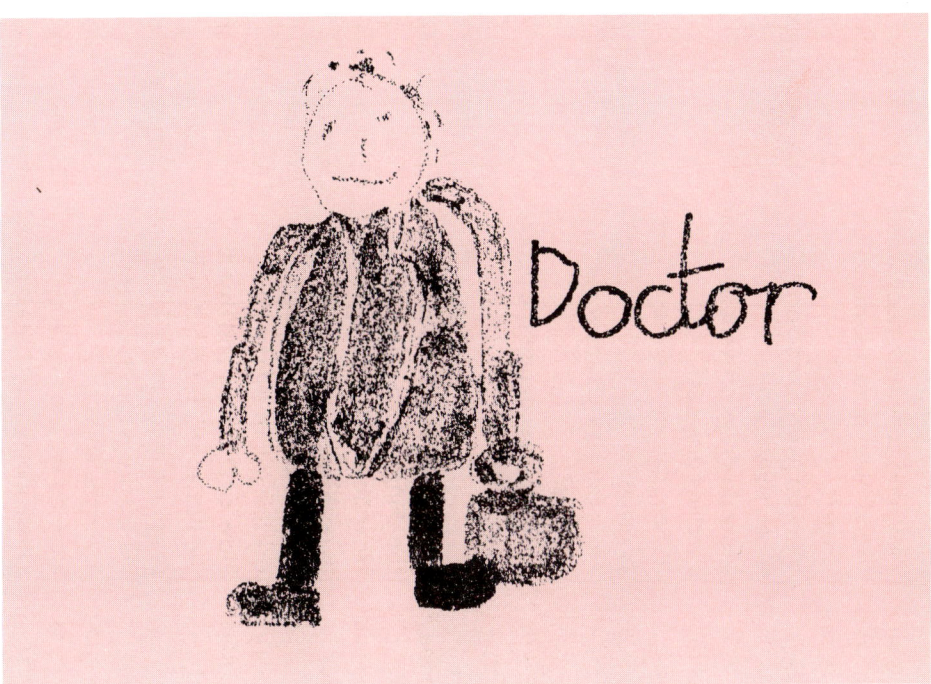

The activities in the following pages are based on the content boxes from the four Action Planners for ages 4 and 5, 6 and 7, 8 and 9 and 10 and 11. There are five or six content boxes in each Action Planner, each of which has a distinctive theme, the main themes are:

- What goes into my body?
- What goes onto my body?
- Who needs drugs and medicines?
- Injections
- Feeling ill and feeling better
- Smoking
- Where are drugs found?

The content boxes suggest questions which are explored in detail in the activities. It is important that you select and modify these activities according to your needs. If you are devising your own drug education programme you may be well aware of the health education priorities of your school and may already have selected the key themes you wish to explore with your pupils. If this is the case, you may find that the following activities are useful as examples, alternatively, you may wish to incorporate them as they stand in your programme.

We are naming more drugs and using words such as 'inject'. We know people sell drugs. We see drugs as dangerous and illegal, and don't mention their legitimate use very much. We think cigarettes are part of the 'drug' scene. We think we would recognise people involved with drugs.

How do I cope with people and friends who persuade me to try drugs?
Why do people need drugs when they are ill?
How do drugs prevent us from catching diseases?
Where can we find these types of drugs?
How can I get to know my feelings?
How can I recognise the people I can trust?

Empathy
Group work
Classroom play
Decision making

8 & 9

We are beginning to learn the 'street names' of drugs. We know that drugs are sniffed and injected and that people buy them from 'pushers' and 'dealers'. We think this is very bad. We have stereotyped ideas of the people involved with drugs.

We know about drug-taking equipment such as needles and syringes, and we know more of the drug-taking language. We are beginning to be aware of the financial gain from drug dealing, addiction and addicts. We think of drug users as sad, depressed people who are usually male, criminal and with a bearded or 'punk' appearance.

How does my body deal with the things which enter it?
How do medicinal drugs make us healthy?
How does my body deal with any dangerous substances?
How can I understand that all medicines are drugs but not all drugs are medicines?
Which drugs can be bought 'over the counter'?
How do we use everyday substances which contain drugs?
Where are medicinal drugs made, tested, prescribed, bought, sold and used?
In which places around us are medicines kept safely, or not so safely?
What kind of people need drugs to live a normal life?
Which drugs help us to recover from or avoid illness?
What kind of people might persuade me to take medicinal or non-medicinal drugs?
What can I say to them?
Who can I trust?
How can I confide in them?

Language Skills:
Talking
Listening
Reading
Writing
Vocabulary
Illustration and presentation
Categorising
Survey interpretation

General skills:
Decision making
Empathy
Coping with peer pressure
Personal responsibility
Role-play
Group skills

feelings?
How can I tell when people use drugs (particularly tobacco or alcohol) to feel grown up?

10 & 11 When asked we can see the possible advantages of drugs as medicines but usually we think of the world of drugs as a bad thing. Seeing two sides of a question is not easy for us. We are becoming aware of the long-term effects of addiction. We know coffee and anti-depressants are addictive, but are not too happy about labelling cigarettes and alcohol in that way. Some of us may fear that our friends will tempt us to try drugs, but most of us cling to our stereotyped view that drug users are older, 'punky' and male.

We are more aware of the long-term effects of drug taking. We still think drugs are illegal, and find it difficult to accept that they can be helpful. We are aware that coffee is a drug of some kind, but don't include cigarettes, alcohol or inhalants.

We think of drug users as stereotyped criminals rather than as sick people who need medical attention.

What goes into my body? How do my body systems deal with these things?

Which of these things could be categorised as 'essential', 'non-essential', 'good', 'dangerous', etc.

How do my brain and body systems work together to affect my feelings and behaviour?

What are the risks involved in using alcohol and cigarettes?

How can addiction affect relationships?

How can I learn to make up my own mind about drugs, and not be persuaded by other people?

Why can some drugs make sick people healthy?

How are drugs invented?

Why do some people misuse drugs?

Who or what can help them?

Who are my role models?

What do they think about drugs?

Who might think of me as their role model?

How do I feel about the world of drugs?

What makes me feel good?

What gives me a kick?

Language skills:
Talking
Listening
Reading
Writing
Investigating
Presenting information
Describing
Categorising
Predicting
Summarising

General skills:
Empathy
Observation
Role-play
Coping with peer pressure
Personal responsibility
Group skills
Decision making
Evaluation
Survey interpretation

Action Planner

The World of Drugs

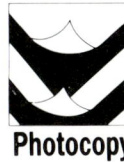

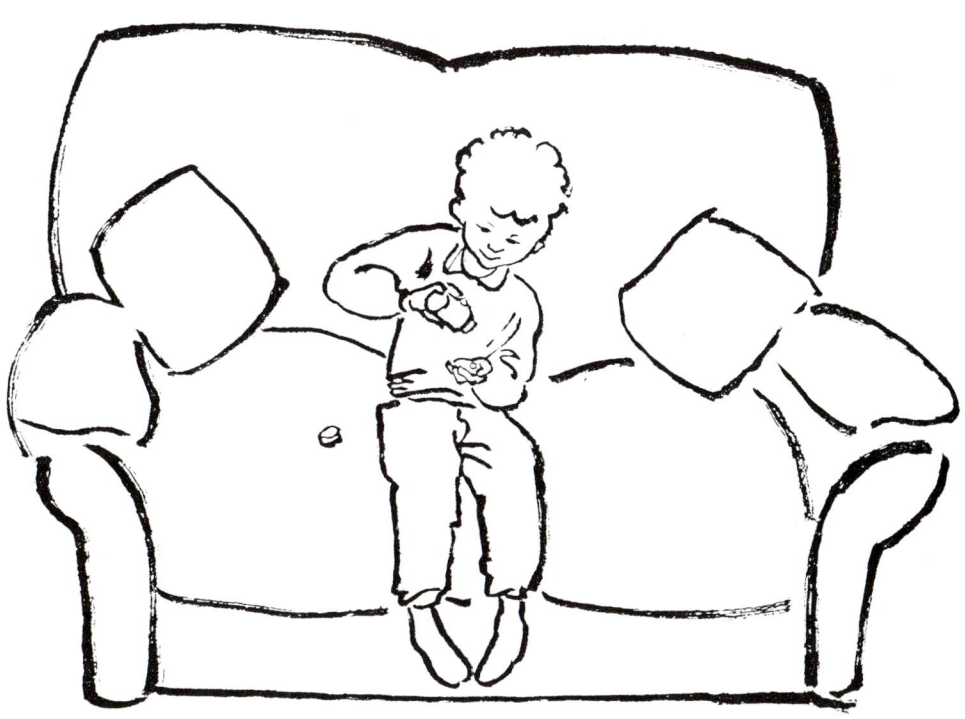

1

What goes onto my body?
How and when does it get there? Who tells me to put it onto my body? What is it for? Which part of my body does it go onto? Do I think it's safe? How does it feel? Do I like it? How do I react? Does it hurt? Should I ask someone about it? Whom do I ask? Whom can I trust? What do I say?

2

What goes into my body?
How does it get in? Who puts it there? Why? Who tells me to put it there? Does it get there on purpose or by accident? How does it feel? taste? look? smell? Do I like it? What do I do if I don't like it, or if it hurts, or if it worries me? What can I say?

3

What is inside my body?
What is under my skin? Where do things go once they get inside me? What happens to them?

4

Who needs medicines?
When have I had to take medicines? Why? Was I ill? Who told me to take the medicine? Was it a safe person? Where did we get the medicine? Was it a safe place? Where did we keep it? Was it a safe place? Who gave it to me? What did it taste like and look like? What did I say? How did I feel at first? How did I feel after a while?

5

What's in here?
Where might medicines and other dangerous things be found? What's under here? What's it for? Who put it there? Do I know what it is? Who does it belong to? Is this a dangerous place to look? What can I say if someone tries to make me touch or taste it? What can I do? Whom can I tell? How do I tell them?

6

How do I feel when I am ill?
How do I look? What do I do? What do I say? What do I ask for? What helps to make me better? Who helps me to get better?

Classroom Strategies and Activities for Ages 4 and 5

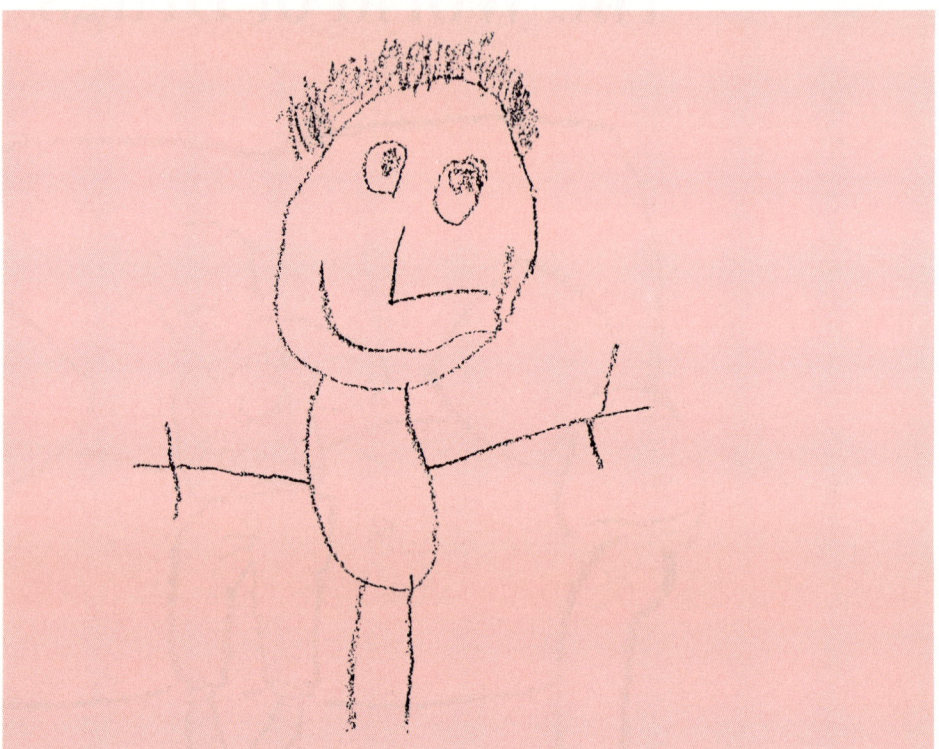

Key messages ● *Learn:*

- what goes onto and into your body.

- when to say 'No' and 'Stop'.

- when to ask for help.

- about medicines, pills and injections.

- about the places where you might find things which aren't safe to touch, taste or sniff.

- about the everyday things which can harm you, for example, tobacco, smoke, sprays, liquids and some drinks.

- about your feelings. Which feelings can you trust?

- who you can trust and confide in.

Content box 1   What goes onto my body?

🔴 How and when does it get there? Who tells me to put it onto my body? What is it for? Which part of my body does it go onto? Do I think it's safe? How does it feel? Do I like it? How do I react? Does it hurt? Should I ask someone about it? Whom do I ask? Whom can I trust? What do I say?

Activity 1 ⚫ ***What goes onto my body?***

- Talking together. Drawing. Writing. Reading.

- Class or group activity.

Make a wall story or large picture of the outline of a child's body. This can either be pinned to the wall or drawn on the blackboard. Write the children's responses to these questions around the outline: 'What goes on my body?', 'Which part of my body do they touch?'

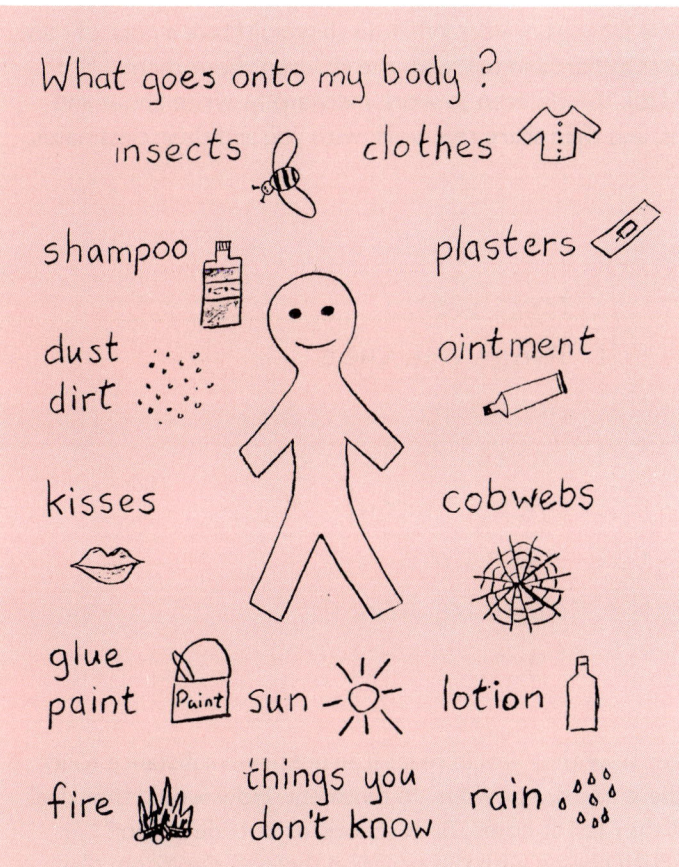

Invite the children to give you their own drawings and pictures cut from magazines which can be added to the larger picture.

Ask the children to categorise (using colour coding) those items which they see in these terms:

– 'OK'.

– 'I'm not sure. I'll ask someone about it'.

– 'It's not OK – so I won't let it touch my body.'

Explore with the children who put these different items onto their bodies. This will involve them in looking for different categories.

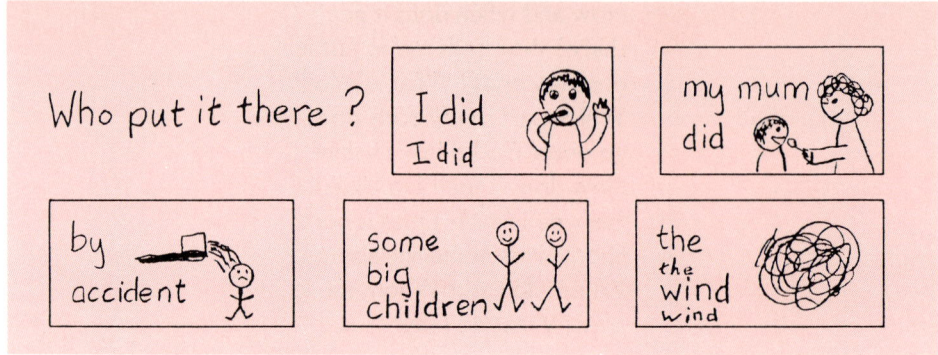

Introduce this type of question to the children: 'If someone tried to force you to put something onto your body what would you do? What would you say?'

Help them to practice saying: 'No.' 'I won't.' 'I'll ask.' 'It's dangerous.'

Activity 2 ● *How does it feel?*

● Talking together. Writing. Drawing. Classroom play

● Class or group activity.

Invite the children to think about how they react to things which touch their bodies. Do they like these feelings or not? What do they do? Make a note of their responses, display them as a chart and talk with the children about them. Alternatively, you could ask the children to work individually, write about and illustrate their reactions, and then share this work with you and their classmates.

> How does it feel ?
> · It feels warm
> · It stings my eyes
> · It tickles
> · It makes me feel good
> · It smells horrid
> · It scares me
> · I rub it in, lick it
> · I cry

Explore with the children how they would react if an unknown substance touched their bodies, for example, a liquid, a powder, an ointment. How would they deal with this? Whom might they tell at home, or at school, or outside school? Encourage them to practice coping with this situation through classroom play.

Content box 2   What goes into my body?

How does it get in? Who puts it there? Why? Who tells me to put it there? Does it get there on purpose or by accident? How does it feel? taste? look? smell? Do I like it? What do I do if I don't like it, or if it hurts, or if it worries me? What can I say?

Activity 1   *What goes into my body?*

- Talking together. Writing. Drawing.
- Class or group activities.

Invite the children to make a second wall picture similar to the one made during the last activity in order to explore 'What goes *into* my body?' Encourage them to include food, drink, dust, smoke, fresh air, sun, sprays, medicines, pills, injections, thorns, splinters, foreign bodies and unknown things. Write the children's responses around the outline.

Invite the children to talk about and illustrate the questions: 'How does it get in?' and 'Who told me to do it?'

Encourage the children to categorise their answers to the question 'How does it get in?' Categories might include:

— the doctor or the nurse;

— by accident;

— on purpose;

— someone told me to.

What goes into my body ?

sweets in my mouth

nose drops in my nose

ear drops in my ears

injections through my skin

Activity 2 ● *How does it feel?*

- Talking together. Drawing. Writing. Classroom play.
- Class or group activities, with some individual work.

Talk with the children about the ways in which they reacted to things entering their bodies.

Did they:

— swallow?

— sniff?

— like it?

— cry?

— sneeze?

— say 'Don't'?

Was it:

— sharp?

— stinging?

— lovely?

— frightening?

Invite the children to illustrate themselves reacting to some of these situations. Add speech bubbles to their pictures in which they can write (or you could write for them) what they said or felt.

Cross-curricular links: you could explore this theme further using language work and classroom play in a similar way to the activities for Content box 1.

Content box 3　What is inside my body?

 What is under my skin? Where do things go once they get inside me? What happens to them?

Activity 1 ● *What is inside my body?*

- Painting and drawing. Talking together.
- Class or group activity.

Ask the children to paint or draw large-sized pictures of themselves which show what they think is under their skin. Talk with them about what they have drawn and how it works.

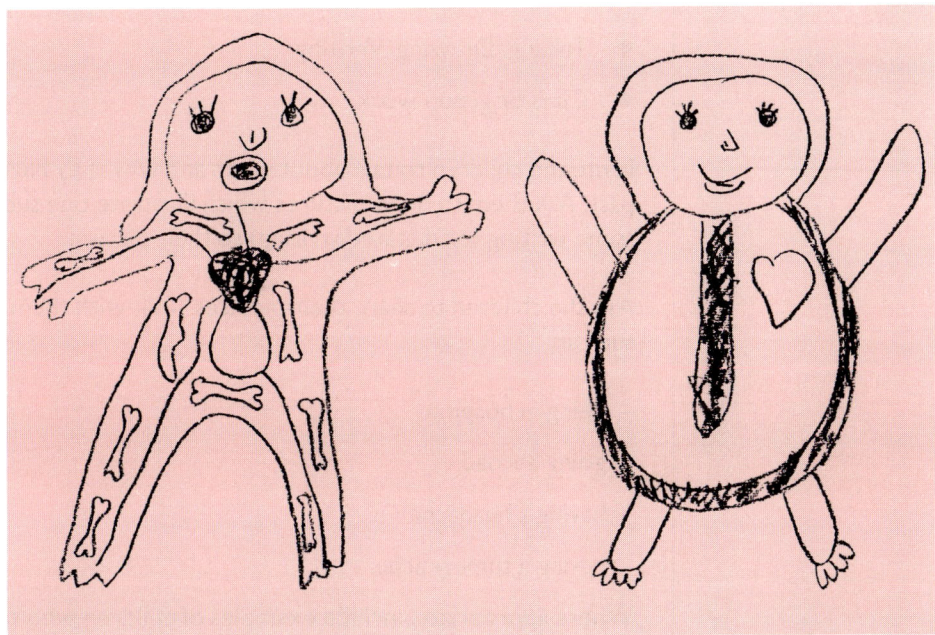

It is particularly interesting to look at their paintings to discover if, and how, they draw the blood circulation system. Does it appear as a single continuous line around the outside of the body? At this stage it is more important to focus on the children's own explanations and drawings, looking closely at what they put in or leave out, rather than to offer them correct diagrams.

Remind the children of the activity in which you all talked about things which entered the body. Ask them to explain or illustrate what they think happens to these things inside their bodies. What do they do? Where do they go?

The children's explanations and the specific words they use could provide you with valuable insights and starting points for offering them new and appropriate information.

Content box 4   Who needs medicines?

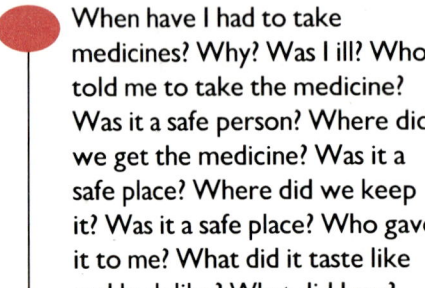 When have I had to take medicines? Why? Was I ill? Who told me to take the medicine? Was it a safe person? Where did we get the medicine? Was it a safe place? Where did we keep it? Was it a safe place? Who gave it to me? What did it taste like and look like? What did I say? How did I feel at first? How did I feel after a while?

Activity 1   *When have I had to take medicines?*

- Talking. Drawing. Writing.
- Class or group work.

Invite the children to talk about when and why they have needed medicines in the past. Ask them to draw pictures which illustrate one such occasion, and to add some writing (or dictated writing) to their picture.

Ask the children to share their pictures. Talk with them about their experiences, such as:

– being in hospital;

– going abroad;

– having a headache;

– having a tummy ache.

Where appropriate, include examples of children who take medicine regularly or who have some medication always on hand, for example, asthmatics.

Activity 2   *Where did the medicines come from?*

- Drawing. Collecting pictures. Writing. Talking.
- Class or group activity with some individual work.

Explore with the children how medicines look, and how they are taken. Ask them to illustrate their responses with their own drawings or using pictures from magazines. Look again at what they said and how they felt and reacted when they had to take medicines.

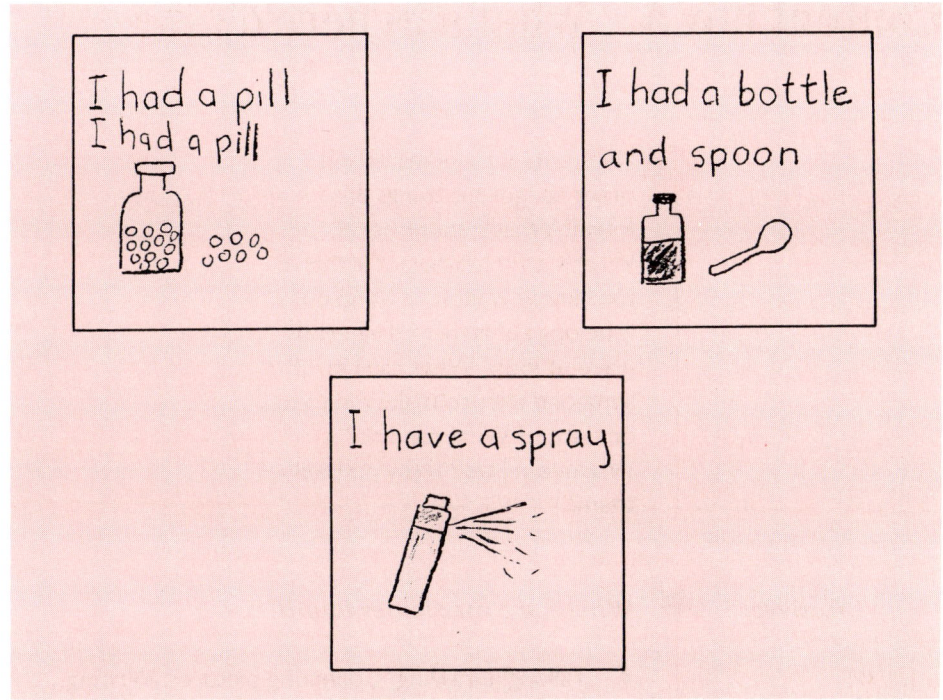

Talk about, and ask them to illustrate and label, their responses to these questions:

— Who gave them the medicines? (For example, my mum, the doctor, the nurse).

— Was this person safe?

— Where did they come from? (For example, the bathroom cupboard, the chemist, my gran's handbag, the shelf in the kitchen, the clinic).

— Are these safe places to keep medicines? You could colour code the children's illustrations to denote which of them represent safe or unsafe situations.

— How did they feel at first when they took the medicine? How did they feel later on?

These activities provide the opportunity to introduce **medicine-wise rules**, such as:

● Don't take any medicines unless they are given to you by your parents, a nurse or a doctor.

● Don't touch other people's medicines.

● Don't touch, taste or take anything just because someone tells you to. If you're not sure, say 'No', 'I won't', 'I'll ask'.

Talk through these rules with the children and help them to learn and practise them. They could then take copies of them home to explain to their **families**. There are **cross-curricular links** with topics which focus on the community and people who help.

Content box 5   What's in here?

 Where might medicines and other dangerous things be found? What's under here? What's it for? Who put it there? Do I know what it is? Who does it belong to? Is this a dangerous place to look? What can I say if someone tries to make me touch or taste it? What can I do? Whom can I tell? How do I tell them?

Activity 1 ● *Where are medicines found?*

- Talking. Drawing. Collecting pictures. Writing.
- Class or group activity.

Talk with the children about the places in and around the home where people put medicines or chemicals. Talk with them about the things they might find:

— on windowsills.

— in bathrooms, in cupboards or on shelves by the side of the bath.

— on tables, bedside shelves or cabinets.

— in handbags, cupboards, first aid boxes, in pockets or glove compartments in cars.

— in garden sheds, garages, storage places and under sinks.

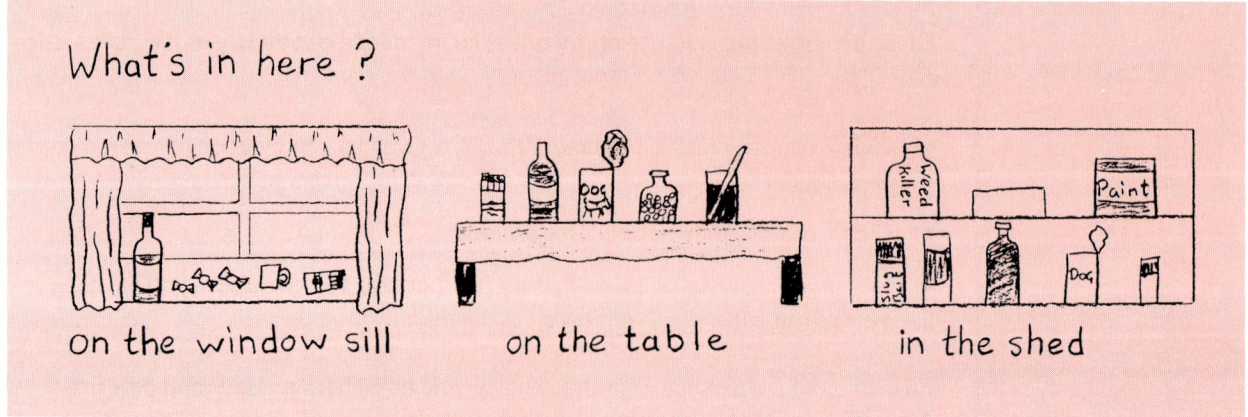

Invite the children to collect pictures of, or to draw pictures of the many things which might be found in these places, and to label them. Add to their responses everyday items such as: sweets, medicines, pills, cigarettes, matches, different kinds of drinks including alcohol, bottles, jars and containers of different kinds, garden and garage materials, sprays, glue, powders, animal food or medication.

Invite the children to explore and categorise these places and items, by answering questions such as:

— 'Who left it there?'

— 'What is it for?'

— 'Is it safe to look in here?'

— 'Is it safe to touch, taste or try this?'

— 'What must I do if I see or find this?'

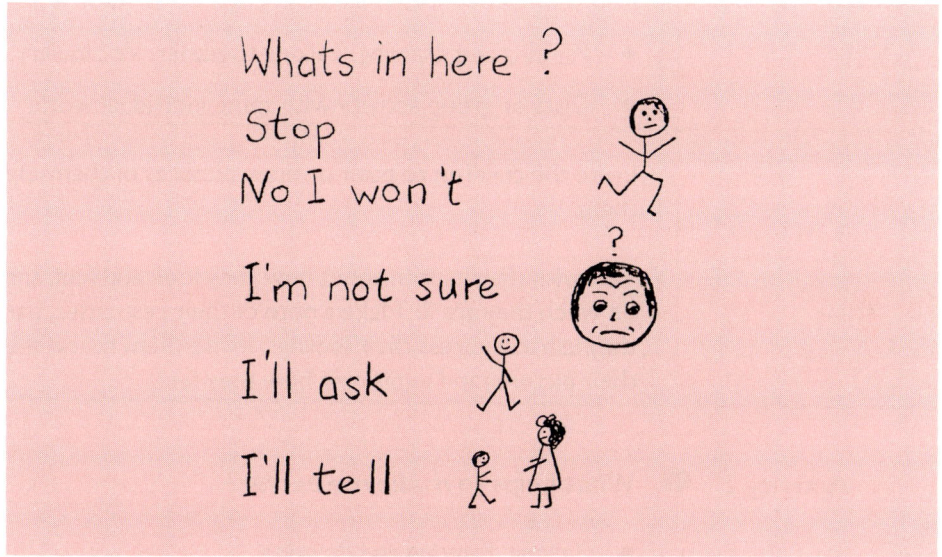

Encourage them to ask of each place and item: 'Is this safe?' 'Should I be careful?', 'Am I sure?', 'Don't touch?', 'Should I ask for help?', 'Should I tell someone?'

Again you could use a simple colour coding system on their pictures to show what is safe and unsafe.

Activity 2 ● *What do I say if someone tries to persuade me?*

● Talking together. Classroom play.

● Class or group activity.

Here it is possible to reinforce the strategies for dealing with persuasion. Ask the children what they think they would say or do if someone tried to pressurize them into touching or tasting something which might not be safe. Help them to practise ways of saying: 'No, I won't'. 'It's dangerous'. 'I'll ask someone'.

The children's work on Content box 5 could be brought together to make a wall story, a class book or individual books which the children could take home to share with their families.

Many of these situations could be explored further using classroom play which is a good way to rehearse coping strategies.

Content box 6   How do I feel when I am ill?

How do I look? What do I do?
What do I say? What do I ask for?
What helps to make me better?
Who helps me to get better?

Activity 1 ● *How do I feel when I am ill?*

- Painting and drawing. Talking together. Vocabulary.

- Class or group activity with some individual work.

Invite the children to paint or draw pictures of themselves feeling ill and to display them.

Talk with the children about how they look and feel, and what they do or cannot do when they are ill. Make a note of their responses, particularly the vocabulary they use to express their feelings. Invite them to use this vocabulary by adding it to their pictures and explaining how they feel.

Activity 2 ● *What helps to make me better?*

- Talking. Painting and drawing.

- Class or group activity.

Explore with the children what they think makes them feel better. What do they ask for apart from medication? For example, love, company and rest. Who provides this? Explore through painting, drawing and talking how the children think they look when they are better. What do they do, say and feel? Again, make a note of their vocabulary. It could be valuable to end by looking at what the children think they did to help themselves get well.

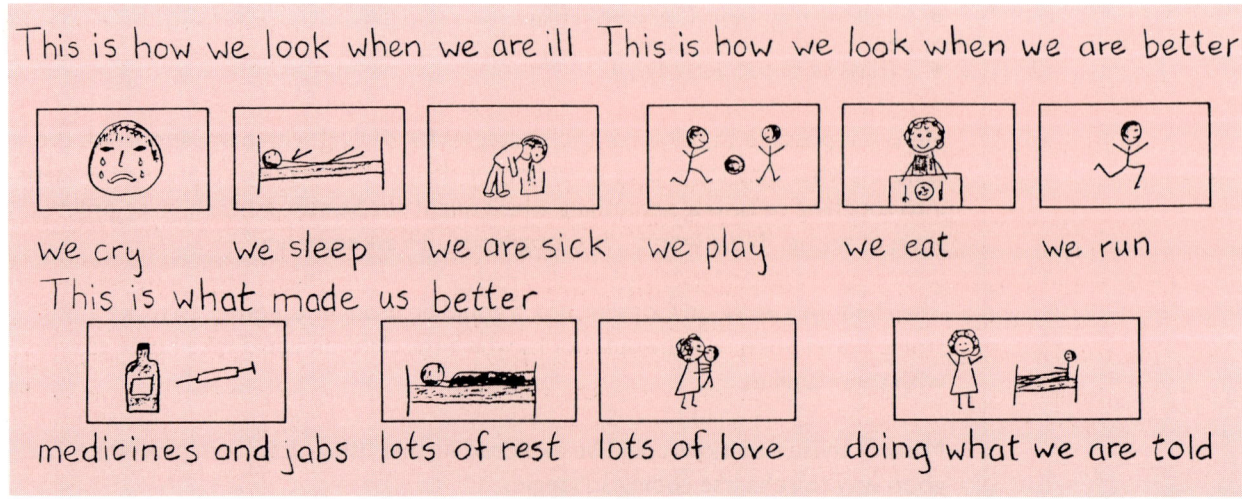

Action Planner
The World of Drugs

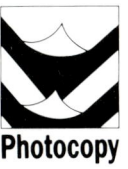

Photocopy

1

What goes into my body?
Can I name these things? Do other people have different names for them? How do they get in? Who puts them there? Who tells me to put them into my body? What is the difference between 'accidently' and 'on purpose'? Which things are safe and not so safe? When should I say 'No, don't' and 'I'll ask someone'? How do all these different things feel, smell and taste, as they go into my body? What do I say? do? think? Do I like it or not? Do I feel worried or unsure?

2

Where do things go when they enter my body
– through my mouth? through my nose? through my skin? What does my body do with the good, not so good and the dangerous things so I will stay healthy? How can I help to keep myself healthy? What should I do when people tell me to take, taste, puff or try things? How do I know who to trust? How best can I say: 'No, I won't, 'I'll ask'. Who are the people I can ask? tell? talk to?

3

Injections.
When and why do I have injections? For example, to prevent me from becoming ill later on? before I visit another country? in an emergency? an accident? at the dentist? the hospital? so it doesn't hurt so much? to extract some of my blood? What do we call the people whose job it is to do this? How do they do it safely? Where inside me do I think the injection fluid goes? How do I think it gets there?

4

Feeling ill and feeling better.
How do I feel when I'm ill? How do I look and sound? What can I and can't I do? Who and what helps me to get well? How can I help? What kinds of medicinal drugs help us to get well? Who decides whether I need to swallow or sniff them, or have injections? Who tells me what to do? How do I know which people are safe? Where do the medicines come from? Are these safe places? Where do we keep our medicines? Are they in safe places? How do I feel when I'm getting better? How do I feel when I'm well again?

5

What can I do when I'm healthy, happy and well?
How do I feel and look? What are the things I can do everyday, or occasionally, to keep myself healthy? Which people have to take medicinal drugs all the time to keep healthy? What do I need to know about them?

26

Classroom Strategies and Activities for Ages 6 and 7

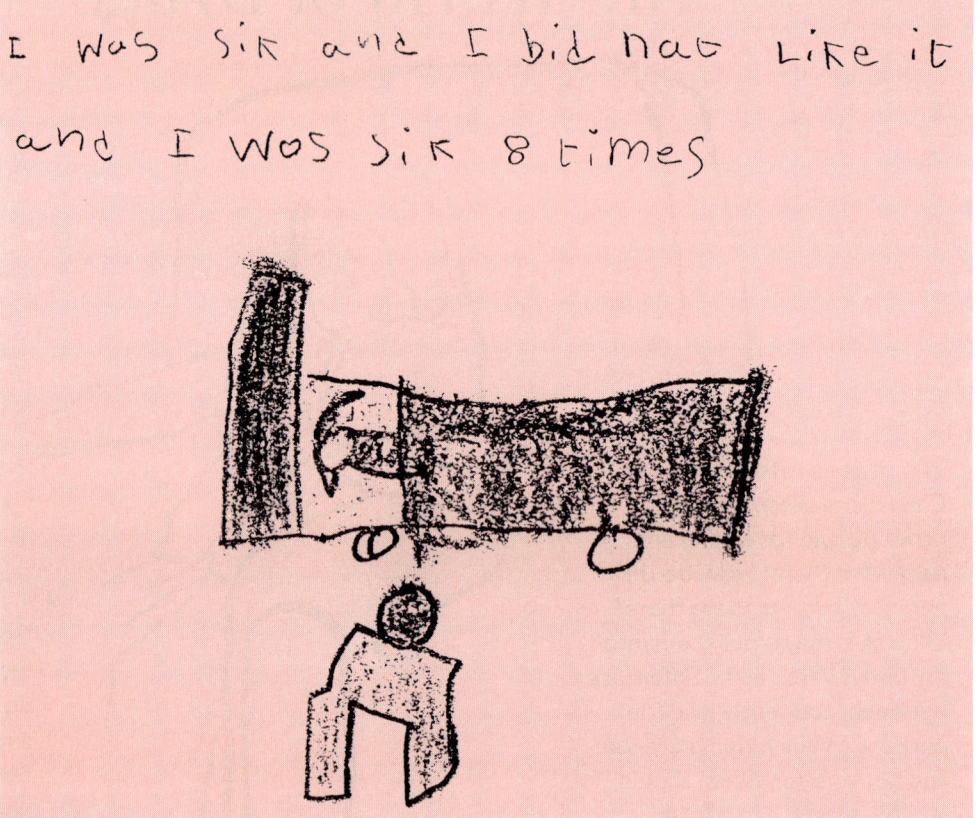

I was sik and I bid nat Like it and I was sik 8 times

Key messages

● *Learn:*

- what goes onto and into your body.

- what happens to things when they enter your body.

- when and how to say: 'No, I won't, 'I'll ask', 'It's OK'.

- about the places where medicines, drugs, dangerous and strange things might be found.

- where and how medicines can be obtained.

- to describe and talk about your feelings.

- which people you can trust.

Understand:

- that cigarettes and alcohol have drugs in them.

- when people or friends are trying to persuade you to touch, taste or sniff strange substances.

- that some people need medicinal drugs to live a normal life or to get well.

- that some drugs prevent us from contracting some diseases.

Content box 1   What goes into my body?

Can I name these things? Do other people have different names for them? How do they get in? Who puts them there? Who tells me to put them into my body? What is the difference between 'accidently' and 'on purpose'? Which things are safe and not so safe? When should I say 'No, don't' and 'I'll ask someone'? How do all these different things feel, smell and taste, as they go into my body? What do I say? do? think? Do I like it or not? Do I feel worried or unsure?

Activity 1

What goes into my body?

- Talking together.
- Class or group activity.

Invite the children, as a class or in groups to suggest as many things as possible which can enter their bodies. Make a note of these as they are suggested. You could talk about items such as: foods, drinks, dirt, dust, germs, cigarette smoke, sunlight, air (fresh and otherwise) sprays, substances which are sniffed or rubbed in, medicines, pills – prescribed and over the counter, injections, thorns, splinters, dirt, foreign bodies from cuts, scratches.

Ask the children to work in small groups, and categorise these items according to the different ways they enter the body, for example, are the items:

– swallowed?

– sniffed or breathed in?

– absorbed or injected through the skin?

The items could be categorised according to the amount of choice the child has. For example, is the item:

– chosen by the child?

– taken into the body automatically?

– chosen by other people who tell the child to take it?

Activity 2 ● *Which things are safe?*

● Talking together. Drawing and writing.

● Class or group activities with some individual work.

The original list of items could be categorised by the children according to whether or not they think they are safe. Ask them to take each item and say whether or not it is:

– good for them?

– not so good for them?

– one which they are not sure about?

– unsafe?

– risky or dangerous?

Children's decisions about the items which belong in any specific category will vary. Encourage them to say why they have categorised the items in a certain way. This will give you an insight into their thinking and provide starting points for introducing new information. The children's ideas can be captured in drawing and writing (or dictated writing) to form:

– a class wall story or display;

– group or class books;

– individual books or folders for the children to explain to their families and add to at home.

Encourage the children to talk about, write about and illustrate their reactions and feelings about all the items which enter their bodies. Write a circle of feelings on the blackboard or large piece of paper which describes their range of reactions.

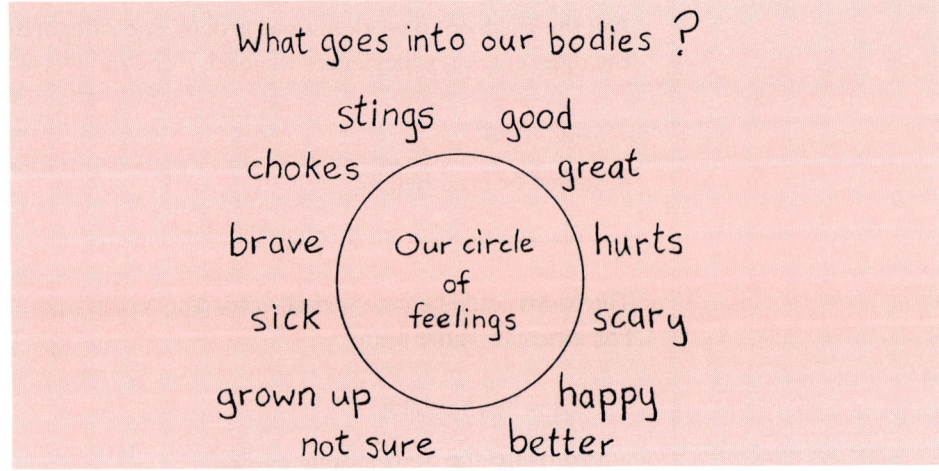

Ask the children to illustrate situations when some of the items mentioned earlier might enter their bodies, for example, mealtimes, outdoor playtimes, parties, snacktimes, visiting friends, taking medicine, after a fall or an accident of some kind.

Suggest they incorporate speech or thought bubbles into their pictures to convey what they said or felt at the time.

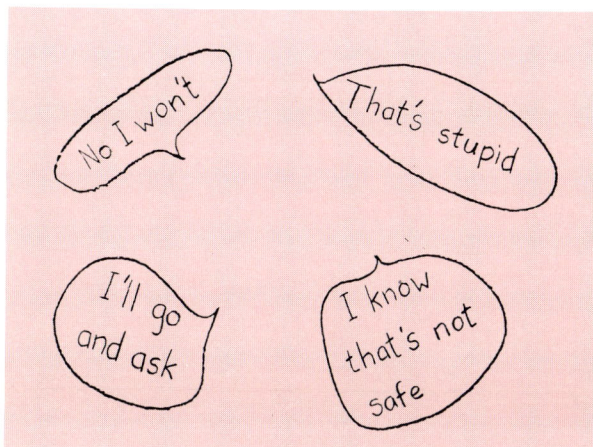

Invite the children to talk about and illustrate in the same way a situation when someone is trying to persuade them to try (taste, smoke or sniff – as appropriate) something dangerous or unknown. What can they say when they are worried, under pressure or unsure?

Make a note of their responses, and display them. Help them to practise them, where possible using the children's own words. Reassure children that telling an adult in these circumstances is a sensible way of behaving.

Encourage the children to explain their work to their **families** and enlist their help.

There are **cross-curricular links** here with:

– science.

– personal safety education.

Content box 2   Where do things go when they enter my body?

Where do things go when they enter through my mouth? through my nose? through my skin? What does my body do with the good, not so good and the dangerous things so I will stay healthy? How can I help to keep myself healthy? What should I do when people tell me to take, taste, puff or try things? How do I know who to trust? How best can I say: 'No, I won't, 'I'll ask'. Who are the people I can ask? tell? talk to?

Activity 1   *Where do things go when they enter my body?*

- Talking. Drawing. Display.
- Individual, and class or group activities.

Remind the children of their previous work on the items which enter their bodies and how they get in. Without further discusssion invite them to draw what they think is inside their bodies.

Invite them to use coloured crayons to show:

— how food or air gets in and where they go.

— how germs from a cut get in and where they go.

— how sunshine gets in and where it goes.

Invite the children to share their ideas with a partner, or in a small group, before coming together as a larger group to pool their ideas and display their pictures.

Investigate in a similar way how the children think their bodies deal with the good and the not so good items which are taken in. You are likely to receive responses such as:

— my body uses the good bits.

— this gives me tummy ache.

— it makes me sick.

— my body fights the germs.

— my body gets rid of the bad bits.

— it makes me cough.

— it makes me feel sleepy.

Children can be asked to illustrate, label and expand on their responses. Once you are aware of the children's perceptions you will be able to see which, and how much, new scientific information is relevant and appropriate.

Some children's concepts of their body systems may be well advanced and they will be ready for a more scientific approach, other children might find such an approach confusing and need more activities.

Activity 2 ● *How can I help to keep myself healthy?*

● Talking. Drawing. Collecting pictures. Classroom play.

● Class or group activities with some individual work.

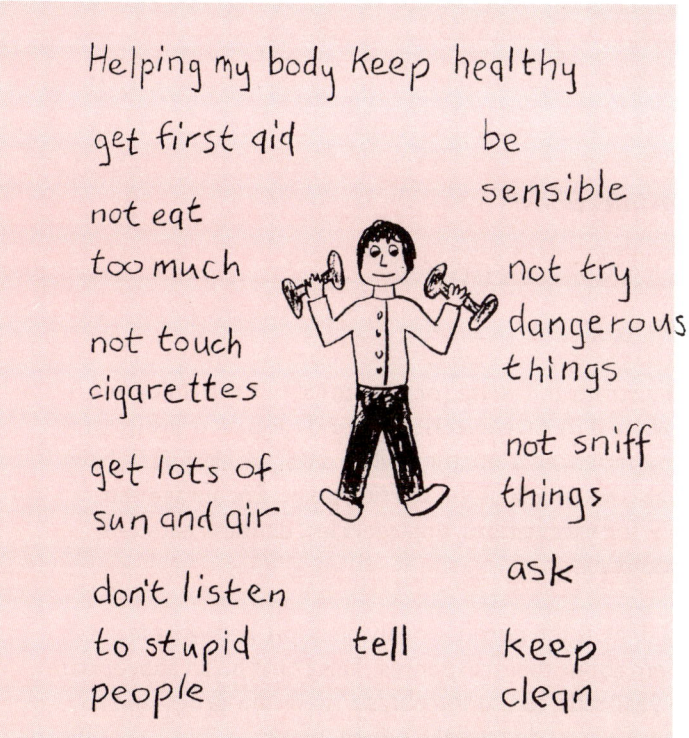

Ask the children to suggest ways in which they can help keep themselves healthy.

Invite them to group their responses into 'do's' and 'don'ts', and to illustrate this with their own drawings or pictures cut from magazines and comics.

Invite the children to think about people who might persuade or force them to touch, taste, sniff or puff strange substances. Who are these people? Ask the children to illustrate and talk about people who might try to persuade them. Look at the children's pictures for stereotyping of strangers or dangerous people.

Ask the children to think about what such people might say, rather than what they look like. Write in speech bubbles, what the children think these people might say (for example, 'Go on', 'Cry baby!', 'It won't hurt') and how they themselves might answer them (for example, 'It's dangerous', 'No, I won't!'). Help them to practise listening to persuasion and giving confident answers. You can also help them to practise telling an adult that they are being persuaded to take something. This is an important coping strategy. Talk with the children about the people who they feel they can trust. Invite them to illustrate and label these people. Explore, where possible, individual's choices and reasons for trust.

There are **cross-curricular links** with:

– personal safety education.

– topics on the home and local community.

32

Content box 3   Injections

When and why do I have injections? For example, to prevent me from becoming ill later on? before I visit another country? in an emergency? an accident? at the dentist? the hospital? so it doesn't hurt so much? to extract some of my blood? What do we call the people whose job it is to do this? How do they do it safely? Where inside me do I think the injection fluid goes? How do I think it gets there?

Activity I

When and why do I have injections?

- Talking. Drawing. Writing. Collecting pictures.
- Class or group activity.

Invite the children to talk, illustrate and write (or dictate) about the times when they, or someone they know, had to have injections, blood tests or transfusions. Some children might have experienced a situation when a dog or cat had to have an injection, and this could also provide a useful starting point. Encourage the children to include injections for vaccinations, emergencies, dental treatment, hospital treatment and blood tests.

Ask the children what they think is the purpose of an injection, and what it puts into the body. Talk with them about their responses. This could be an appropriate time, especially with seven year olds, to use the phrase 'medicine-drugs' and to remind the children that these are made to make people better.

Where appropriate, talk about people who need an injection daily (such as diabetics) and emphasise that injections can be used in a positive and controlled way. It would be valuable to involve the school nurse and parents at this stage, and to talk about your own experiences.

Display the children's work and emphasise both how important these kinds of injections are to these people, and the careful way they should be handled.

Talk with the children about their reactions to injections. What did they do, say or think? Invite them to write what they said or thought on speech bubbles, and then glue them onto their own drawings or relevant pictures cut from magazines.

Activity 2 ● *Whose job is it to give me injections?*

- Talking. Classroom play.

- Class, group or pair activity.

Ask the children to think of all the safe people whose job it is to use syringes and needles of this kind, for example, doctors, nurses, dentists and vets. Talk about how they use syringes safely. Emphasise the dangers of playing with any kind of needle or syringe. Ask them to say how they recognise safe people such as doctors and nurses. Can they be recognised by what they wear? Or is it by what they say? Look at ways of being sure, for example, being with or asking a known adult, and look at ways of saying: 'No, I won't', 'I'm not sure', 'I'll ask'. Help them to practise asking and telling using classroom play or role-play.

Remind the children of the work they did exploring where things go once they enter the body. Where do injections go? Where did the blood sample come from? You could try to find out the children's perceptions of blood circulation and its purpose so you will know what additional and appropriate information to give them.

There are **cross-curricular links** with:

- science.

- topic work.

- safety education.

34

Content box 4   Feeling ill and feeling better

How do I feel when I am ill? How do I look and sound? What can I and can't I do? Who and what helps me to get well? How can I help? What kinds of medicinal drugs help us to get well? Who decides whether I need to swallow or sniff them, or have injections? Who tells me what to do? How do I know which people are safe? Where do the medicines come from? Are these safe places? Where do we keep our medicines? Are they in safe places? How do I feel when I'm getting better? How do I feel when I'm well again?

Activity I   ● *How do I feel when I am ill?*

- Talking together. Painting and drawing.
- Class or group activity with some individual work.

Invite the children to help you write a circle of feelings to describe how they look, sound and feel when they are not well.

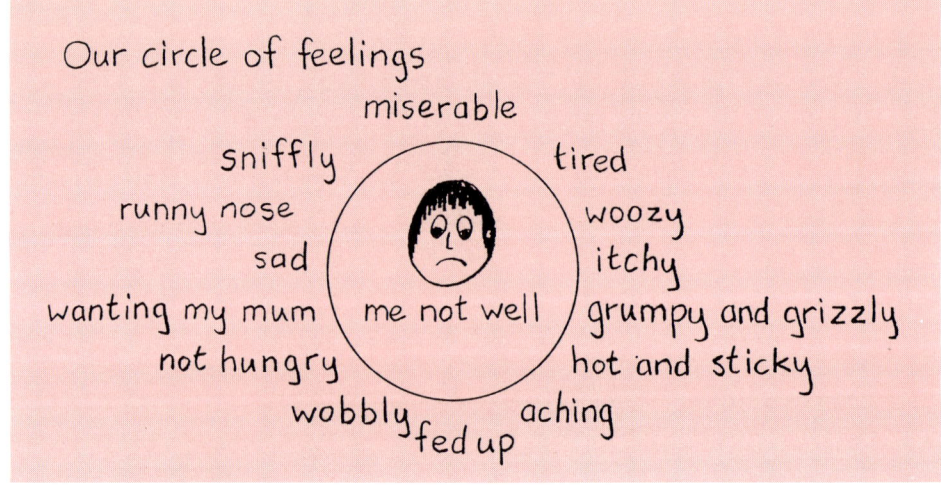

Suggest that they paint or draw portraits of themselves feeling unwell, and include some of this vocabulary in their pictures.

Invite them to group the vocabulary into two categories: 'feelings in my head' and 'feelings in my body'.

Activity 2 ● *Who and what helps me to get well?*

- Talking. Drawing. Role-play.

- Class or group activity and family work.

Talk with them about who and what helps them to get better:

- *the people:* doctor, nurse, chemist, shopkeeper, mum, dad, gran, the dentist etc.

- *the medicines:* creams, lotions, sprays, injections, powders, throat sweets etc.

- *the source of medicines:* the chemist's shop, the clinic, the hospital, the supermarket, other shops, around the house.

Encourage the children to talk about, illustrate or role-play some of these people, places and situations. Focus on: 'Who decides on the treatment – who tells me what to do and take?'

This would be an opportunity both to revise the **medicine-wise rules** introduced at ages **4** and **5** (see page 21) and to look at the rules for ages **6** and **7** and talk about the reasons behind them:

- Don't take any medicines unless they are given to you by your parents, a nurse or a doctor.

- Only take the right dose – don't take any extra.

- Don't touch, taste or take anything just because someone tells you to. If you are not sure, say 'No', 'I won't', 'I'll ask'.

- Don't play with medicines or leave them about.

Help the children to practise these rules. Display them and invite the children to take copies home and explain them to their **families**.

More **family work** could involve:

- looking at the different kinds of medicinal drugs found around the home.

- looking at other hazardous substances such as tobacco and alcohol.

- assessing the safety of the places where these are found.

Activity 3 ● *Feeling better*

- Painting. Talking together.

- Class or group activity and individual work.

Invite the children to paint a second portrait of themselves feeling well (see Activity 1).

Make a circle of feelings as before, but this time with the aim of enlarging their vocabulary of feeling better and feeling good. Explore with the children what they think helped, or could help, them to get better when they have been ill. Encourage the children to identify how they helped to make themselves well. How did medication help? How did other caring activities help?

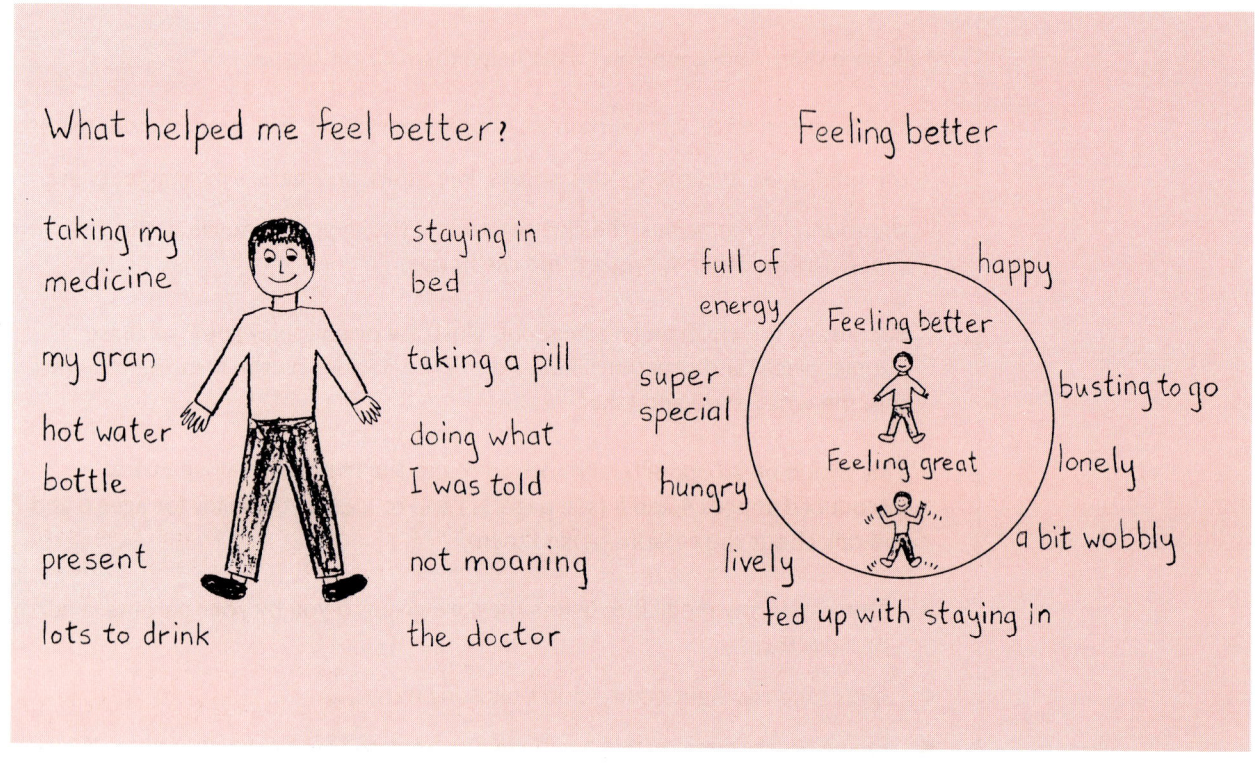

Content box 5 What can I do when I am healthy, happy and well?

 How do I feel and look? What are the things I can do everyday, or occasionally, to keep myself healthy? Which people have to take medicinal drugs all the time to keep healthy? What do I need to know about them?

Activity 1 ● *What can I do when I am feeling healthy, happy and well?*

- Drawing. Writing. Talking together.
- Class or group activity.

Invite the children to draw and label the things they can do when they are feeling healthy and happy without prior discussion. For example, 'I can run fast', 'I play with my friends', 'I don't grumble much'.

Make a note of their ideas and, with the children's help, group them into categories such as play, exercise, eating and being with friends. Suggest other categories such as: work, sleep, helping others, enjoying ourselves.

Activity 2 ● *What can I do to keep myself healthy?*

- Talking together.
- Class or group activity.

Ask the children to explain how their activities can help keep them healthy. Suggest that healthy activities also mean sensible activities, and that it is important to know:

– which things not to touch, taste or try.

– which people might try to persuade them to try drugs or other substances.

– which people to trust and how to tell them you need help.

Ask them to think about people who have to take medicines which are drugs either all of the time, or part of the time, to lead a healthy or near healthy life. Who looks after them and their medicinal drugs? This work could be extended where appropriate to include the problems of the physically and mentally handicapped.

8 & 9 Action Planner
The World of Drugs

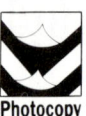
Photocopy

1 What goes into my body?
Who decides? Which things are taken in automatically? How do things get into my body systems? What stops things getting in? How do all the systems work together? How do I feel when I've eaten or drunk too much, or tried something strange or unpleasant, or tried alcohol or cigarettes? What makes me feel better? What does my body do with dangerous things if they get in? Can it always cope?

2 Who uses drugs? Who needs drugs?
When are drugs medicines? Who needs drugs occasionally? Who needs drugs all the time? Who needs drugs to avoid catching diseases? Where do these drugs come from? Who else uses drugs? Why do people use them when they are anxious, or when they can't sleep? Why do people think drugs make them confident? What kinds of drugs are these? Do people know that cigarettes, alcohol and coffee contain drugs? Where do people buy these drugs? Why do some people think they can't manage without them?

3 Who handles drugs at work?
Doctors, nurses, dentists, chemists, vets. Where do they use them? How do they keep them safe? Which drugs can we find in our school, our home, and the places we go? Which drugs are medicines? Which are not? How safely are they kept? How can we help to keep them and ourselves and others safe? What are the drug-wise rules?

4 Feeling better – feeling great.
When I'm ill and have to take medicinal drugs what can I do to help myself get well? What are the drug-wise rules? What makes me feel better when I'm low, bothered, lonely or bored? Who or what makes me feel confident and on top of the world? Where are the safe places I can go for help? Who can I trust? How can my family and friends help?

5 Why do people think that cigarettes, alcohol and other drugs make them look and feel grown up?
Do they know the risks? Do we? What can we do if people try to persuade us to try drugs of any kind? What do we do if they are our friends? What do we say to them?

6 Focus on smoking.
What are the facts about smoking? Who smokes and why? What do I need to know, and do, to be a non-smoker?

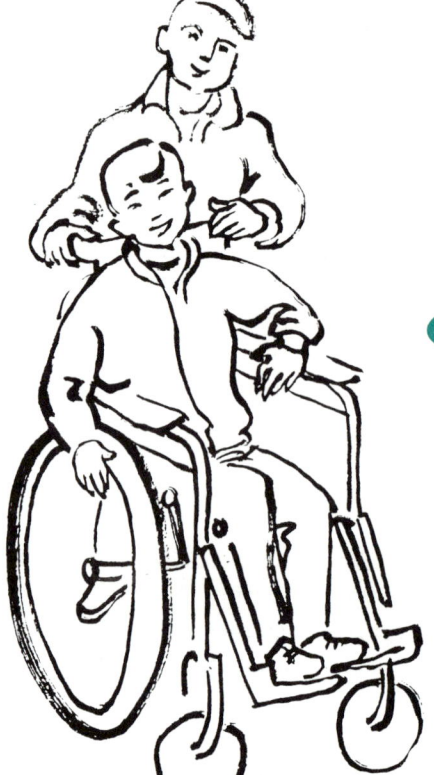

Classroom Strategies and Activities for Ages 8 and 9

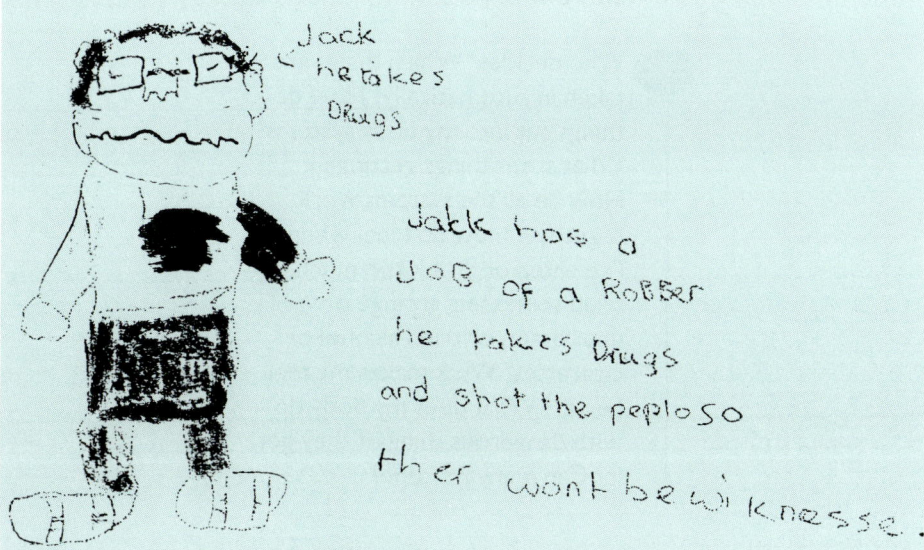

Key messages

Learn:

- what can, and does, go into your body.

- how medicinal drugs work for our health.

- how your body deals with any dangerous things which enter it.

- about 'over the counter' drugs such as aspirin and 'everyday' drugs, such as tobacco, alcohol, tea and coffee.

- where medicinal drugs are made, tested, prescribed, bought, sold and used.

- about the places at home and school where medicines are kept safely and not so safely.

- how to recognise 'persuaders' by what they say and do.

- to be wary of those who use drugs carelessly or abuse them.

- who you can trust. How can you confide in them?

- to know, and talk about, your feelings. What makes you feel better?

Practise:

- saying 'No, I won't', 'I won't take that risk', 'I'll ask'.

Understand:

- that all medicines are drugs but not all drugs are medicines.

- that some people need drugs to live a normal life and to recover from or avoid illness.

- that some people might persuade you to take drugs.

- that some people use drugs, especially tobacco and alcohol, to feel grown up.

Content box 1   What goes into my body?

Who decides? Which things are taken in automatically? How do things get into my body systems? What stops things getting in? How do all the systems work together? How do I feel when I've eaten or drunk too much, or tried something strange or unpleasant, or tried alcohol or cigarettes? What makes me feel better? What does my body do with dangerous things if they get in? Can it always cope?

Activity 1

What goes into my body?

- Brainstorming. Talking together.
- Individual and group activity.

Invite the children individually or in small groups to think about this question and 'brainstorm', making a note of their responses. Ask them to group their responses into different categories. For example include things which:

— I can't stop or avoid taking in.

— people tell me to take.

— are dangerous and could make me ill.

— make and keep me healthy.

— get into my body by accident.

— could change the way I think and act.

Invite the children to share their responses and to talk about them. Some children may include items such as sounds, noise, sights and good and bad feelings. (This work combines well with the *My Body* project (Heinemann Educational Books, see Appendix, page 423.)

Activity 2

How do things get into my body systems?

- Talking together.
- Class or group activity.

Use the range of items resulting from the children's brainstorming session and invite them to regroup these according to *how* they can, or do, get into the body.

Categories such as the nose, mouth, skin, ears and eyes may be given, and after discussion other categories may emerge, such as: eating, drinking, swallowing, sniffing, cuts and injections.

Encourage the children to think of categories such as: deliberate, accidental, avoidable, unavoidable, told to, persuaded to, my choice, someone else's choice.

Suggest to the children that they review the ways things get into their bodies by deciding whether they result from a safe situation, a risky situation or an occasionally risky situation.

There are **cross-curricular links** here: you can help and encourage the children to display the results of their categorisation using different forms of mathematical or pictorial representation and to explain these to other people.

Activity 3

● *Where do things go once they are in my body?*

- ● Drawing. Writing. Talking together.
- ● Individual and class or group activity.

This question can provide a way into a more scientific approach to the body systems and how they interact. It would be useful to explore the children's perceptions first, using their answers to this question and the drawings or diagrams they produce to illustrate their answers. This could be done by asking each child to choose one item from the list produced in response to the question asked in the previous activity: 'What goes into my body?', and to illustrate where it goes and what happens when it gets into the body.

Ask the children to come together to share their perceptions and look at the differences in their answers. This will provide you with opportunities to talk about:

- how sunlight gets into the body.

- how dust, smoke and nicotine get into the lungs.

- the body's defences against substances which get in through the mouth, nose, ears, eyes and skin.

- the impact of some of the items on the way people think and act.

- the body's own immune system.

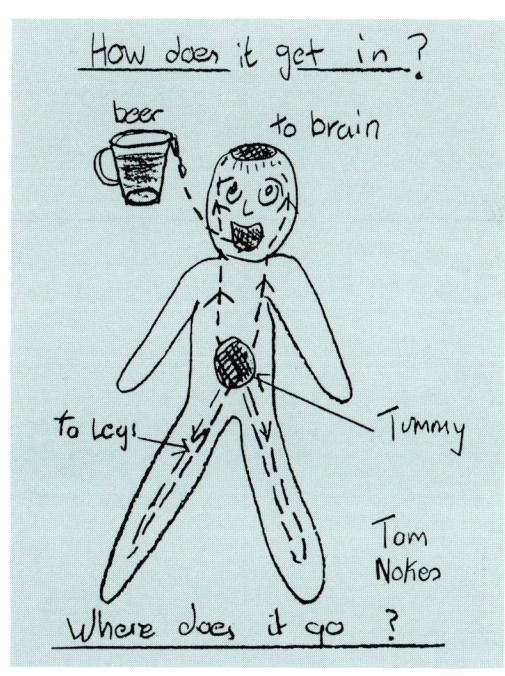

Activity 4 ● *How do I feel when I have had too much?*

- ● Talking together. Vocabulary.

- ● Class or group activity.

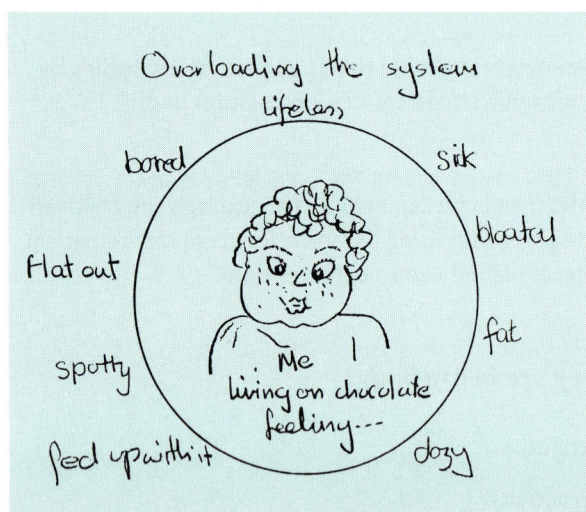

Invite the children to choose a favourite food or drink and to imagine having to eat or drink only that (and in larger and larger amounts).

With the children, make a circle of feelings which describes how the children think they would feel. Make a note of the resulting words and phrases. Invite the children to make their own versions.

Ask the children to give you their own ideas of how their bodies deal with overloading, and dangerous substances resulting from eating, drinking, sniffing, puffing, or injection.

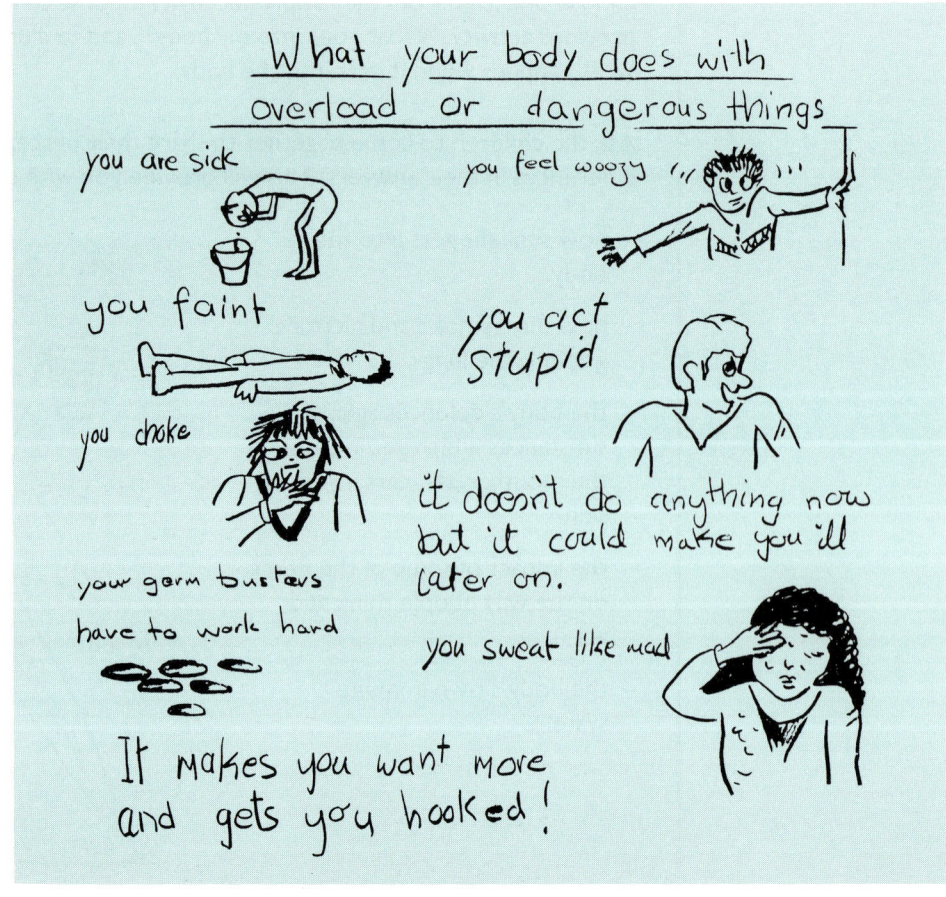

Provide the children with the information to supplement their knowledge where appropriate. Help them to understand how the body copes both in the short and the long term with overloading and dangerous substances.

Opportunities will arise to introduce or focus on:

– aspects of smoking, drinking, alcohol and substance abuse, including glue sniffing.

– careless use of medicines and of unknown or illegal pills, capsules, powders and injections as appropriate to the group.

– the link between the body's physical reaction and the way people think and act.

– scientific explanations of short-term and long-term effects.

Activity 5　　　*What makes me feel better?*

●　Talking together. Vocabulary. Drawing. Writing.

●　Individual and class or group activity.

Encourage the children to talk about, explore the vocabulary of, and record in drawing and writing, their perceptions of getting better and the stages they go through.

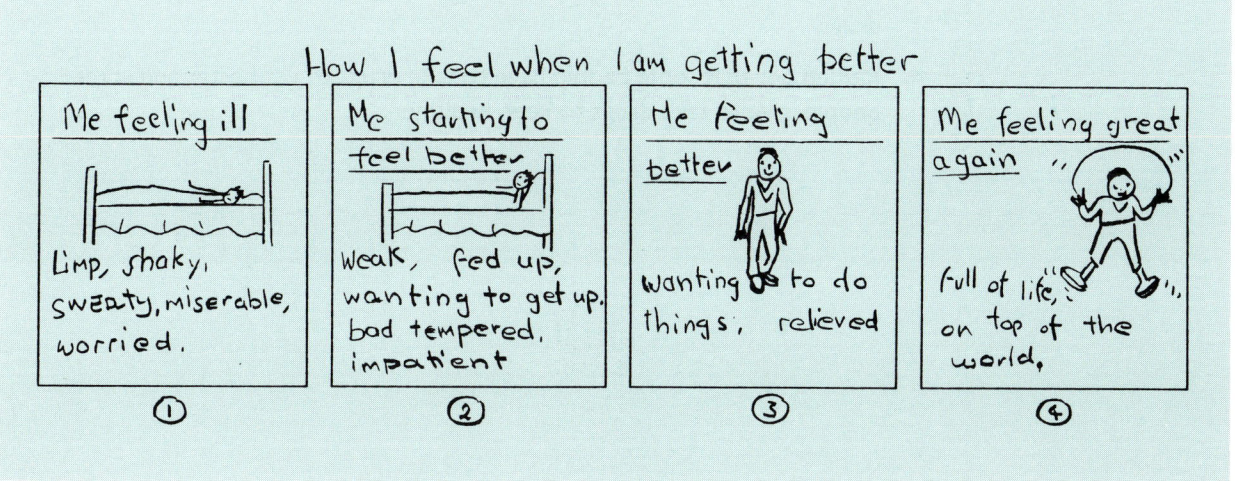

Invite the children to focus on what makes them better, or helps them to get better, and to sort their random responses into different categories, such as:

Things *I* can do:

●　rest, sleep

●　stay in

●　take care of myself

●　listen to what I'm told

●　ask myself if I could have stopped myself from getting ill

Things *other people* can do:

- tell me what to do

- give me medicines

- take me to the doctor

- look after me

- warn me about doing things which make me ill

Things *my body* can do:

- fight off the illness

- slow me down

- try and sort out the trouble

This could be an appropriate point to revise the earlier **drug-wise rules** especially those which relate to taking medicines. The drug-wise rules for ages 8 and 9 are:

- Remember *all* medicines are *drugs*, but not all drugs are medicines. If in doubt, say 'No', 'I won't take that risk', 'I'll ask'.

- Remember everyday things such as cigarettes, alcohol and coffee contain drugs.

- Remember that some people have to take drugs to get better and some people have to take drugs to keep healthy.

Content box 2   Who uses drugs? Who needs drugs?

When are drugs medicines? Who needs drugs occasionally? Who needs drugs all the time? Who needs drugs to avoid catching diseases? Where do these drugs come from? Who else uses drugs? Why do people use them when they are anxious, or when they can't sleep? Why do people think drugs make them confident? What kinds of drugs are these? Do people know that cigarettes, alcohol and coffee contain drugs? Where do people buy these drugs? Why do some people think they can't manage without them?

Activity 1

What do we know about drugs?

- Drawing. Writing. Mathematical representation. Talking together.

- Individual and class or group activity.

It could be useful, before working through Content box 2, to use the draw and write technique (see Appendix, page 410) to discover, or rediscover, how far the children's perceptions of the world of drugs have progressed. You should also be able to ascertain to what extent their perceptions now include, or fail to include:

— drugs which are medicines.

— illegal drugs.

— socially acceptable drugs such as, tobacco and alcohol.

The children could be invited to share their perceptions and to present their shared views in different ways. **Cross-curricular link:** this could be an opportunity to use mathematical representation.

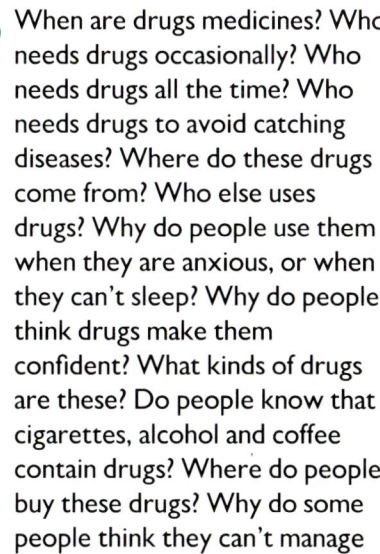

The lost bag of drugs – What was in it?

12 of us thought it would have medicines in it.

4 of us thought it would have cigarettes in it.

5 of us thought it would have alcohol in it.

15 of us thought it would have drugs which aren't medicines in it.

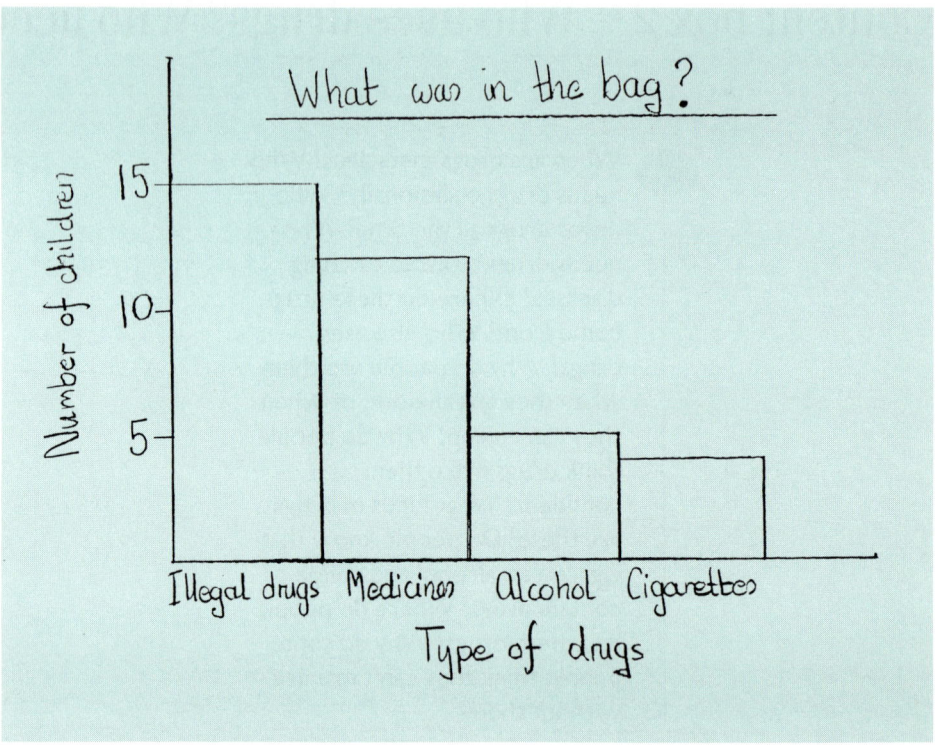

Encourage the children to reflect on narrow views and stereotyped attitudes towards drugs and drug users.

Activity 2 ● ***When do people need drugs?***

● Talking together. Drawing.

● Class or group activity.

Invite the children to recall and share, in a small group or as a class, times when they, or someone they know (including pets) needed to take drugs which were medicines.

Ask them to make a note of their random answers (or you could act as a reporter for them). Review their answers and encourage them to think about the prevention of illness, vaccination for travel abroad, curing illness, emergencies and pain killing.

Invite the children to describe:

– *the kinds of drug* which were taken, for example: pills, medicines, inhalants, injections.

– *the source of these drugs:* for example doctor, nurse, dentist, chemist, supermarket, local shop, medicine cupboard, bathroom shelf.

It is possible that the children will include, or you may want to suggest they think about drugs given to, or taken by people to help them through shock, distress, depression, loss and grief.

The children's responses could be presented pictorially to demonstrate for others the wider meaning of the word drugs.

It may be that children know of someone who is able to lead a comparatively normal life only through the regular use of drugs. There may be children in school who are diabetics or who are affected by asthma or epilepsy or other conditions. It is important that children become aware of and sensitive to the needs of these people and the important role of drugs and other therapies in their lives.
The Health Education Officer, school nurse, local groups and branches of national organisations can provide valuable input and resources to teach the children more about this aspect of drugs, drug users and the help available to them.

Activity 3 ● *Where do drugs come from?*

- Topic work.

- Individual or group activity.

This question could provide children with a broad-based topic to investigate and present. They could work outwards from the local doctor's surgery, chemist's shop, supermarket, local shop and medicine cabinet, to investigate the source of present-day drugs as well as the history of medicine. Their topics could explore:

— major landmarks in the discovery of new drugs.

— women's fight to become doctors.

— natural remedies.

— how drugs are developed, tested and controlled.

Activity 4 ● *Who thinks they need drugs when they are not ill?*

- Talking together.

- Class or group work.

Remind the children of their work on people who need drugs.

Invite them to think and talk about people who only *think* they need drugs:

— What kinds of drugs do they think they need?

— Are they medicinal or not?

— Are they social drugs such as cigarettes and alcohol?

Look with the children at different categories of these people. For example, people who:

— always feel ill or think they are going to be ill (hypochondriacs);

— prescribe drugs for themselves, or take other people's drugs;

— are anxious, worried or not able to sleep;

— can't wake up or relax;

— want to get thinner, fatter or stronger;

— think that drugs make them perform better in their work, particularly in the fields of sport and entertainment;

— think drugs make them feel or look grown up;

— think drugs make them feel great.

The children could look at the sources of some of the drugs these people think they need. Do they get them on prescription? Over the counter? From other people? Around the house? By mail order? Are there warnings about the drugs on the packaging?

Ask the children how they would describe people who think they *need* to have:

— a cigarette.

— an alcoholic drink.

— a cup of tea or coffee

Are these people taking drugs? Do they know about the drugs contained in these things? Are there warnings on the packets, jars or bottles in which the drugs are kept? Suggest the children look out for such warnings.

This would be a good time to revise the **drug-wise rules** and to emphasise the risks involved in the misuse of medicines, and accepting cigarettes, alcohol, drugs or unknown substances from other people.

Activity 5 ● *Why do some people think they cannot manage without drugs?*

● Talking together. Writing.

● Individual and class or group activity.

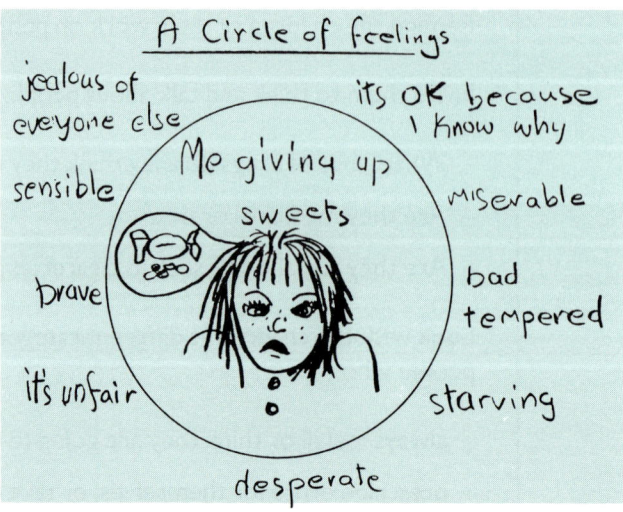

Invite the children to imagine that they have to give up a favourite food or drink, for example, sweets, crisps, chips, ice cream. Talk with them about how they would feel at first, and then as they got used to it.

Invite them, individually or in groups, to make a circle of feelings around a picture of themselves. You could ask the children to try to give up something for a day or two, so that they are more aware of how it can feel.

Invite the children to think of ways in which they would try to help themselves give up this special treat. For example, ask the family to help, tell myself I can do it, go for a swim, save the money I would have spent on something special. Emphasise the interaction between body and brain, mind and feelings.

It is possible to lead on from this work, where appropriate, and explore 'getting hooked', with reference to over-the-counter medicines, nicotine and alcohol, and to introduce the misuse of glue and other inhalants and illegal drugs. You could also look at how the body and brain can seem to become used to and dependent on substances such as nicotine, alcohol and drugs.

Content box 3   Who handles drugs at work?

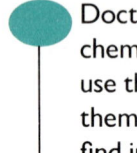

Doctors, nurses, dentists, chemists, vets. Where do they use them? How do they keep them safe? Which drugs can we find in our school, our home, and the places we go? Which drugs are medicines? Which are not? How safely are they kept? How can we help to keep them and ourselves and others safe? What are the drug-wise rules?

Activity 1   *Who handles drugs at work?*

- Collecting pictures. Painting. Collage. Talking together. Making a classbook or wall story.
- Individual, pair or group activities.

Ask the children to collect magazine pictures, advertisements and photographs of people who handle drugs for other's benefit. For example, doctors, dentists, nurses, chemists, shopkeepers, vets and scientists and all their assistants. It would be possible to use this theme for creative activities, inviting the children to paint their own pictures, and make a collage of these and the pictures they collected.

Invite the children to work in pairs or small groups to explore how these people handle, prescribe, experiment with, use or store drugs safely, protecting other people and themselves. It would be valuable, where possible, to involve the school health and dental education services and people in the community.

The discussion, illustration and interpretation of these legitimate, responsible drug related activities could be explored further as part of a topic or presented as a wall story or class book.

Activity 2   *Are there drugs in our school?*

- Survey work. Writing. Family work.
- Class or group and pair activities.

Invite the children (and staff) to plan and take part in a survey on drugs in school. Why they are kept? Which drugs can be found? Where are they? How safely are they kept? It would be important to have the full cooperation of all the adults in the school.

<u>We have been doing a survey of drugs in our school.</u>

<u>This is what we found:</u>

6 people who had headache pills in their handbags or pockets.

1 person who had cigarettes, but he didn't smoke in school.

4 people who had indigestion tablets to suck.

2 people who had cough medicines in a cupboard.

A first aid box in an unlocked drawer.

2 asthma sprays in a locked cupboard.

Lots of : tea and coffee in the staff room.

Invite the children to work in pairs to write their own drug-wise rules for the school, for the children and for the staff. Compare the different sets of rules and invite the children to develop one set of rules incorporating all their ideas.

Family work: where appropriate, invite the children to share the survey, the results and the rules with their families. You could invite the children's families to conduct their own surveys at home and apply or adapt the drug-wise rules.

Content box 4   Feeling better – feeling great

When I'm ill and have to take medicinal drugs what can I do to help myself get well? What are the drug-wise rules? What makes me feel better when I'm low, bothered, lonely or bored? Who or what makes me feel confident and on top of the world? Where are the safe places I can go for help? Who can I trust? How can my family and friends help?

Activity I

What helps me to get better?

- Talking together. Survey work. presentation.
- Class or group activity.

Remind the children of the activities connected with Content box I when they explored their feelings about being ill and recovering. Invite them to recall times when they were ill and needed medicinal drugs. Ask the children to think of the types of drugs they had to take and how they took them. You could make this into a survey.

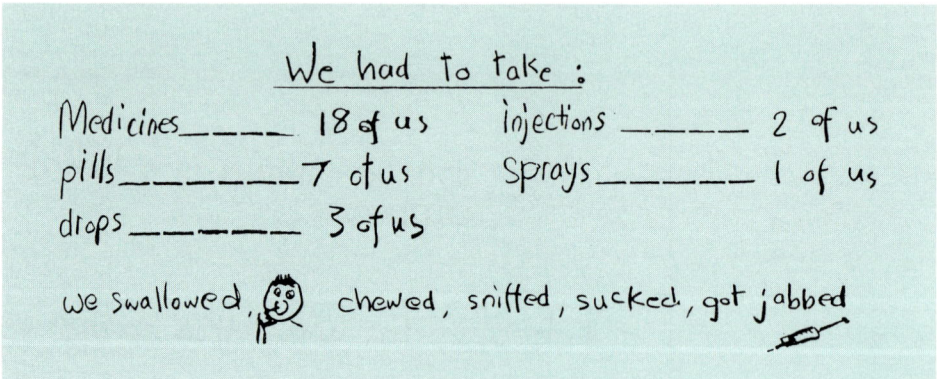

This could be a good time to revise body systems with the children. You could also explore:

– how the body deals with germs;

– the role of drugs in helping to deal with germs, and to introduce (as a basis for later work) the important role of the immune system or 'germ busters' which the body produces to protect itself;

– the quickest and slowest ways in which drugs work in the body and why;

– the fact that drugs are substances which change the way people feel and behave.

Remind the children of the activities based on Content box 1, when they looked at ways in which they thought they could help themselves to get better. Ask the children to think in particular of ways in which they could help the medicinal drugs to work. Help them to focus on:

— following instructions;

— only taking the right dosage at the right time;

— only taking drugs with adult supervision.

This would be a good time to revise the **medicine-wise rules** introduced at the earlier stages, and to ask the children to think of ways of presenting and explaining these to families, friends and younger children.

Activity 2 ● *Feeling low*

● Talking together. Vocabulary. Role-play. Writing. Tape recording.

● Individual, pair and group activities.

Children will have different experiences of feeling upset, lonely, bored, bothered by other people, pressured by friends and older children. They often need help in finding the language with which to communicate this. Encourage them to talk about their feelings and share them with others, trying out new vocabulary.

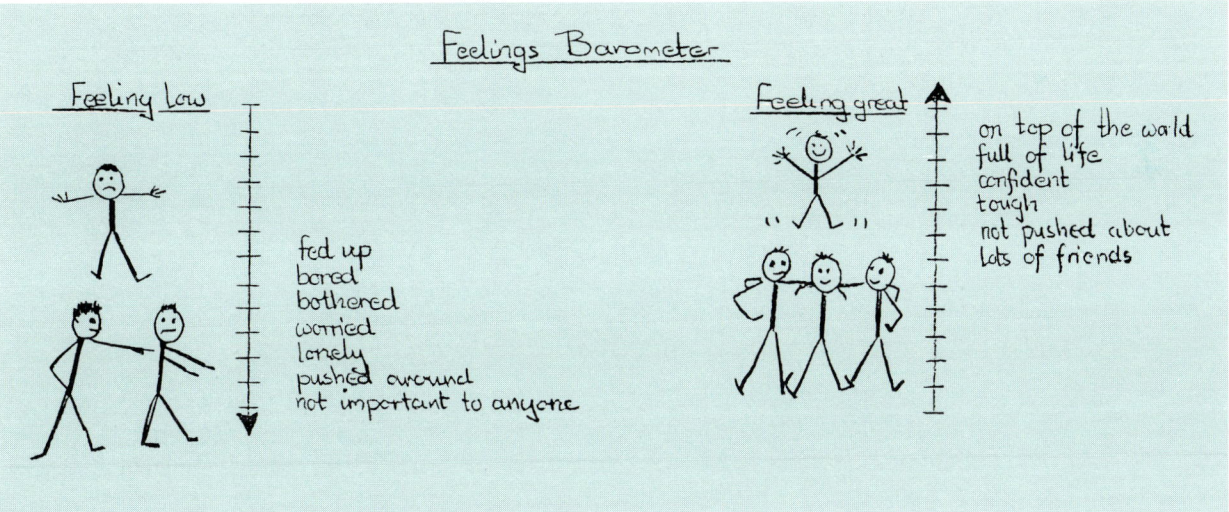

Explore with the children who and what makes them feel better and how it works. Encourage them to focus on things which they themselves can do. Look at physical exercise, changes of interest and routine, the role of friends, pets and the family. Invite the children to work individually or in pairs and group their responses into categories such as:

— What can I do to make myself feel happier?

— What can my family do?

— What can my friends do?

Ask the children to share their ideas, and to try to regroup these under other headings, such as:

— What can I do?

— What can I say?

— What can people do?

— What can people say?

Encourage them to see the difference between support in terms of practical help and caring and the importance of both.

The activities based on Content box 4 lend themselves to role-play, both structured and improvised. Children can be encouraged to choose a situation, explore it and play through its potential outcomes.

It is useful sometimes to invite the children to record the role-play situation, the characters and outcomes, and to note any problems they have met and how these were solved. This can be done during, or at the end of the session. Different methods of recording, can be used, for example, using adults as 'scribes' or using a tape recorder. The 'reports' can be edited, illustrated, presented by the group and used as a further resource.

Content box 5 Why do people think that using cigarettes and alcohol makes them grown-up?

Do they know the risks? Do we? What can we do if people try to persuade us to try drugs of any kind? What do we do if they are our friends? What do we say to them?

Activity 1 *What is it like to be grown-up?*

- Drawing and painting. Talking together. Writing. Tape recording.

- Individual and class or group activities.

Invite the children to draw or paint themselves going to a fancy dress parade looking like a grown-up man or woman. Ask them to depict and label specific things which they could wear to make themselves look like a grown up, for example, certain clothes, make-up etc.

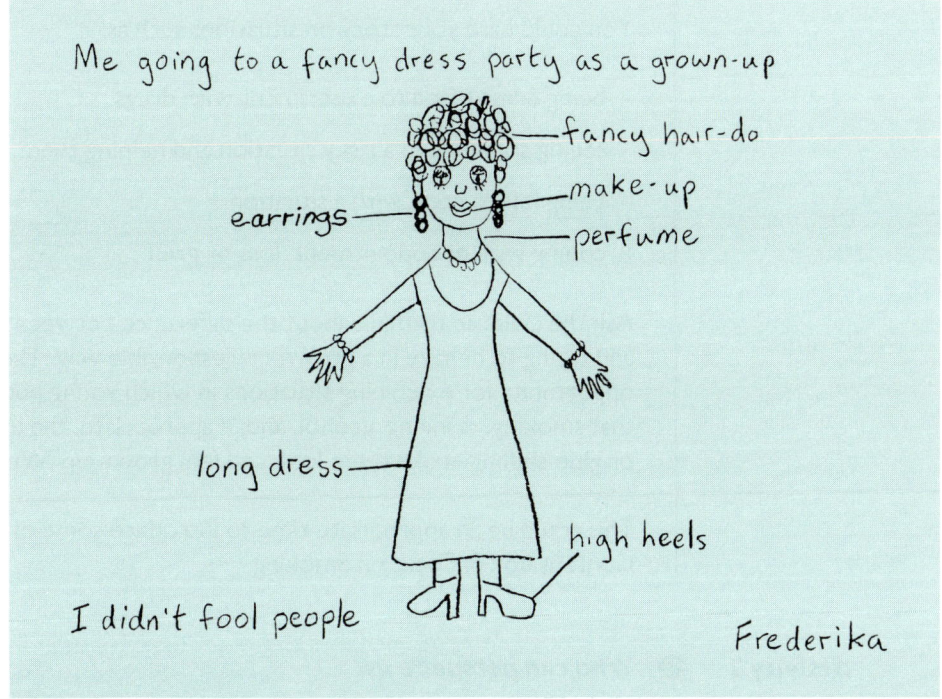

Collect up and talk about their work. Are all the pictures concerned with appearance? Do cigarettes, and alcohol appear?

Ask the children if their fancy dress could fool anyone into thinking they really are grown-up. Invite them to record their responses in some way, for example, using shared writing or tape recordings.

Outline to the children a story in which a child deals with a difficult situation in a responsible and mature way. Invite the children to illustrate the character behaving in a grown-up, responsible way, asking them as before to label the responsible behaviour.

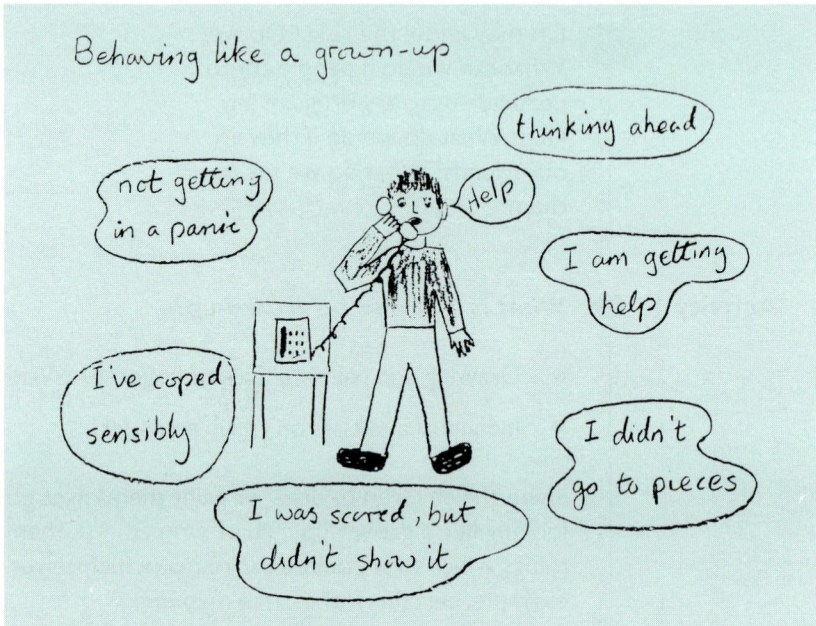

You could base your story on situations such as:

— being pressurised to experiment with drugs.

— seeing someone in a risky situation and helping them.

— being left to cope with a situation.

— coping with disappointment, loss or grief.

Ask the children to think about the difference between dressing like a grown-up and trying to behave in a grown-up responsible way. This could provide an opportunity for examining situations in which young people have been persuaded that smoking, drinking alcohol, and, if appropriate, the use of non-medicinal drugs or glue-sniffing, make them look and feel grown-up. What are the risks?

This could be an appropriate time to introduce some of the activities based on Content box 6: Focus on Smoking.

Activity 2 ● *Who can persuade us?*

• Talking together. Drawing and painting. Role-play. Family work.

• Individual, pair and class or group activities.

With the children, consider the possibility that someone might try to persuade them to experiment with, or take risks with, drugs. What does a persuader look like?

Ask the children to construct, draw or paint a robot who is designed to persuade people to do all sorts of things. Invite the children to think of some techniques which the robot might use.

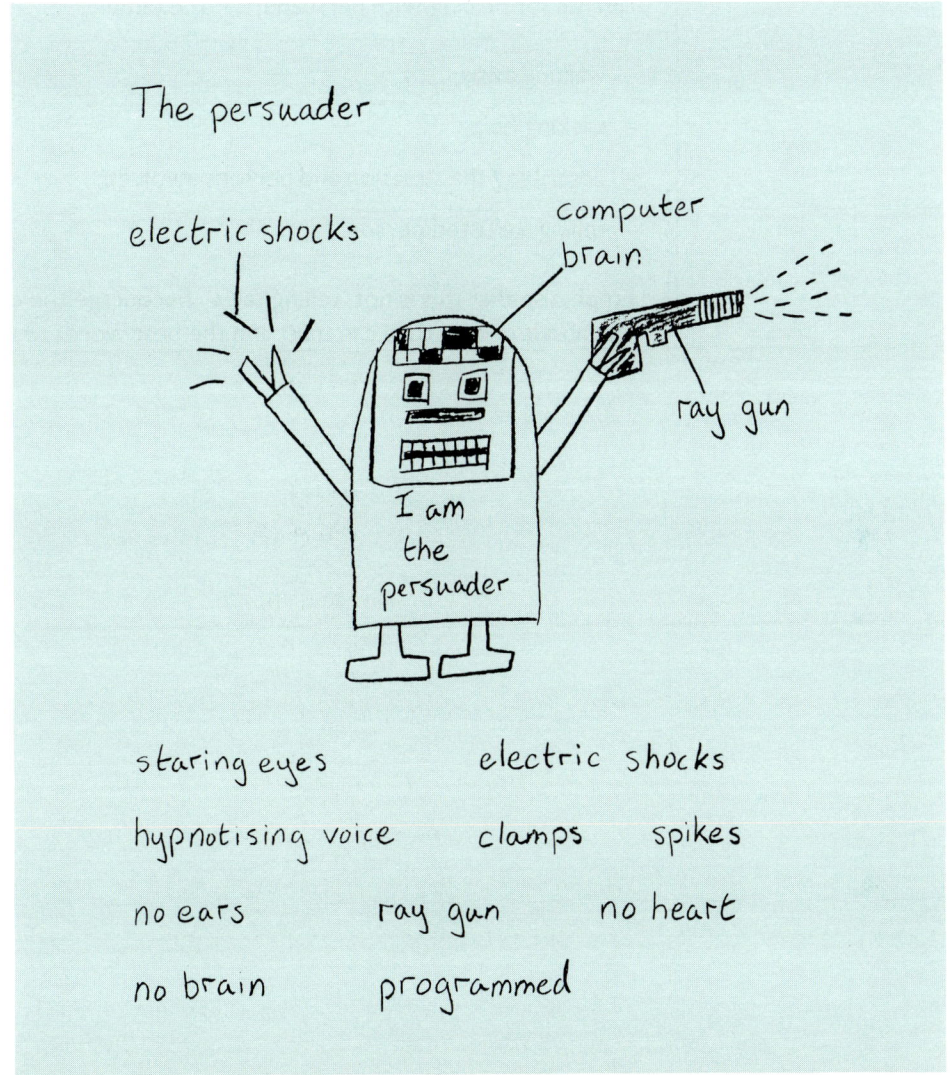

Ask the children: would they give in to this persuader? How would they know it was a persuader? How could they deal with it? How could they resist persuasion?

Invite the children to draw, paint, label or describe a *human* persuader who might encourage them to touch, taste, puff or sniff strange substances. Ask them to suggest ways in which persuaders of this kind could be recognised, if not by their appearance, by the things that they say. For example, 'It makes you feel great', 'Don't be a baby', 'Everyone else does it', 'You can't be in our gang if you don't', 'It's fun'.

Ask the children how they would deal with the robot persuader. How would they deal with a human persuader? What could they say? For example, 'I won't take the risk', 'It's stupid', 'You're not much of a friend if you say that?', 'I'm going'. Write these responses on the board or on a chart, so that the children can discuss them, and practise using them.

Organise role-playing activities in pairs or small groups to help the children to practise and reinforce these responses and other coping strategies.

Talk with the children, and if possible, with their families, about the strategies they can use for dealing with persuaders. For example,

— walking away;

— seeking help;

— describing the situation and persons involved;

— telling a trusted person.

Emphasise that this is not 'telling tales'. Encourage the children and their families to talk about people they can trust and the best words to use.

Content box 6   Focus on smoking

 What are the facts about
smoking? Who smokes and why?
What do I need to know, and do,
to be a non-smoker?

Activity 1   ● *Advertising*

- Collecting advertisements. Talking together.

- Class or group activity.

It would be useful to explore some of the other content boxes, especially box 5,
before working through the ideas in this one.

Ask the children to look out for advertisements for cigarettes, cigars and tobacco,
and to note the wording of the advertisement and the government health warning.

Make a collection of advertisements from papers and magazines, and add to these
the children's own illustrations of advertisements they may have seen on television
and billboards.

Invite the children to recall the people shown in the advertisements. Are they
young? old? healthy? sick? sad? happy? tired? energetic? well-dressed? shabby?
Why are they shown in the way that they are? What size print is used for the
advertisement, and for the warning? What do the warnings say? Collect as many as
possible. Do people who smoke look at the warnings?

Activity 2   ● *What are the facts about smoking?*

- Brainstorming. Talking together. Writing and drawing.

- Class or group activity.

Ask the children to brainstorm, as a class, or in groups, what they know, or think
they know, about smoking. What have they heard, read and learned about
smoking? For example, it stops you growing, it can kill you, it won't hurt you if you
only smoke a little, it costs a lot of money, it's bad for pregnant mothers.

You could show the children a simple smoking 'fact sheet', like the one on page 61
to help them. Children could be helped to categorise their responses into two or
three groups, for example,

- Smoking facts.

- What people say.

- What nobody really knows – yet.

Invite the children to devise messages for people who might be thinking of taking up smoking to appear grown-up, and to present these as advertisements.

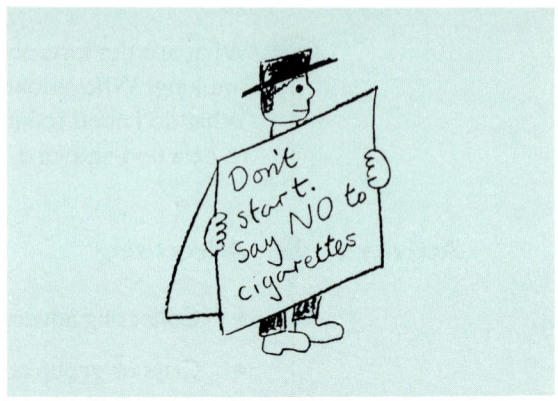

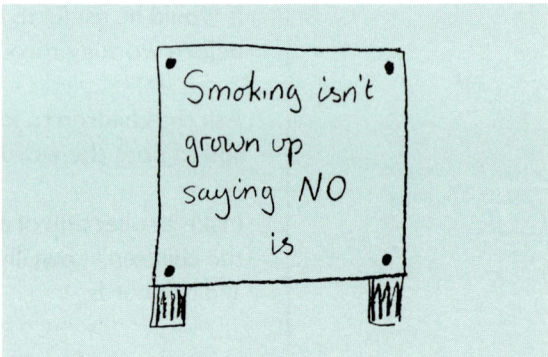

Activity 3 ● *Why do people smoke?*

- Talking together.
- Class or group activity.

Explore with the children their explanations of why some people smoke – especially young people. Encourage them to think about reasons such as:

– they see other people doing it.

– they want to know what it's like.

– they think it is grown-up.

– people persuade them.

– they don't know how dangerous it can be.

Emphasise how important it is for the children to know:

– the facts about smoking.

– how nicotine gets into the body.

– what it does to the body.

– how to say 'No', 'It's not for me', 'I know the facts'.

A smoking fact sheet

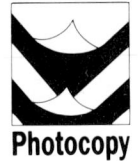
Photocopy

- Cigarettes contain a substance called nicotine.

- Nicotine is a drug. People who smoke say it helps them to feel calmer and more relaxed.

- Nicotine is also a poison.

- When a cigarette burns it produces dangerous substances:

  - a gas called carbon monoxide;

  - a sticky material called tar.

- Nicotine, tar and carbon monoxide can damage your health.

- Smoking causes or helps to cause:

  - lung and chest diseases, for example, chronic cough, bronchitis;

  - heart diseases;

  - diseases in other parts of the body.

- Smoking can also stain fingers and make a person's breath and clothing smell.

- Other people's smoke can harm people around them who breathe it in.

- If a woman smokes and she is expecting a baby the nicotine can go into her blood and affect her baby.

- Now that people in this country know about the dangers of smoking, more and more people are giving it up. There are many places where people are not allowed to smoke.

- BUT: many young people are *still* taking up smoking.

IT IS IMPORTANT TO KNOW ALL THE FACTS ABOUT SMOKING

10 & 11

Action Planner
The World of Drugs

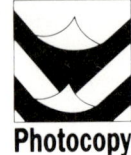

Photocopy

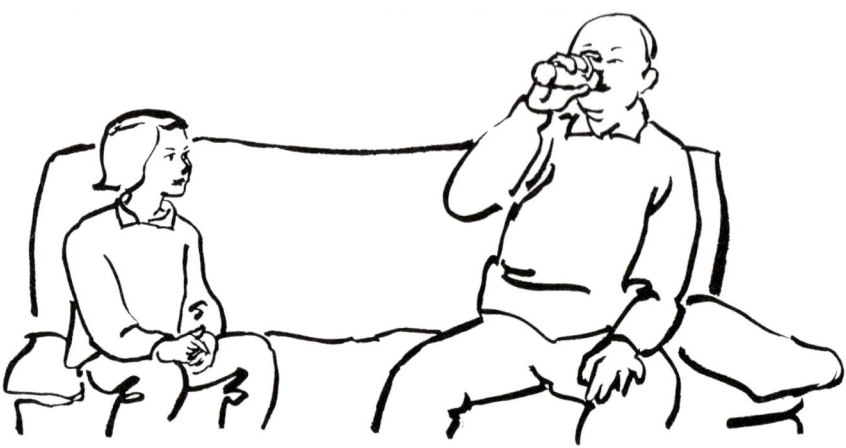

1

What goes into my body?
Who chooses what goes in?
Who tells me to do it? Whose
responsibility is it? What is
useful, non-essential, accidental,
avoidable, deliberate, legal and
illegal? How do drugs of all kinds
make me feel, look and behave?
How do they affect my energy,
judgement, control and moods?
What are the risks of using
drugs? What facts do I need to
know to help me decide,
especially about the 'everyday'
drugs people use, such as
tobacco and alcohol?

2

Drug users.
Do they know the difference
between drugs which are
medicines and drugs which are
not? Do we? Which drugs seem
to be part of everyday life, for
example, in cigarettes, alcohol,
coffee and tea? Why can these
become addictive? Which drugs
are illegal to use, buy and sell?
How are these used? What are
the risks? Who invents new
drugs?

3

Where are drugs found?
What kind of drugs do we find at
home, at school, in places we
visit alone or in groups? Are
these safe places? Where do
people keep drugs safely? How
can we help? What does it mean
to be 'hooked' on drugs,
dependent or addicted? Can
children become dependent on
drugs such as cigarettes? What
helps people not to become
dependent?

4

Taking risks.
What does this mean? Is it the
same for everybody? Who warns
people about the risks of drugs?
Why are there *no* warnings on
some drugs? How do I assess the
risks? What would life be like
with no risk? What makes risk-
taking satisfying? Does it vary
depending on whom I'm with?
What do I need to know in
order to make a healthy choice?
How do I recognise opinion?
Where can I find out the facts?
How can I keep the drug-wise
rules?

5

Smoking and the persuaders.
Where are the warnings against
smoking? Why do some people
smoke despite the warnings?
Why do some people find it
difficult to stop? What is our
school's policy on smoking at
school? Why have some people
never smoked? Why have others
given up? Who and what are the
persuaders? How do they tempt
me to try tobacco? How do I
recognise the persuaders in
person, on TV and advertising?
How do I know what they are
really trying to say and do? Who
are my models? What is my self-
image? How can I achieve it and
be healthy?

6

Feeling good.
When have I wished for the
ground to open up and swallow
me? When have I felt on top of
the world? What can I learn from
these experiences? What can I
learn about drug-free ways of
coping, and about being in
control?

Classroom Strategies and Activities for Ages 10 and 11

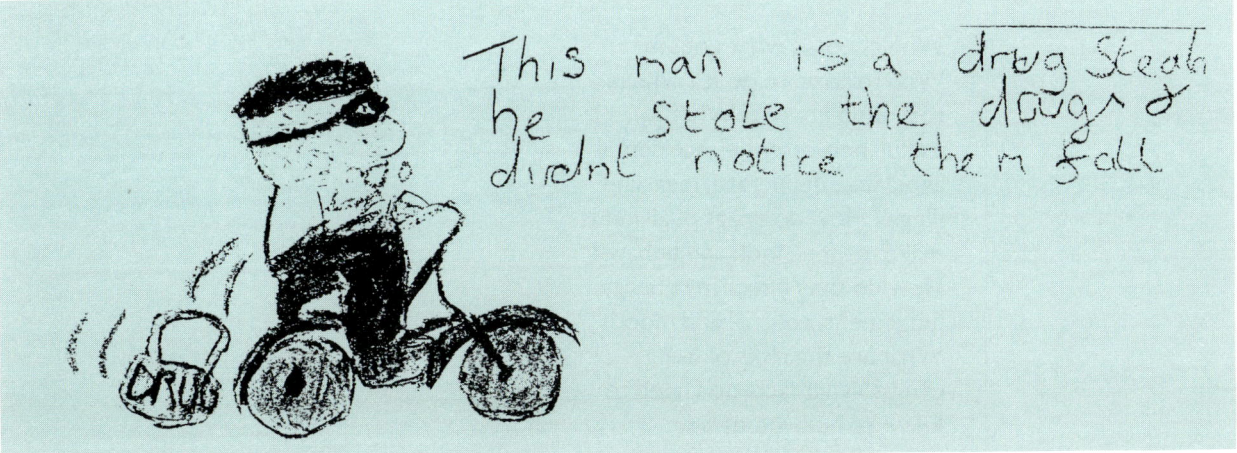

Key messages

Learn:

- what can, and does, go into your body and how your body systems cope.

- how your brain and other systems work together and affect how you feel and behave.

- to categorise what goes into your body as 'essential', 'non-essential'. etc.

- about the risks of using everyday drugs socially, such as cigarettes and alcohol.

- how to recognise persuaders and persuasion.

- about the people who need and use drugs for their health.

- who controls drugs and how new ones are invented.

- to talk about your feelings about the world of drugs.

Practise:

- saying 'No', it's not for me.' 'I won't take that risk.' 'I'll ask.'

Understand:

- the effects these drugs can have on friendships and relationships.

- what addiction can mean.

- that some people use drugs to appear grown-up or confident.

- that you are a role model to younger children.

- that you have your own role models. Look at them – do they keep the drug-wise rules (see page 68)

- what makes you feel good, what makes you feel better, what gives you a 'kick', and what makes you feel confident.

- when to say: 'That's OK', and when to say 'No'. Be aware of how difficult this can be.

Content box 1   What goes into my body?

Who chooses what goes in? Who tells me to do it? Whose responsibility is it? What is useful, non-essential, accidental, avoidable, deliberate, legal and illegal? How do drugs of all kinds make me feel, look and behave? How do they effect my energy, judgement, control and moods? What are the risks of using drugs? What facts do I need to know to help me decide, especially about the 'everyday' drugs people use, such as tobacco and alcohol?

Activity 1   *What goes into my body?*

- Writing. Drawing. Talking together. Making a wall story or chart. Vocabulary.

- Class or group and pair activities.

Ask the children to keep a record of, or to try to recall, everything they can remember having taken into their bodies in the previous day, or weekend, or week. The children could work in pairs or small groups to make a record of this using both writing and drawing, and devise their own ways of presenting their results. (You could keep your own record and make your own contribution.)

Invite the class to bring together and share their work. Ask them to extend their lists if possible. Encourage them to include:

– drugs of different kinds, for example, lotions, ointments, injections, sprays, eye drops, nose and ear drops.

– smoke, dust, germs, sunshine.

– sights, sounds, feelings, ideas, new learning.

Invite the children to look at the extended list and, working in pairs or small groups, to group their responses into different categories, such as:

– things which can be seen, touched, tasted, and felt.

– things which cannot be seen, touched, tasted and felt.

    or

– things which enter the body.

– things which enter the mind, or affect feelings.

They could present and explain these activities as a display, a wall story, a chart or a file. They could also include an exploration of how these things were taken into the body, for example, sniffed, swallowed, absorbed or injected.

Ask the children to explore how they might, or did, react to each of these items as they were taken in. Use this as a vocabulary-extending activity. For example;

— loved it

— gulped it down

— soothed

— tickled

— stung

— hurt

— choked

— improved

— relaxed

— got angry about it

— wanted some more

-- coughed

Ask the children to regroup the items on their lists into categories such as:

— these are necessary, useful or essential.

— these are inessential.

— these can be avoided.

— these cannot be avoided.

— these can be taken accidently.

— these can be taken on purpose.

— these are safe to take.

— these are risky.

— these are dangerous.

— these are illegal to take.

It is very important that the children explain why they have put each of the items into a particular category, and to reflect on and question other children's decisions and explanations.

Activity 2 ● *Whose responsibility is it?*

- Talking together.
- Class or group activity.

The children could then review their list in terms of who made the decision to take the item into the body. They could consider the decisions that they made or were able to control, and evaluate these decisions by asking: 'Was it, or would it be, sensible/safe/risky/dangerous?' In this way, they could build up their own evaluation framework.

Activity 3 ● *How do drugs make me feel?*

- Talking together.
- Class or group activity.

Ask the children, in groups or as a class, to go through their lists again and pick out items which contain, or could contain:

- drugs which are medicines.
- drugs which are not medicines.

Explore with them the reasons for their responses and relate these to other previously explored categories, particularly those relating to personal responsibility.

This would be an appropriate time to revise the children's knowledge of the body systems and to introduce or focus more closely on:

— the immune system and some of the activities which endanger it (where appropriate this could provide an introduction to the AIDS – drugs link).

— the nervous system.

— the impact of drugs of all kinds on mood, emotions, judgement and control.

Discuss this statement with the children: 'Cass wanted to look grown up, so she or he tried smoking a cigarette and drinking some beer'.

Explore with the children the likely impact on Cass's body, mood, behaviour and feelings. Work as a class or in groups. Collect all their responses and group them, for example,

What did it do to Cass's body?	*What did it do to Cass's brain?*
It made him/her:	It made him/her:

– wobbly	– feel clever
– woozy	– act stupid
– cough	– get violent
– sick	– have an accident
– dizzy	– let the dog out
– choke	– get his/her words muddled up
– turn green	– say stupid things
– sweat	– get into more trouble
– fall over	– want some more

Ask the children to recall a time when they, or someone else (include pets) had to take medicinal drugs. Encourage them to include times when they visited the doctor, dentist, hospital and veterinary surgeon, and to take account of immunisation, anaesthetics, injections, medicines, pills and sprays. Ask the children to differentiate between prescribed medicines and medicines bought over-the-counter and in supermarkets.

Ask them to remember the effect on the person or the pet, looking at the immediate effect of some drugs and the slower effect of others. How do they explain this?

Group their responses in this way:

These acted quickly:	*These acted slowly:*
– anaesthetic	– immunisation injection
– asthma spray	– pain killing pill
– cough linctus	– ointment

Explore further the way these drugs can affect both body and mind. Discuss with the children how medicinal drugs can make you feel, for example,

– slowed down	– sore
– unconscious	– better
– sleepy	– not so itchy
– numb	– more confident
– hot at first	– you want some more
– miserable	– glad it's stopped hurting
– babyish	

This is the time when the children should apply what they have learned about the effect of medicinal drugs to:

— nicotine, alcohol and caffeine;

— mood-changing substances;

— illegally obtained drugs;

and to ask again:

— how they affect the body, mood and behaviour,

— how they can make you feel.

This would be an appropriate time to revise the earlier **medicine-wise** and **drug-wise rules** in the light of what the children have learned. The **drug-wise rules** for ages 10 and 11 are:

- Learn about the way drugs can affect your body, your brain and the way you behave.

- Try to understand the reasons why people take drugs.

- Know what it means when you say: 'All medicines are drugs, but not all drugs are medicines'.

- Do not take any medicines except those given to you by a parent, nurse or doctor.

- Take the exact dose, never take any extra.

- Never take anyone else's medicine.

- Never try something just because someone tells you to.

- Never play with medicines or leave them lying around.

Content box 2   Drug users

Do they know the difference between drugs which are medicines and drugs which are not? Do we? Which drugs seem to be part of everyday life, for example, in cigarettes, alcohol, coffee and tea? Why can these become addictive? Which drugs are illegal to use, buy and sell? How are these used? What are the risks? Who invents new drugs?

Activity 1   *Who uses drugs?*

- Talking together. Drawing. Collecting pictures. Using reference material. Family work.

- Class or group activity with opportunities for individual work.

Revise with the children their exploration of the times when they, or someone they knew, needed or took drugs of different kinds (see Content box 1). Help them to remember how they said they felt, or might have felt.

The focus could now be shifted to drug users. Invite the children to extend their awareness of the wide range of people who use and handle drugs. Offer the children a range of categories (you could write these up on the blackboard) and invite them to suggest, and illustrate, groups of people who fit each category.

— These people use drugs in their *work:*
  for example scientists, pathologists, chemists, dentists, vets, nurses, ambulance people.

— These people need to take drugs *regularly to live a normal life:*
  for example, diabetics or epileptics.

— These people need to take bought or prescribed drugs *sometimes:*
  for example, people who become ill or catch diseases.

— These people get drugs given to them in an *emergency:*
  for example, people who have accidents.

— These people *mistakenly think* they need to take drugs:
  for example, people who think they are ill, or addicts.

— These people take drugs, but *don't know* they are drugs:
  for example, people who smoke, drink alcohol, coffee and tea.

Encourage the children to cover the widest possible range of groups. Invite them to write their own descriptions of drug users, illustrations from magazines and newspapers, consult reference material (in and out of school), and to talk with their families.

There are **cross-curricular links** with environmental and community studies here. This is also an opportunity to use the wide range of resources provided by national organisations and regional and local services.

Family work: where there are good school–family links, children could take home their work on drug users and explain it to their families. The families could be asked to describe their own experiences of drug use. They could start from themes such as:

— people we know who need drugs sometimes.

— times when we have taken drugs.

— the drugs we have in our house – and where we keep them.

Activity 2   ●   *What are the risks?*

- Talking together. Topic work.

- Class or group activity with opportunities for individual work.

Invite the children to review their work to look at the risks and dangers involved in using drugs for different groups of people. Suggest that they devise a simple risk measure and apply it to each group, or individual, who uses drugs.

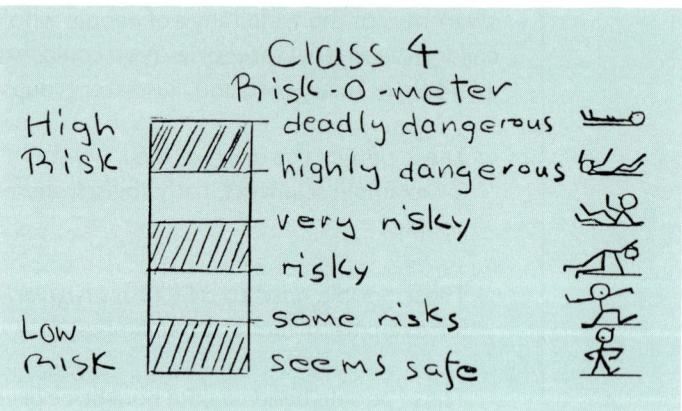

Discover with the children the precautions which different drug users feel compelled to take, or are advised to take. When is the decision left to them? You could ask them to talk about, or list, drugs which they themselves take, or have taken. Help them to recall the risks, the precautions and who made the decisions in each case.

There are opportunities here to develop topic work which explores present-day and historical landmarks in the discovery of drugs and which enables the children to discover how new drugs are invented and tested.

Content box 3   Where are drugs found?

What kind of drugs do we find at home, at school, in places we visit alone or in groups? Are these safe places? Where do people keep drugs safely? How can we help? What does it mean to be 'hooked' on drugs, dependent or addicted? Can children become dependent on drugs such as cigarettes? What helps people not to become dependent?

Activity 1   *Where are drugs found?*

- Family work. Writing. Making a chart. Topic work.

- Individual and group or class activities.

Invite the children (with the help of their families where appropriate) to make a note of where they think drugs might be found. Ask them to share their perceptions.

Invite the children to work individually, or in small groups, and devise and make a chart which shows the variety of places where drugs are found. Afterwards they could present their findings to others. Encourage the children to include:

— hospitals, clinics, surgeries, veterinary clinics, first aid stations.

— chemists's shops, supermarkets, corner shops.

— laboratories, scientific establishments.

— factories, lorries, trains, aeroplanes.

— zoos, animal and bird sanctuaries.

— briefcases, handbags, pockets, shopping bags.

— school, home, cupboards, shelves, bedside tables

— police cars, ambulances.

— refrigerators, sheds, car glove compartments, kitchens.

— pubs, clubs, cafés, restaurants and snack bars.

It would be possible to develop a wide-ranging topic exploring the places where drugs are found, used, made, stored, transported, exchanged, bought, sold, prescribed, dispensed, given and taken. Issues such as control, safety, testing, community concerns and environmental health could also be included and both local and national sources could be used.

Activity 2 ● ***Are there any drugs in our school?***

- Survey work. Family work. Research.

- Class or group and individual activities.

Invite children to ask members of the teaching staff and other adults in the school community to take part in a survey of the drugs which can be found in the school, and to present and explain their findings.

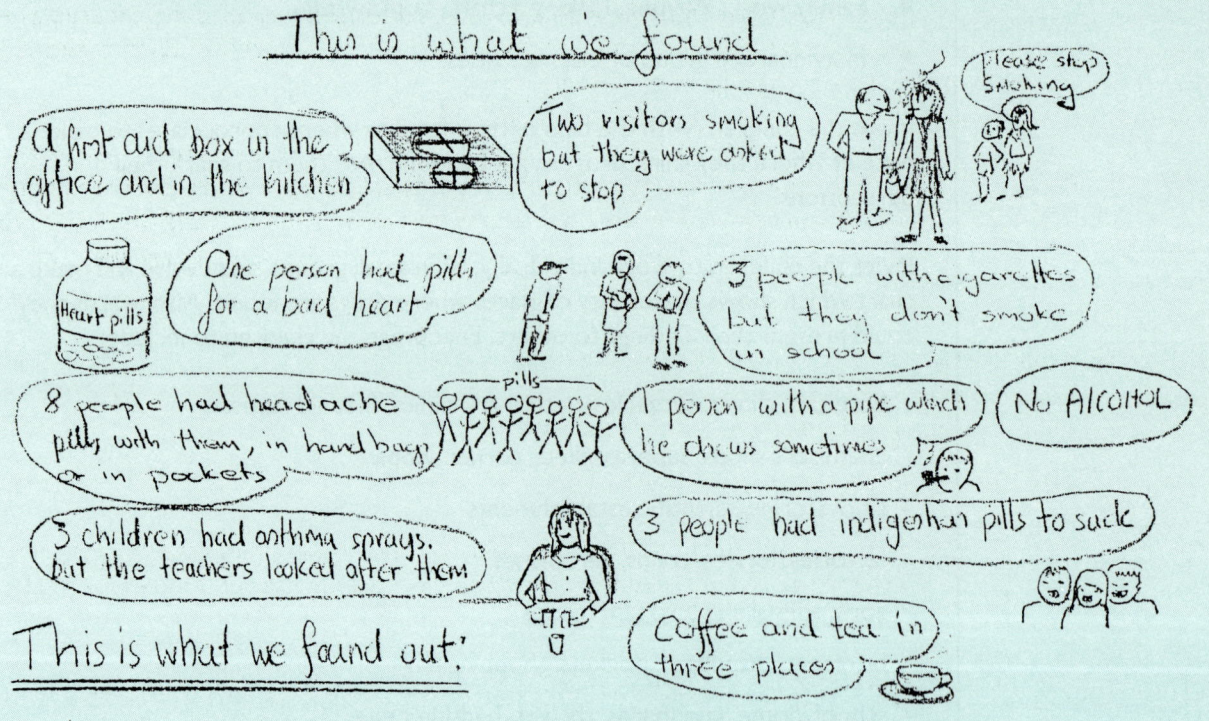

Drugs in school - survey by class (6)

We have conducted a survey of drugs in our school. We inspected eight rooms and interviewed eighteen people: teachers, caretaker, dinner Ladies, a cleaner, the school nurse and a visitor.

This is what we found

- A first aid box in the office and in the kitchen
- Two visitors smoking but they were asked to stop
- Please stop smoking
- One person had pills for a bad heart
- Heart pills
- 3 people with cigarettes but they don't smoke in school
- 8 people had headache pills with them, in handbags or in pockets
- pills
- 1 person with a pipe which he chews sometimes
- No Alcohol
- 3 children had asthma sprays, but the teachers looked after them
- 3 people had indigestion pills to suck
- Coffee and tea in three places

This is what we found out:

* The heart pills and the sprays were prescribed by a doctor.
* People with headache pills had prescribed them for themselves and bought them in the shop
* Some people didn't think nicotine in cigarettes, alcohol and caffeine in coffee and tea were drugs.
* The visitors didn't know we had a no smoking bargain at our school.
* People kept doctor's medicines locked up, but not other drugs.

Ask the children to ask people why they used these drugs and to record their answers.

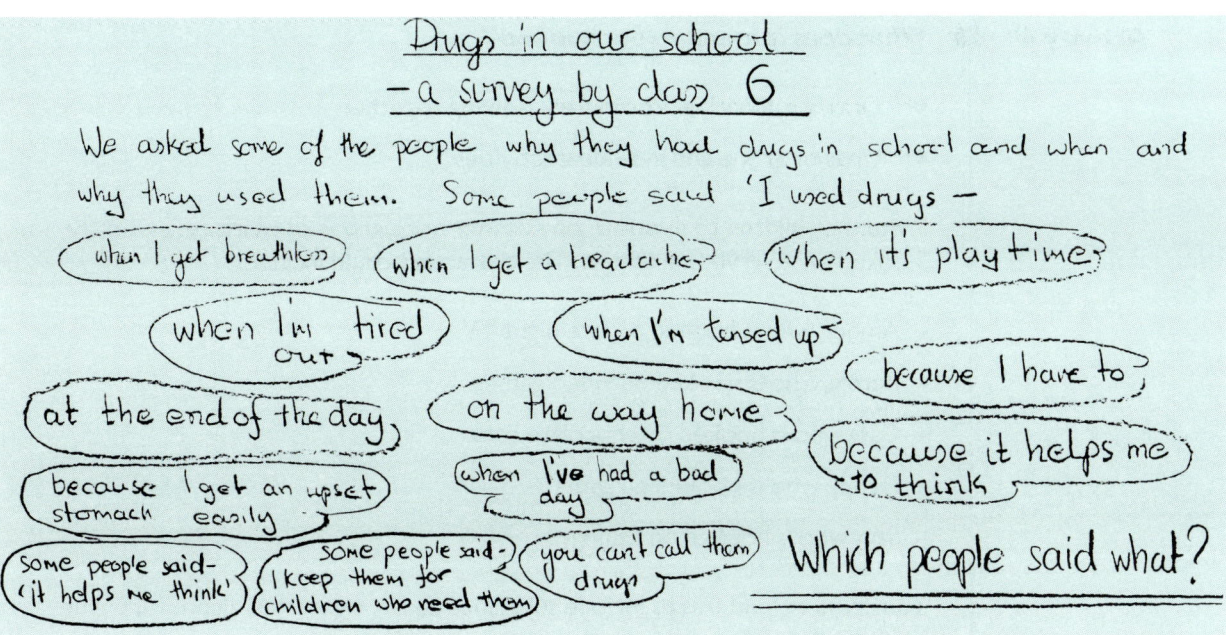

Drugs in our school
— a survey by class 6

We asked some of the people why they had drugs in school and when and why they used them. Some people said 'I used drugs —

when I get breathless   when I get a headache?   when it's play time?

when I'm tired out   when I'm tensed up   because I have to

at the end of the day   on the way home   because it helps me to think

because I get an upset stomach easily   when I've had a bad day

Some people said 'it helps me think'   Some people said 'I keep them for children who need them'   you can't call them drugs   Which people said what?

The children could share the findings of the survey with their families and look with them at the location of drugs in their homes. They could classify the drugs as doctor-prescribed or bought over the counter, and look at how safely they are kept, and the degree of risk involved.

You could ask the children to be observant about the kinds of drugs available in shops, cafés, youth clubs, parties, discos and public houses with children's rooms and off sales service. Invite them to look for and/or collect notices which refer to legal age limits for the sale of cigarettes and alcohol. Are these being followed?

Activity 3 ● ***How can we help to keep drugs safe?***

- Talking together. Planning a 'campaign'.

- Class or group activity.

Ask the children to talk about and think of ideas in response to this question. What can they do to help others see the dangers? What can they do to keep themselves safe? Suggestions could include:

– reminding people that there are different kinds of drugs, some which are medicines, some which are not, some which can do good, some which are dangerous or deadly.

– reminding people to keep drugs of all kinds in safe places.

– setting a good example to younger children.

– learning, or finding out, all the *facts* about drugs and the risks of using and taking them and not listening to opinion.

– being aware of the people, programmes, advertisements and articles which try to persuade people that using drugs is a good thing.

– planning a 'Keep Drugs Safe' campaign for the school, class or club.

Activity 4 ● *What does it mean to be 'hooked'?*

- Drawing. Writing. Vocabulary. Talking together.

- Class or group and individual activities.

Invite the children to illustrate one or more of a group of characters who are 'hooked on' everyday activities. The characters could include:

— Amber who is hooked on late night TV.

— Bernie who is hooked on video games.

— Cass who is hooked on chocolate bars.

— Denny who is hooked on sport.

— Sam who is hooked on fishing(!)

You could extend this to include substance abuse, cigarettes, alcohol and glue sniffing, where these are appropriate.

Ask the children to convey in their pictures, and by adding words and phrases:

— what being hooked can mean.

— how the character looks, feels and behaves.

— the possible outcomes of being hooked.

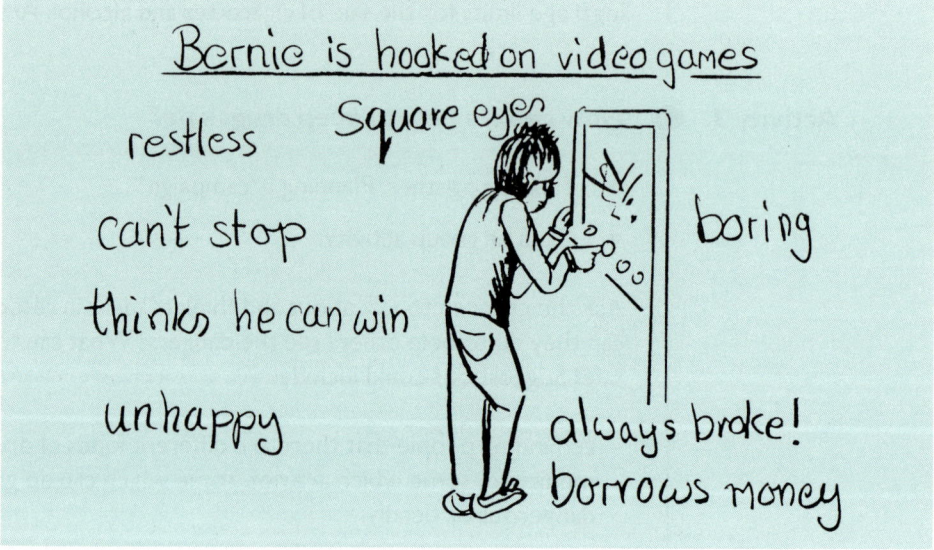

Ask the children to share their work and extend their vocabulary which describes 'being hooked', for example, 'think they can't get by without', 'dependent', 'addicted'.

Ask the children to imagine that the same group of characters, for reasons which they can invent, are forced to stop 'being hooked'. How would the characters feel? Help the children make a circle of feelings which include both physical and mental feelings.

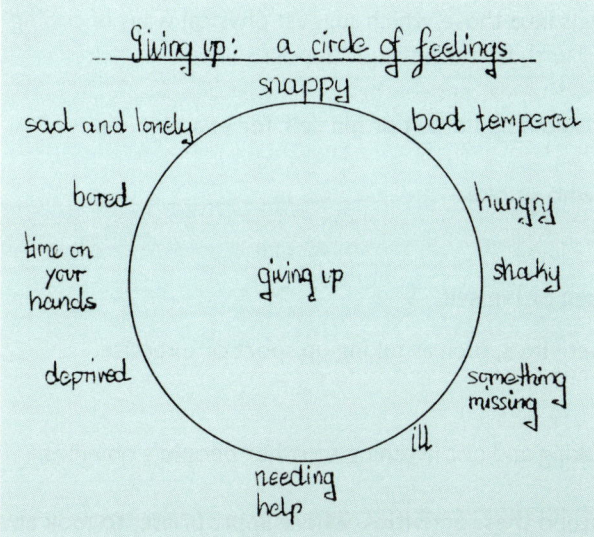

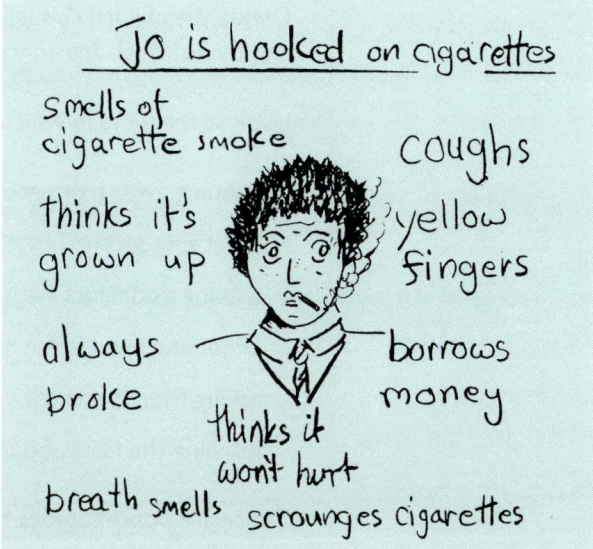

Extend this activity to explore the case of Jo who is hooked on cigarettes. Explore how Jo looks, feels, thinks, behaves, and the consequences of being hooked.

Explore, or revise, the effects of nicotine on the body systems, and on the brain, consider both the short-term and long-term effects.

Explore with the children the notion of dependency, or thinking we can't do without something, and the way that body and brain can become used to believing they need certain substances.

Activity 5 ● *Jo wants to give up smoking*

● Talking together.

● Class or group activity.

Ask the children to plan how they would help Jo to give up smoking. Recall the activity (page 74) where they drew a circle of feelings connected with giving up. Make a note of their random suggestions. These could include:

— Say, 'Don't listen to people who try to get you to smoke'.

— Suggest Jo makes a contract with herself or himself.

— Keep Jo busy with other interests.

— Persuade Jo to do some exercise or to take up a sport.

— Take no notice if Jo is snappy.

— Explain to Jo that her/his body has become temporarily dependent on nicotine.

— Say, 'Well done!' lots of times.

— Tell Jo to chew chewing gum instead of smoking.

— Say, 'You look better and you don't smell of smoke'.

— Say 'You *know* it's going to work'.

Divide the children's suggestions into those which suggest physical ways of coping and those which are concerned with friendship and support.

Look at the ways in which Jo could help herself or himself, for example, by

- keeping away from groups who smoke.

- practising saying 'No'.

- making a contract with herself or himself.

- becoming involved in new activities, such as taking up sport or exercise.

- asking friends to help.

- learning the facts about smoking and not listening to other people's opinions.

There are opportunities to extend these activities, where appropriate, to look at other types of dependence:

- on alcohol;

- on tranquilisers or anti-depressants;

- on over-the-counter drugs;

- on illegal drugs.

Content box 4   Taking risks

What does this mean? Is it the same for everybody? Who warns people about the risks of drugs? Why are there *no* warnings on some drugs? How do I assess the risks? What would life be like with no risk? What makes risk-taking satisfying? Does it vary depending on whom I'm with? What do I need to know in order to make a healthy choice? How do I recognise opinion? Where can I find out the facts? How can I keep the drug-wise rules?

Activity I   *Are risks the same for everybody?*

- Talking together. Family work.

- Class or group and individual activity.

Invite the children, with family help where appropriate, to look at what they and other people think are the health and safety risks for children at different ages.

What's the risk?

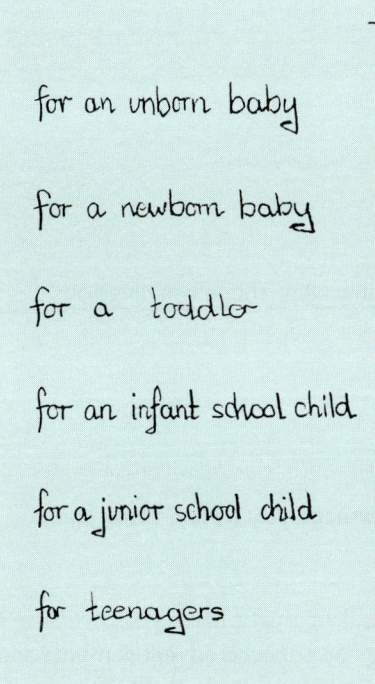 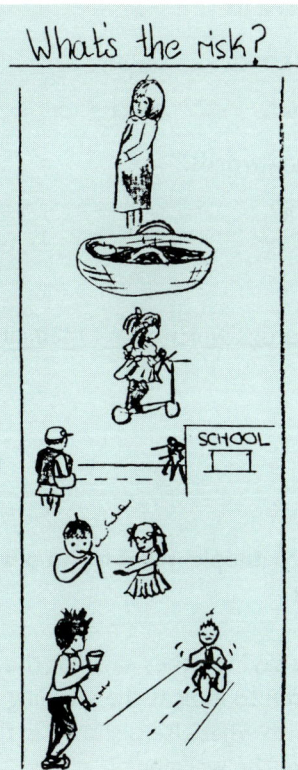

for an unborn baby	the mother not looking after herself, eating the wrong food
for a newborn baby	being left, becoming ill
for a toddler	busy roads, running away, being taken away not knowing things are dangerous
for an infant school child	going to school, big children, busy roads people may hurt them
for a junior school child	starting to smoke, lungs become damaged, smelly breath, fire
for teenagers	starting to drink alcohol, can't control body when cycling etc

Ask the children to extend this and say what they think are the risks for grown ups and old people.

Invite the children to share their perceptions of risk, and compare their views with those of their families. Ask them to explain how what is thought to be risky changes as they grow up. Return to the risk list above and ask the children to say who decides what is risky for each age group. It is likely that their responses will vary and often begin: 'It depends . . . .' Encourage them to enlarge on their replies.

Activity 2 ● *Advertising the risk*

- Collecting advertisements. Talking together. Drawing. Writing.
- Class or group activity.

Ask the children to collect, or make a note of, all the advertisements they see for medicinal drugs with warnings, and all the advertisements they see with no warnings. Ask them to look at advertisements in a variety of media. The children could ask their parents to join them in this activity.

Ask the children to look critically at the warnings. Where in the advertisement are they placed? In what size print are the warnings set? Ask them to think about these questions also:

What will happen if

- you are a little child and can't read?

- it's so small you can't see it?

- your eyes aren't very good?

- it's in another language?

- it's all expressed in long words?

- you can't understand it?

- *there isn't a warning?*

Remind the children of drugs which aren't medicines. Are there warnings on:

- cigarettes?

- alcohol?

- coffee, tea, etc?

- other substances which people might try to persuade you to try, taste, sniff, smoke, drink or inject?

What do these warnings say? Do they say that the drug might harm you, or cause a disease? Invite the children to look at the warnings on tobacco advertisements and compare their impact with what else is shown in the advertisement. How important does this make the warning?

Invite the children to devise their own warnings for:

— cigarette packets;

— bottles and tins of alcohol;

— jars of coffee and packets of tea.

Ask the children to talk about the important messages they would want to put across. Would they warn people about how these things make us feel and behave or what they might do to damage our health? Would they put: 'This can kill you' in the warning? How would the people who produce or make a living out of these goods react?

Activity 3 ● ***Assessing the risk***

● Talking together. Vocabulary. Writing. Using reference material. Role-play. Tape-recording. Photography. Drawing.

● Class or group and individual activities.

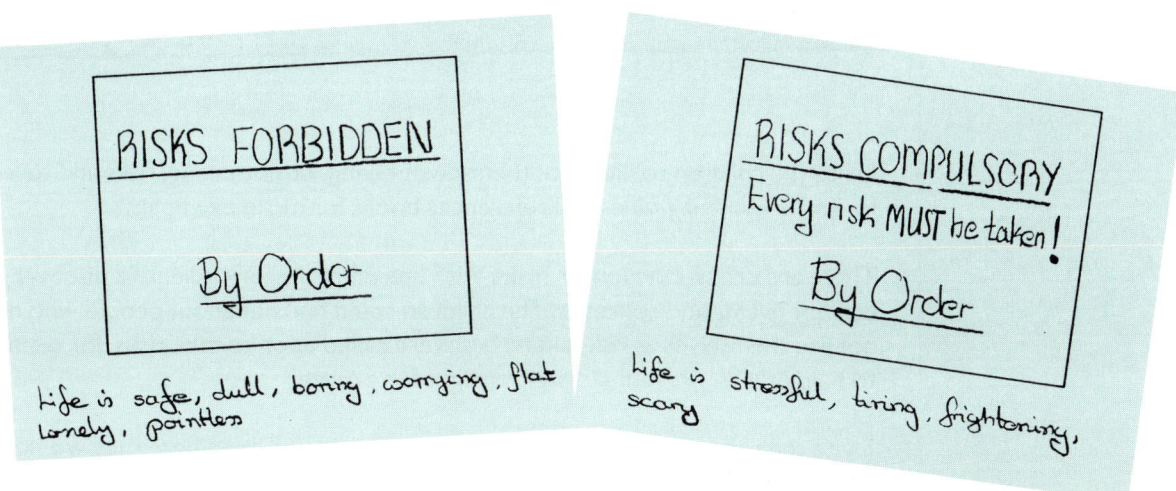

Ask the children to imagine they are living in a world where risk taking is forbidden. Ask them to describe the kind of life they think it would be. Make a list of the vocabulary they use.

Invite the children to write a one-day entry in the diary of a person (it could be themselves or another person) living in the world in which risks are forbidden. Would they feel satisfied with their lifestyles?

Ask the children to imagine a world in which people had to take risks all the time. Invite them to write a one-day entry in the diary of someone living in that world. Would that lifestyle be satisfying?

Invite the children to remember situations when they took risks and had the skills to cope, for example, swimming without armbands, riding a bicycle, being lost, being frightened.

Develop a personality chart with the children. To do this the children need to ask themselves about their attitude to risks. Do they take risks? Do they like or dislike taking risks?

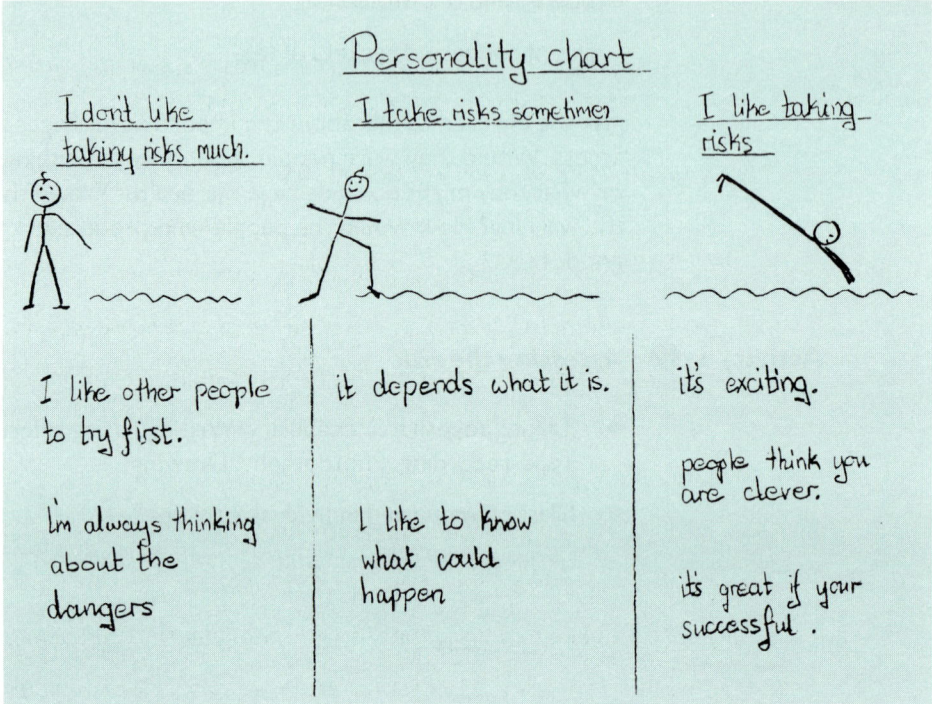

Invite the children to illustrate themselves taking, or not taking, risks and to look for pictures in magazines and references books for more examples.

There are **cross-curricular links** with literature, history, scientific discovery, and current events and concerns. The children could find out about people who did not see themselves as risk takers, but were called upon to take risks, for example, to help others, prevent disaster, or fight for a cause.

Invite the children to look at the personality chart and say where they would put themselves. Is it possible to be at one point on the chart in one situation and at another point in another situation? Suggest some situations to the children and ask them how they would react. Include situations in which they are persuaded to try, or experiment with, cigarettes, alcohol, solvents or other drugs.

Emphasise to the children that they need to be able to assess the risks. Stress the importance of:

— knowing as many facts as possible.

— being able to recognise opinion.

— knowing that the satisfaction which comes from taking risks successfully depends on having the skills with which to cope.

These situations could provide children with starting points for role-play and for devising and recording playlets. You could use tape recorders, drawing, writing and photography to help with this activity.

Activity 4 ● *Finding out about the risks*

- Talking together. Writing.
- Class or group work.

Ask the children to make a list of ways in which they could find out about the risks of taking drugs of all kinds. For example,

- learn all you can about drugs;
- listen to what your teachers, parents and families keep telling you;
- watch the television health advertisements;
- look at advertisements in papers, posters and leaflets;
- listen to what older children tell you about it;
- listen to what your friends tell you;
- listen to what other people say;
- you might find out by accident;
- you might see people using drugs;
- you might take the risk of trying something and find out that way;
- find out the facts about drugs and don't just accept people's opinions.

Invite the children in small groups to take this list, or their own lists, and put the items in what they think is their order of importance. Ask them to be prepared to explain the way they have ordered them.

Activity 5 ● *Fact or opinion?*

- Media study. Talking together.
- Class or group and individual activity.

Invite the children to explore the difference between fact and opinion by looking at different reports of news items, or reviews of television programmes.

They could try summarising a nursery rhyme, for example, Little Miss Muffet, retelling it from the point of view of the spider (who found it amusing) or Miss Muffet (who found it frightening). Or they could take a traditional story, for example, Three Billy Goats Gruff, and retell it from the point of view of the Troll.

Help the children to revise the drugwise rules.

Activity 6 ⬤ *Why is it difficult to keep the rules?*

- Talking together.

- Class or group activity.

Invite the children to think about the rule: 'Keep off the grass'. Ask the children to talk about times when they would, or would be tempted, to break that rule and why. For example they may break it

- as a dare.

- because all the others did.

- in an emergency.

- to rescue someone or something.

- to escape from someone or something.

- because others do it and don't get caught.

- for fun.

- because it's not dangerous.

- because someone makes you do it.

- because someone says it's a stupid rule.

- because you're not thinking and you do it by accident.

Ask the children to use their risk measure (see page 80). Ask them:
'What is the risk involved in breaking this rule?'
'What's the worst thing that could happen?'
'Why would you keep the rule, or not keep it?'

Invite the children to repeat this activity, this time exploring a situation where the rule is known about but not written up for all to see.

This would provide opportunities for the children:

- to explore situations involving the use of cigarettes, alcohol, unknown substances or illegally-acquired drugs.

- to look at reasons why people might be tempted to break the rules.

- to assess the risks in each situation, and hypothesise what their decision would be.

- to practise ways of dealing with the situation which would be of help to them.

Activity 7 ● *What helps me to keep the rules?*

- Talking together. Role-play. Writing. Drawing and painting.

- Class or group and individual activities.

Invite the children to suggest ways in which they could help themselves, or be helped, to keep the rules.

Review this list of strategies, looking at what makes each one easy or difficult to put into practice:

— say 'No, I won't take the risk.'

— stay with friends who back you up.

— learn the facts about drugs and what they can do to you.

— learn the rules.

— see what's happening and have the sense to keep away.

— walk away.

— tell someone.

Suggest to the children they think through situations in different settings, such as, the school playground, the street, the youth club, at home, in a group, alone. The children could explore these situations using:

— role-play or playlets.

— comic strips, using speech bubbles and a written commentary.

— drawing and painting.

Come together to share and review the coping skills. Emphasise the importance of talking an experience through with others, one's family, friends and other adults.

It would be possible at this stage for some groups to explore the importance of setting good examples to younger children and being able to explain the **drug-wise rules** to them.

Invite the children to recall the kinds of warnings which accompany some drugs. Which warnings are intended to shock or scare people? Which warnings explain the risk? Why do some drugs carry no warnings? Which warnings do the children think work best for them? Which would work for younger children? Ask the children to design a poster for a class of 7 year olds. List the main points they would make when explaining it to the class.

Content box 5   Smoking and the persuaders

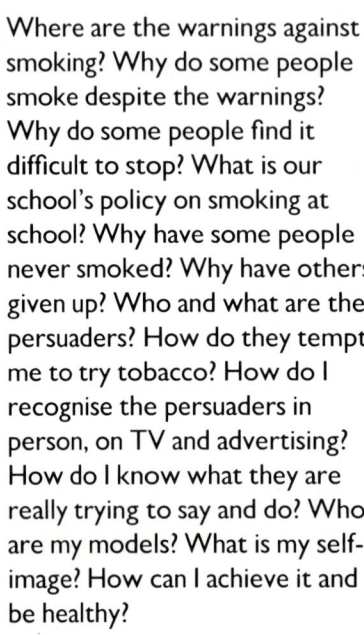

Where are the warnings against smoking? Why do some people smoke despite the warnings? Why do some people find it difficult to stop? What is our school's policy on smoking at school? Why have some people never smoked? Why have others given up? Who and what are the persuaders? How do they tempt me to try tobacco? How do I recognise the persuaders in person, on TV and advertising? How do I know what they are really trying to say and do? Who are my models? What is my self-image? How can I achieve it and be healthy?

Activity I

What are the warnings against smoking?

- Media study. Display. Talking together.
- Class or group activity.

Ask the children to make a collection of the warnings which are printed on advertisements for cigarettes and to note where these advertisements are usually seen, for example, on posters, bill boards, in magazines, on television programmes.

Look at and classify the warnings under different headings, for example,

- those which refer to unborn babies;

- those which refer to the risk of disease;

- those which mention death;

- those which give facts and figures, and

- those which don't.

At the same time it could be interesting to explore the advertisements to see which show cigarettes, or packets of cigarettes, which don't, and which contain hidden messages. The advertisements and the children's findings could be displayed along a continuum, for example, from very frightening to not very frightening.

Invite the children to tackle these questions: 'If there are warnings . . . why do people start smoking? . . . go on smoking? . . . find it difficult to stop?' (You could revise Content box 3 here.)

Responses to these questions might include: 'Because they –'

- 'think it's grown up.'

- 'don't know the facts.'

- 'think it makes them look good.'

- 'are curious to know what it's like.'

- 'see other people enjoying it.'

- 'become hooked.'

- 'like it.'

- 'are persuaded by other people.'

- 'think they need it to feel better.'

- 'don't believe it will hurt them.'

- 'don't care what happens later on.'

Activity 2   ● **What is smoking?**

- Talking together. Writing. Drawing.
- Class or group activity.

Ask the children to explain, for the benefit of a Rip Van Wynkle character, or a being from another planet, what smoking is. Help them to include:

- illustrated descriptions of a cigarette and a cigarette packet (including the health warning).

- an account of how cigarettes are advertised, sold and bought, explaining the restrictions on television advertising and sales to children.

- an explanation of why people do it and find it difficult to stop, and the help they can get.

This work could be shared among small groups who could display it in the form of wall stories and posters.

Invite the children to devise messages for other children who might be tempted to experiment with smoking. Recall the warnings on cigarette packets which focus on the negative reasons for not smoking. Do the children think this kind of warning works?

Ask the children to look for positive reasons for not smoking and to include these in their messages. For example,

- Non-smokers don't puff.

- Non-smokers aren't broke.

- Let chimneys smoke – don't join them.

- A fool at one end, a fire on the other.

Activity 3 ● *Smoking and school*

- Survey work. Family work. Presentation.
- Class or group activity.

With the co-operation of the school staff, it would be possible for the children to organise a survey on aspects of smoking in school. They could develop their investigation and presentation skills, and look at questions such as:

— Has our school got a policy about smoking?

— How does the staff let people (including visitors) know? Are there signs or notices?

— Where are the notices?

— Where (if anywhere) is smoking allowed?

— Are there any warnings about the dangers of smoking?

— Has any one given up smoking? How did they do it?

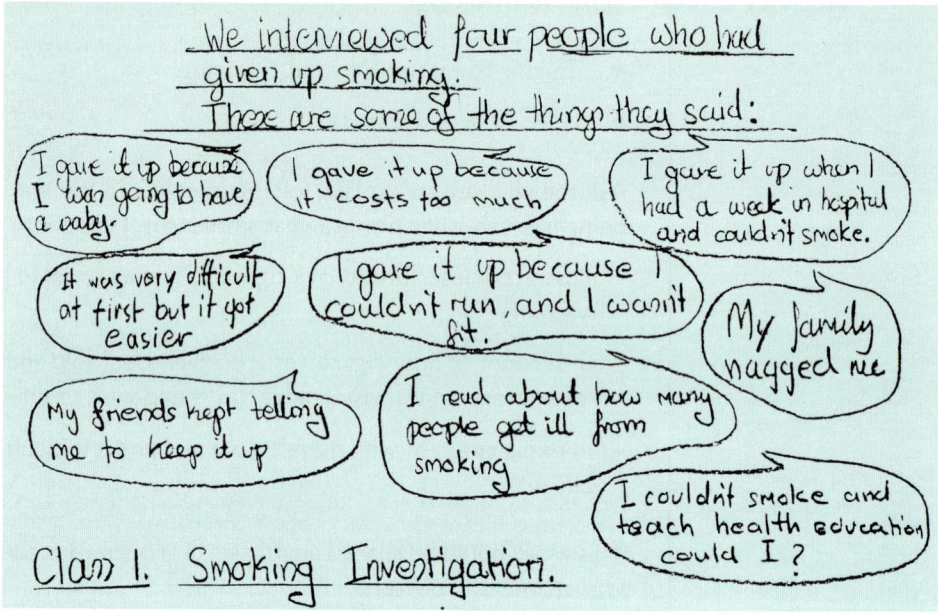

Where there is good parent-school involvement, children could use their survey and interview techniques to ask their families and relatives about their smoking and non-smoking careers. Ask them to try to find out:

— why some people didn't ever start smoking.

— who tried it at a very early age and gave it up after one try.

— who began smoking early, and who began later, and why.

— who has tried to give up, and succeeded, and what helped them.

— who has tried to give up and failed.

— who would like to give up.

Cross-curricular links: the devising of a simple questionnaire, and the analysis and presentation of findings can provide opportunities for mathematical analysis and presentation.

There might be an opportunity for an investigation to discover if children in the class have tried smoking, and why. The children themselves may feel that they could take part (anonymously) in a simple survey by questionnaire about their views on smoking and experimentation.

Activity 4

The persuaders

- Talking together. Drawing. Writing. Role-play.
- Class or group and pair activities.

Revise the activity on persuaders for ages 8 and 9 (page 57), in which the children were asked to invent a robot persuader which could force people to do what it wanted. Emphasise how easy it would be to recognise such a robot as it went around wearing the label *Persuader*.

Talk with the children about the persuaders they are likely to meet. How might they look? How might they disguise themselves to blend in with the scene? Might they become 'undercover' people in order to tempt children to experiment with non-medicinal drugs (such as cigarettes, alcohol, unknown substances and illegally obtained drugs)?

Invite the children to work in pairs or small groups, and imagine and then draw persuaders who are trying to persuade them to try one or more of the following:

- cigarettes.
- alcohol.
- an unknown substance.
- illegally obtained drugs.

Ask the children to add to their pictures by writing around their drawings, how they would recognise the persuader. Look for reasons based solely on appearance, especially stereotyped responses showing easily recognisable characters. Invite the children to think about these and the dangers involved.

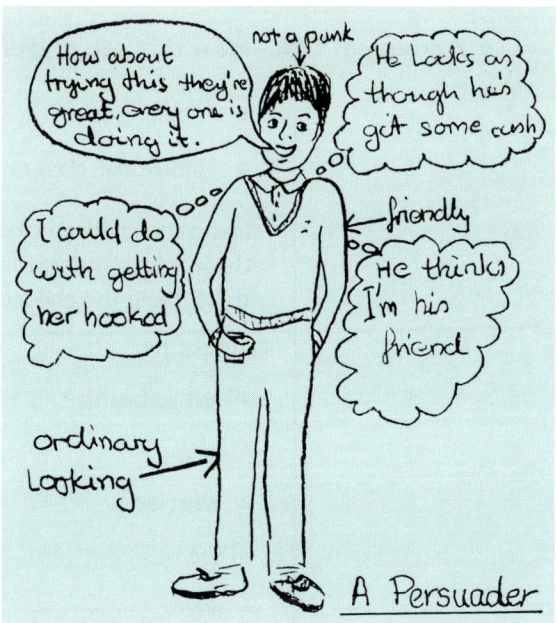

Ask the children to add to their pictures speech bubbles showing what the persuader might be saying.

Encourage the children to include thought bubbles showing what the persuader might be thinking or planning, and to comment on the difference between what is being said and what is being thought.

Invite the children to remember the strategies for keeping rules, for assessing risk and for sticking to a decision. Ask them to look at those they might choose and the help they might need when confronted by a persuader like this.

This situation can be enacted through role-play. The children could explore alternative endings to the situation and talk about the role-play with other groups.

Invite the children to think about the other persuaders they might find among:

— the people they see around them.

— the people they see on television and in other media.

— the people they see in advertisements.

Talk with the children about how these people might try to persuade them to try drugs, and why they themselves might be talked into trying something?

This is a good time to look at role models: family, older school children, young adults, pop stars, local heroes, television personalities, sports personalities, characters in television series and comic strips. Ask the children:

'What is it about their lifestyle that we like?'
'Why do we admire these people?'
'Why do some of them resist using drugs?'
'Why do some of them use cigarettes, alcohol and other substances?'

Activity 5 ● *How do I see myself?*

● Collecting pictures. Writing. Drawing. Talking together.

● Individual, class or group activities.

Invite the children to collect pictures of people from magazines, with emphasis on those which portray faces clearly. Display the pictures, it might help to number them. Help the children to group the pictures into categories such as:

— healthy

— not so healthy

— happy

— worried

— sad

— angry

— confident

— kind

— wicked

Ask the children to write about their individual views on the different images people have, and present them to the others.

This could be a good moment to remind the children of how narrowly some people see drugs and drug users, and to emphasise how much *they* know about the world in which drugs are used – and sometimes misused.

Invite the children to write about themselves using the miminum of words and adding a picture if they wish. Ask them to focus on the kind of person they see themselves to be, their lifestyle, awareness of drugs, interests and their ambitions for themselves.

Ask them to extend the activity by portraying themselves as they think they will be in ten years time. Will they have different role models?

Invite them to complete the activity by thinking about and describing (orally, in pictures, or in writing) one or more role models: characters whom they would to imitate and whose lifestyles they think they would like. Invite them to ask themselves:

'What do I admire about *them*?' (Not just their lifestyles.)
'What would I need to know before I decide to imitate them?'
'Is their lifestyle healthy? Is it drug-wise?'

Activity 6 ● *Are all persuaders trying to harm our lifestyles?*

- Collecting pictures and advertisements. Talking together.

- Class or group activity.

Invite the children to observe, note down and bring into class examples of healthy lifestyle promotion. These might include posters, leaflets, advertisements on television, in magazines, on food packaging and in shops. (Your local Health Education Officers could provide you with resources.) Encourage them to categorise what they find under headings such as:

– healthy eating

– healthy heart

– exercise

– healthy pregnancy

– infant care

– parenthood

– personal hygiene

– dental care

– caring relationships

Extend their thinking to healthy persuasion in the form of love, care and support from families, friends, school, health professionals, church and community groups.

Content box 6   Feeling good

When have I wished for the ground to open up and swallow me? When have I felt on top of the world? What can I learn from these experiences? What can I learn about drug-free ways of coping, and about being in control?

Activity 1   *When have I wished for the floor to open up and swallow me?*

- Talking together.

- Individual and group activity.

Invite the children to work individually or in groups to explore times when, because of something which happened, they wished the floor could have opened up and allowed them to disappear.

Encourage them to share their feelings by asking questions such as:

— Was it something said or done by you or to you?

— Was it something which was threatened or forced on you?

— Was it something that you felt you couldn't cope with?

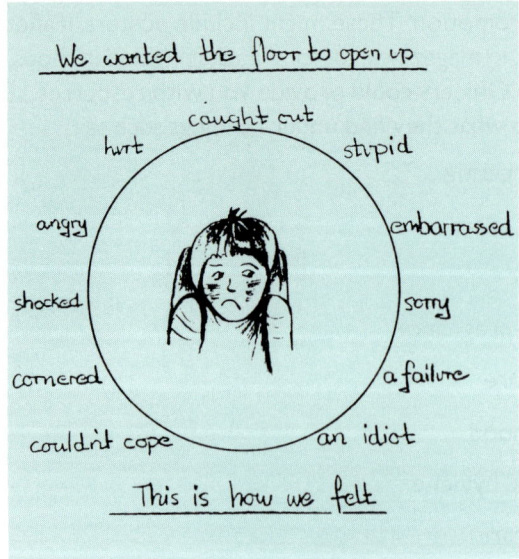

Emphasise that everyone has times like these and shares these feelings. How did the children cope? Invite them to share their strategies, or lack of strategies, and to pick out ones which might have helped. You could make a circle of feelings to identify the feelings more clearly.

Ask the children what would have helped them (apart from disappearance!) Would a drug have helped? A medicinal drug? A non-medicinal drug, such as a cigarette, a drink, a cup of coffee or tea?

Activity 2 | ***When have I felt on top of the world?***

- Talking together. Writing.
- Class or group activity.

Ask the children, for contrast, to recall times when they felt on top of the world because of something which had happened. Ask them to draw a circle of feelings to describe this. Invite them to review the different occasions when they felt like this by asking these questions:

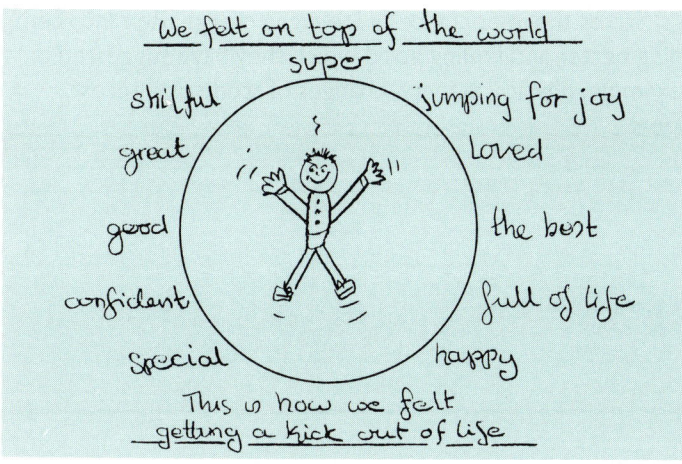

'Was it because of something I did?'
'Was it because of something someone else did or said?'

Ask them to write about and illustrate the reasons why they felt this way.

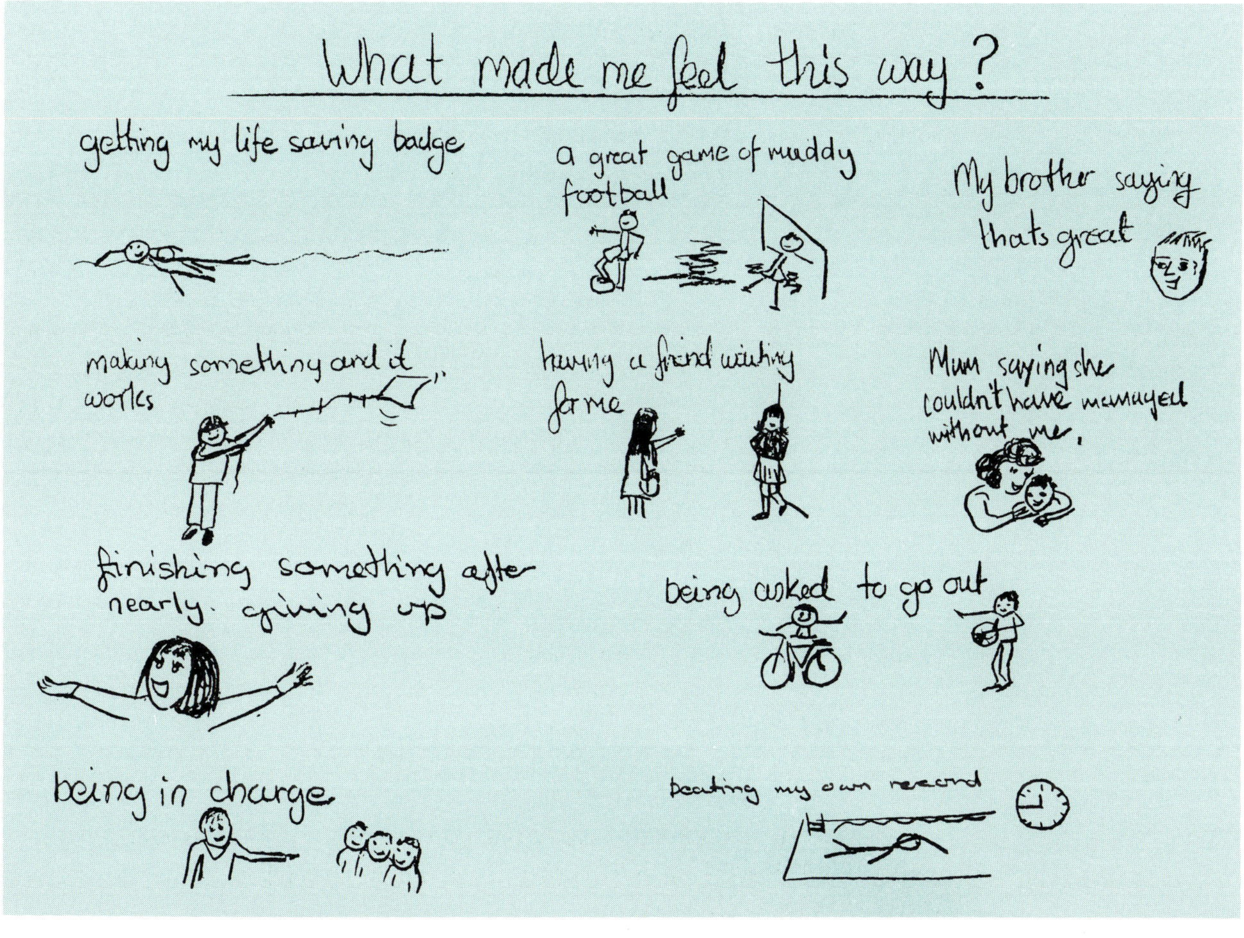

Ask the children to try to pin down where the 'on top of the world feeling' comes from. Is it something you can capture, put in a bottle, sell or keep? Explore with the children the difference between this kind of good inner feeling and the good effects of:

— medicinal drugs, taken in a controlled way to cure or cope with illness.

— non-medicinal drugs, which are not needed for illness, and give a temporary 'lift' or 'kick', but can become addictive.

Help the children to weigh up the difference between drug induced good feelings and natural good feelings. Stress the importance of feeling in charge. Remind them of the strategies for feeling better and feeling good which they have suggested in previous activities, for example, physical activity, changes of scene or interest, sharing and seeking support.

Family Worksheet Masters

The worksheet masters in the following pages are photocopiable so you can give them to the children to take home and work through with their families. The worksheets can also be used by the children with the teacher in a one-to-one session, or in group work. However, home use brings to your health education programme the important benefit of family involvement.

The worksheets vary in difficulty, and begin with worksheets for the younger children. They have not been age-graded as you will probably prefer to select them according to the needs of your class.

A photocopiable letter has also been provided which you can send home with the worksheets. This explains to the parent, or family, the purpose of the worksheets and suggests ways in which they could be used. You may wish to adapt this letter to your own needs.

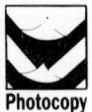

Dear

Family Worksheets

These worksheets are an important part of your child's health education. We would like you and your child to work on them together. They will show you some of the ways in which the children are learning about the world of drugs. We are trying to stress that there are drugs which make people healthy and drugs which are harmful. One important message they will meet is, 'All medicines are drugs *but* some drugs are NOT medicines'. Many of the worksheets ask the children to think about understanding risks and making decisions.

The children are bringing these worksheets home so you can share in the work they have been doing at school. You can help them to get the most out of what they have learned. This is not the kind of homework which is taken back to school and marked, it is family work, everyone can share in it. We think you will learn a great deal from the way your child thinks about health and explains it all to you.

When you sit down with your child to start a worksheet, one way to start is to ask your child to explain what has been happening in health education sessions at school. The next step is to work together through the activities on the worksheet. Remember that there are no right and wrong answers. The important thing is to talk together. Don't worry if your child's drawings are not very clear, you can always ask her, or him, to tell you about them. Read the worksheet *with* your child or read it *to* your child, but don't make the reading a struggle. Write for your child if that is what she or he would like you to do. Most importantly, feel free to contribute some questions of your own, and think of other things to talk, draw and write about.

This school is working to promote health and your child is sharing that with you at home. This is your chance to help bring important health messages home to your child.

We hope you enjoy sharing these worksheets with your child.

© Health Education Authority 1989

The World of Drugs

Family Worksheet 1

Photocopy

My name is ....

What goes onto your body?

Talk about all the things that go onto your body.

Can you draw some of them? We have done two for you.

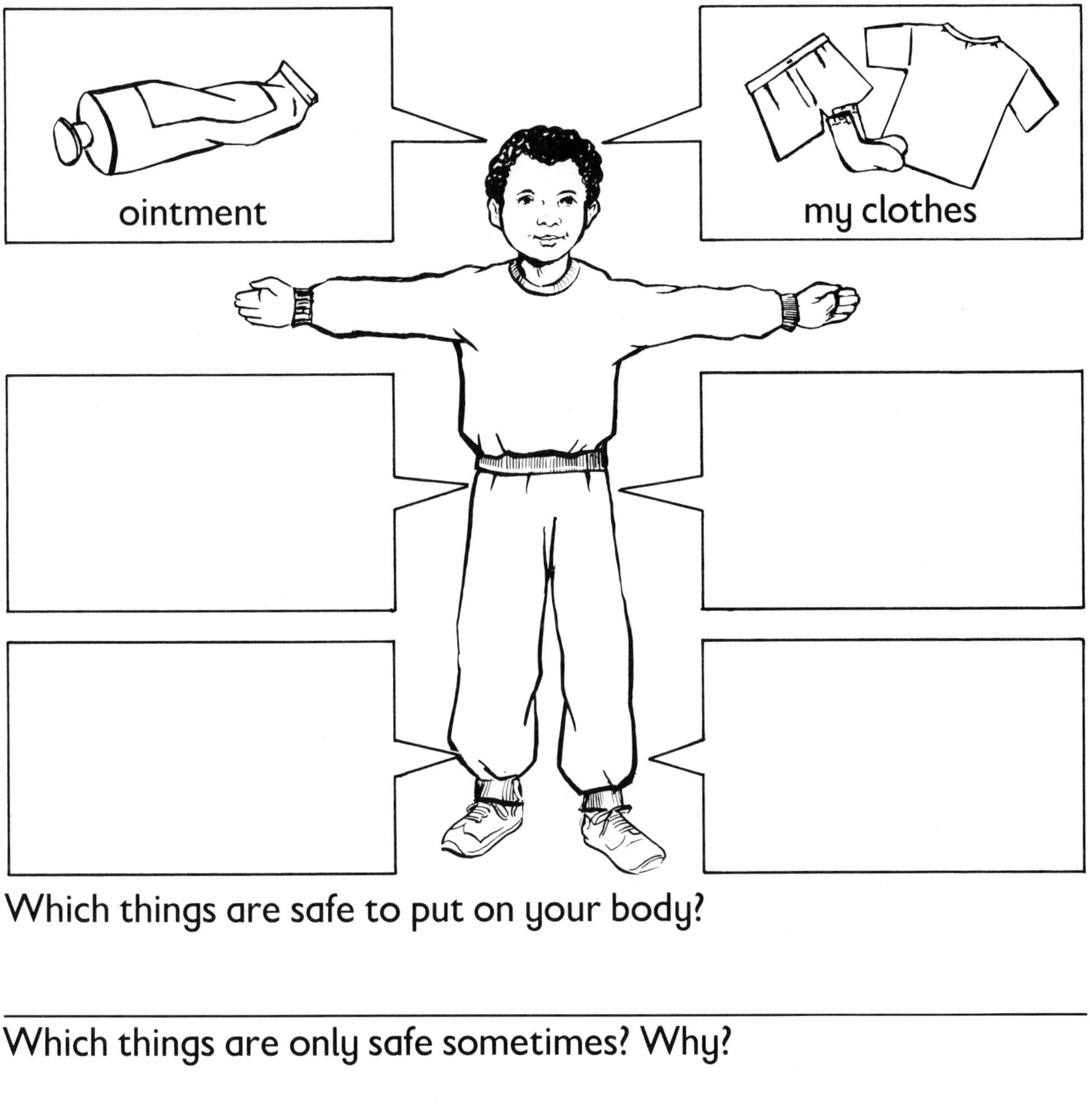
ointment
my clothes

Which things are safe to put on your body?

____

Which things are only safe sometimes? Why?

____

Which things are NOT safe? Why?

____

Photocopy

The World of Drugs

Family Worksheet 2

My name is ....

What do I do when things go onto my body?

Here are some things which could go onto your body

What would you do if they did go onto your body?

Draw a line to show what you would do. We have done one for you.

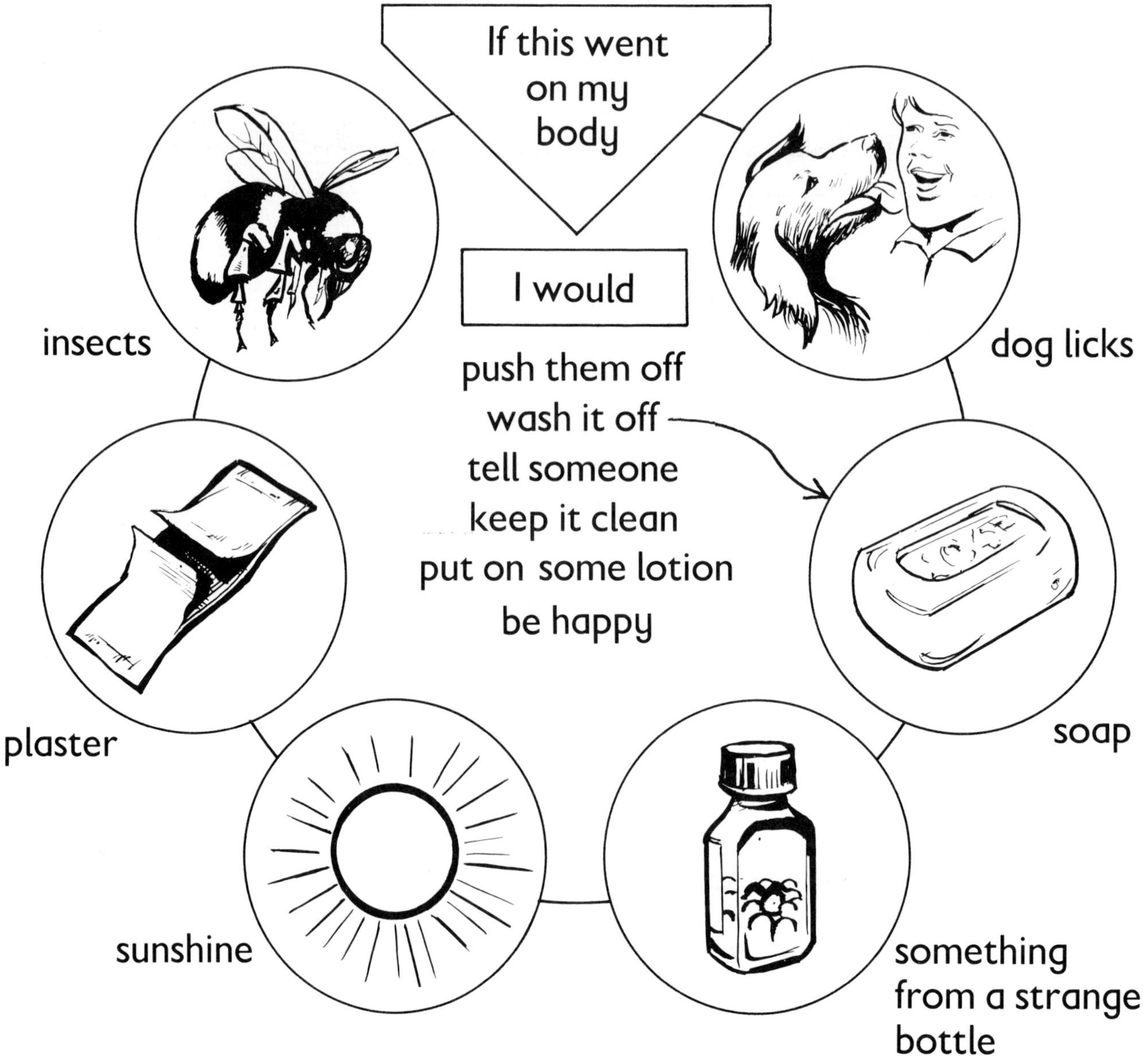

If this went on my body
I would
push them off
wash it off
tell someone
keep it clean
put on some lotion
be happy
insects
dog licks
plaster
soap
sunshine
something from a strange bottle

Can you think of some more?

The World of Drugs

 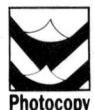
My name is ....

What is safe for me to touch? 1

Talk about all the things on this table.
Can you sort them out? We have done one for you.

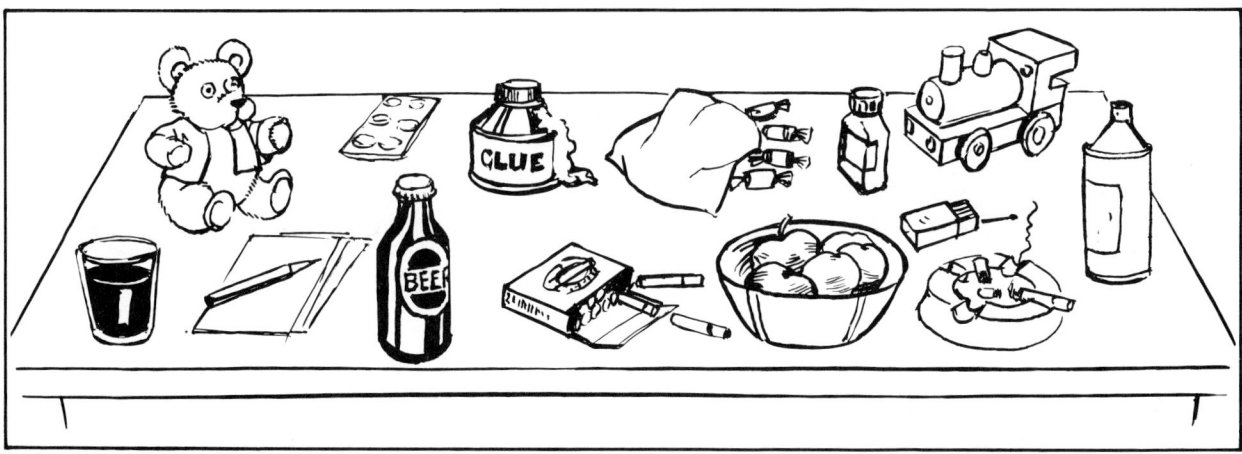

Draw things which are safe to touch in this box

Draw the things which are NOT safe to touch in this box.

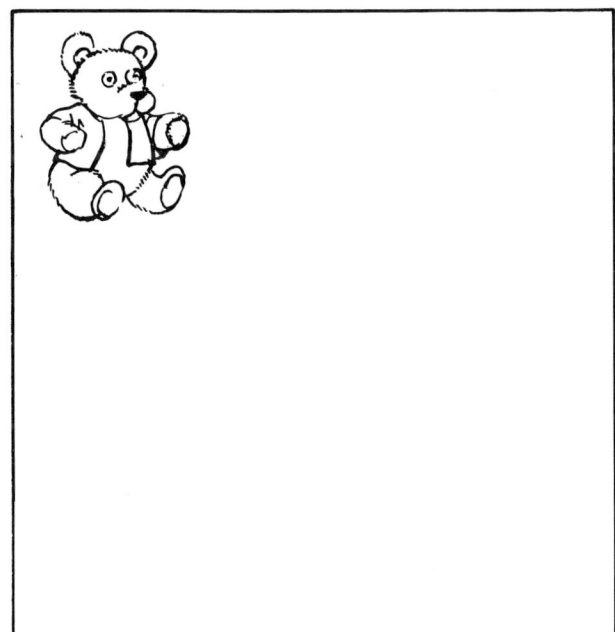

Can you think of some more things you might find here which are NOT safe to touch?

Talk about why they are not safe to touch.

When would you go and ask someone for help?

The World of Drugs

My name is ....

What is safe for me to touch? 2

Talk about the things here.

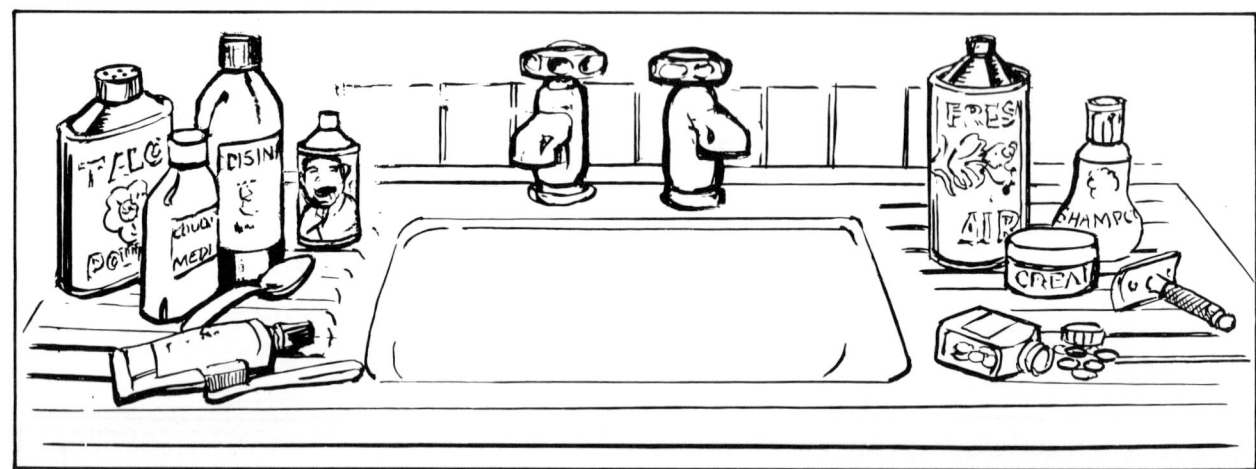

Draw things which are safe to touch in this box

Draw the things which are NOT safe to touch in this box.

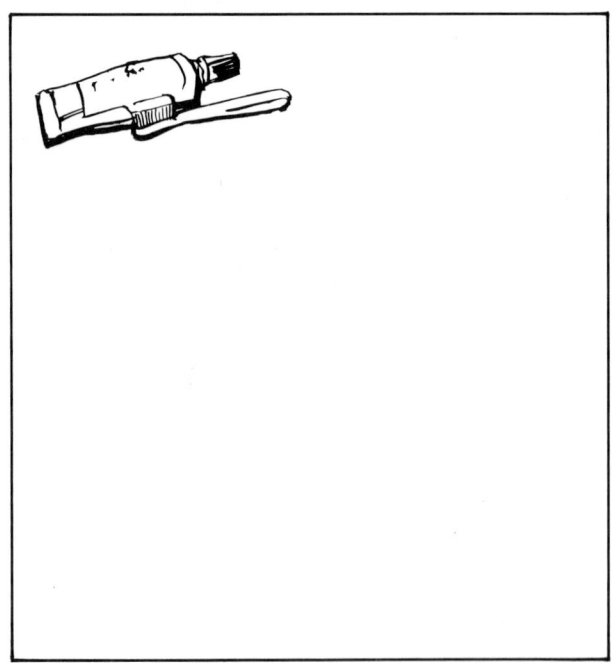

Can you think of some more things you might find here which are NOT safe to touch?

Talk about why they are not safe to touch.

When would you ask someone to help?

The World of Drugs

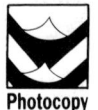
Photocopy

My name is ....

Feeling ill and feeling better

Draw yourself feeling ill.
Talk about:
What is making you feel ill?

What are you doing?

_____

This is me feeling ill.

Draw yourself feeling better.
Talk about:
What you are doing now.

_____

This is me feeling better

Draw some of the things that
helped you to get better.

Talk about:
The things which made you get
better.

What must you remember
about medicines?

_____

The World of Drugs

My name is ....

Which things are safe to put on my body?

These are some of the things Tammy says go on her body.

Talk about them. Do any of them go on *your* body?

Can you think of any more?

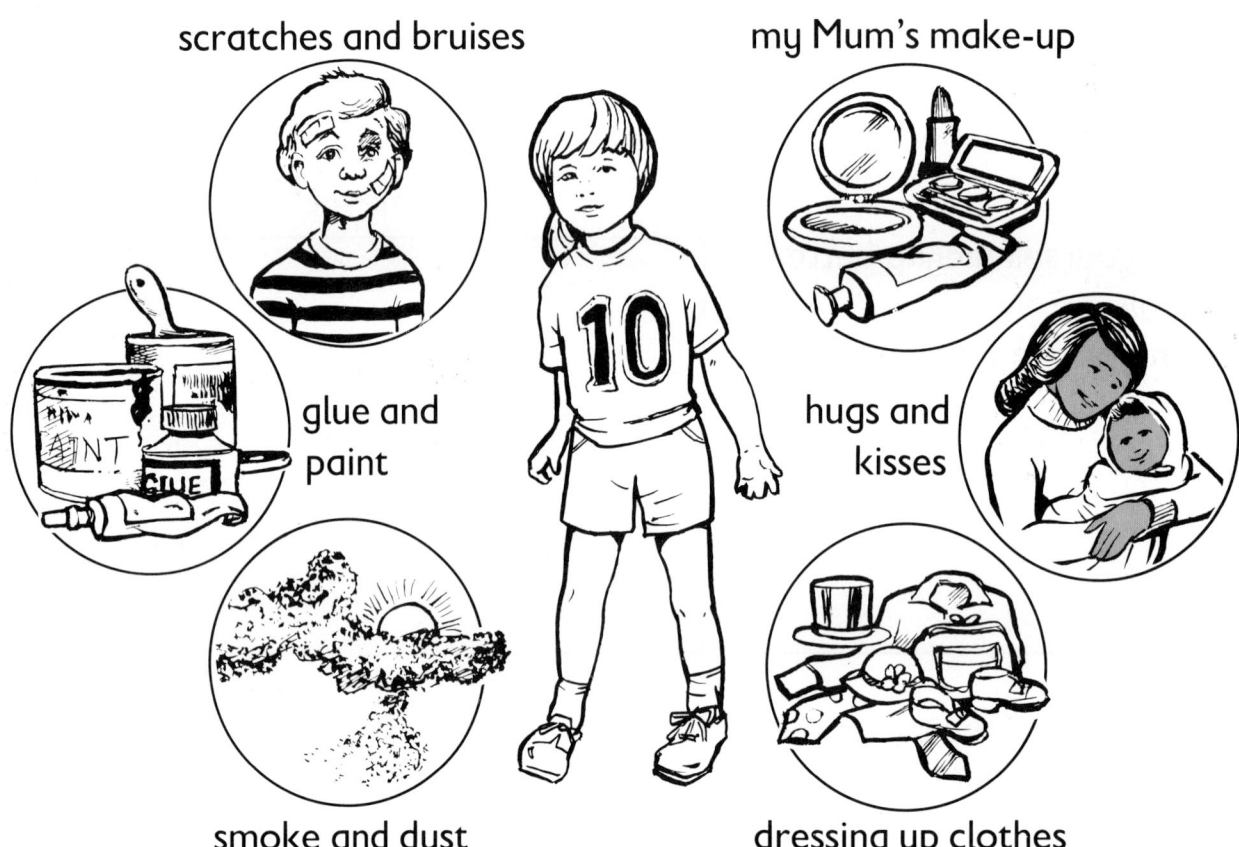

scratches and bruises

my Mum's make-up

glue and paint

hugs and kisses

smoke and dust

dressing up clothes

Which things do you think are safe?

_____

Which things do you think Tammy should ask someone about? Why?

_____

Which things do you think are NOT safe? Why?

_____

The World of Drugs

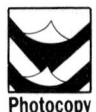

My name is ....

Which things are safe to put in my body?

These are some of the things Sammy says go *in* his body.

Talk about them. Do any of them go in *your* body?

Can you think of any more things?

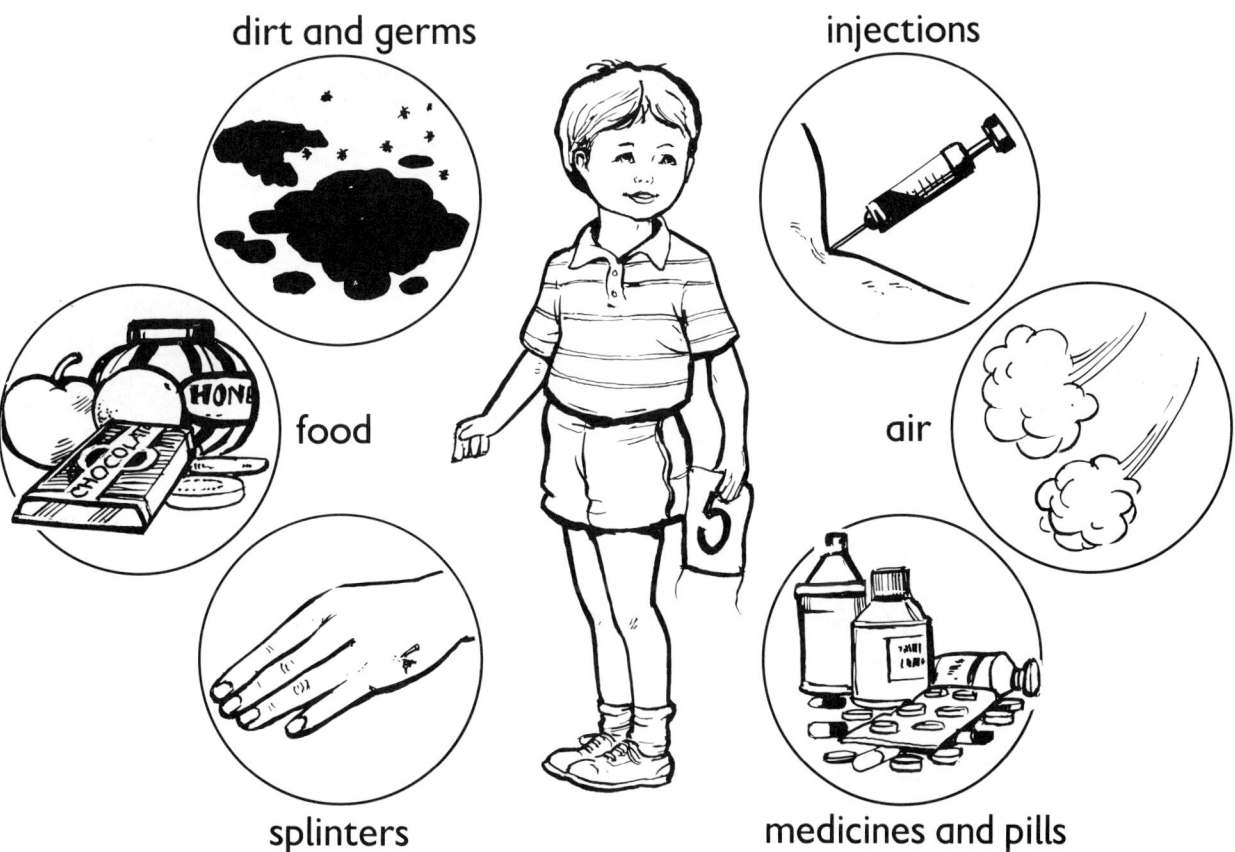

dirt and germs

injections

food

air

splinters

medicines and pills

Which things do you think are safe?

_____

Which things do you think Sammy should ask someone about? Why?

_____

Which things do you think are dangerous? Why?

_____

Photocopy

The World of Drugs

My name is ....

Who decides what goes into my body?

Here are some things which could go in your body.
Talk about them. Can you think of some more?

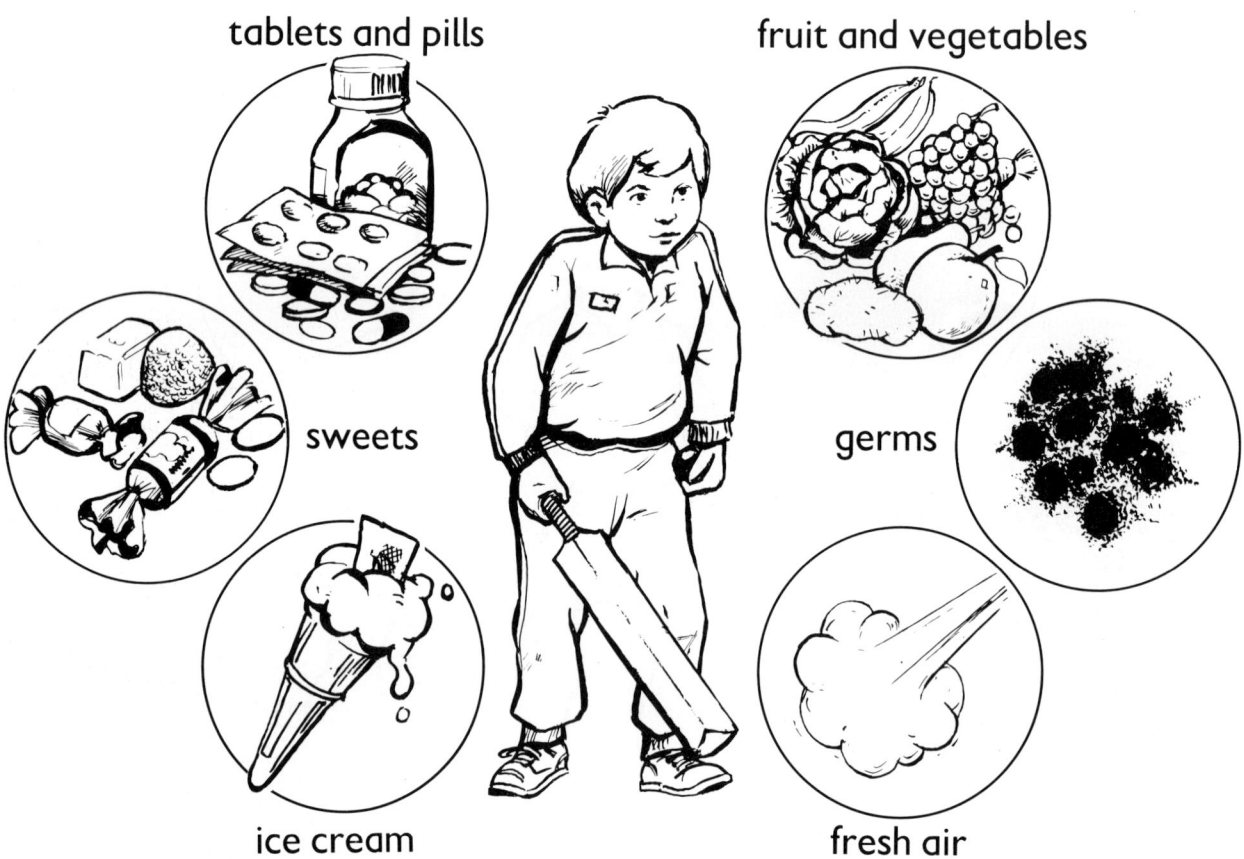

tablets and pills

fruit and vegetables

sweets

germs

ice cream

fresh air

Can you sort them into these three boxes?
We have done one for you.

Things which I put into my body.	Things which other people tell me to take.	Things which get in by themselves.
sweets		

Talk about the things which you think are safe, the things which you
should ask or tell people about, and the things which could be dangerous.

© Health Education Authority 1989

The World of Drugs

Photocopy

My name is ....

How do things get into my body?

Look at these things.
Talk about how they get into your body.
Now fill in the boxes showing how things get into your body.
We have done one for you.

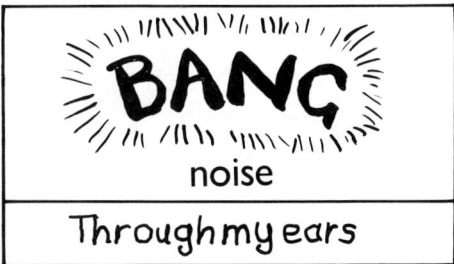
noise

Through my ears

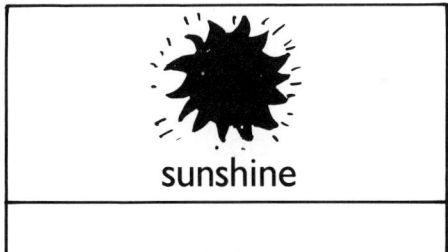
sunshine

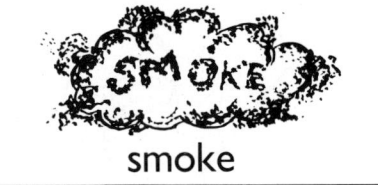
smoke

– through your nose?
– through your mouth?
– through your skin?
– through your eyes?
– through your ears?

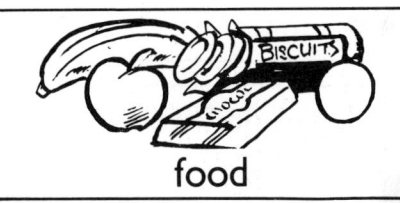
food

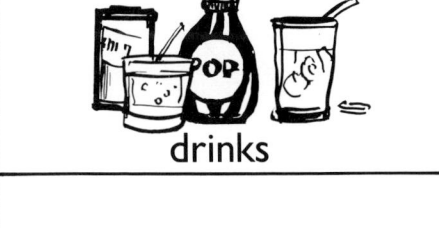
drinks

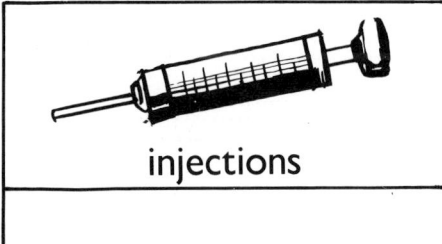
injections

Can you draw some more?

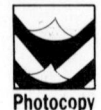

The World of Drugs

My name is ....

What goes into my body through my mouth, nose and skin?

Think about all the things which go into your body?
Can you finish these lists? We have started them for you.

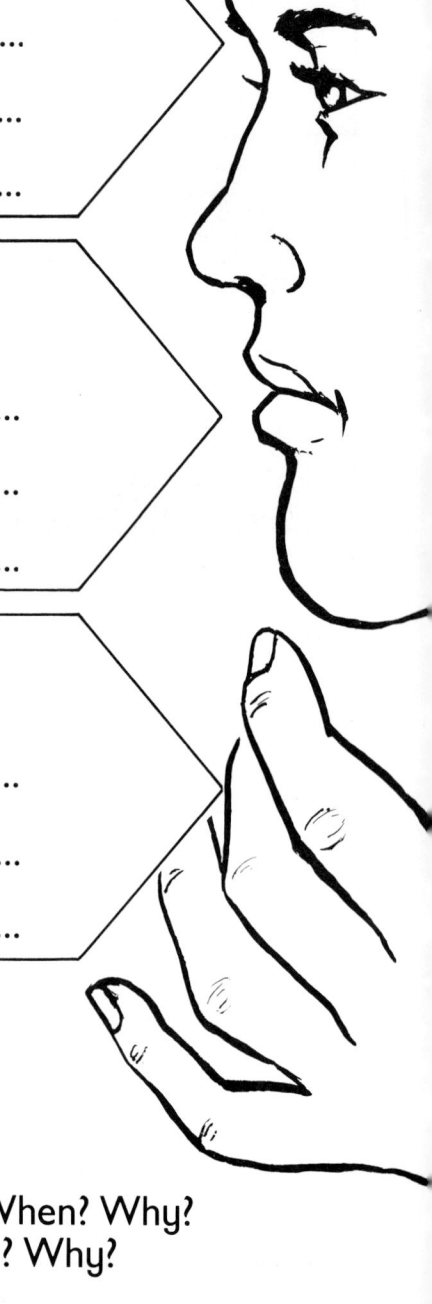

These go into my body through my
nose:

- nose drops ....
- ....
- ....
- ....
- ....
- ....

These go into my body through my
mouth:

- food ....
- ....
- ....
- ....
- ....
- ....

These go into my body through my
skin:

- insect bites ....
- ....
- ....
- ....
- ....
- ....

Talk with your family.
Can they think of any more things?

Now talk about:
– the ones which you think are safe.
– the ones which you think are only safe sometimes. When? Why?
– the ones which you think could be dangerous. When? Why?

The World of Drugs

 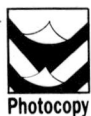
My name is ....

Body systems

Here are four ways in which things can get into your body.
Can you give some examples? Ask your family to help you.

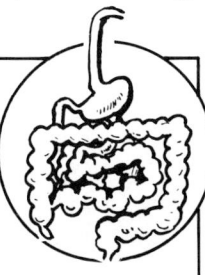

These things go into my
digestive system and
are absorbed by my
body:

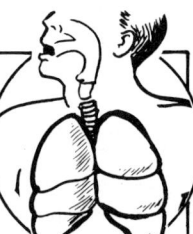

These things go into my
lungs and are absorbed
by my bloodstream:

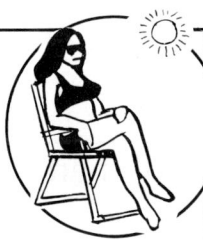

These things are
absorbed through
my skin into my body:

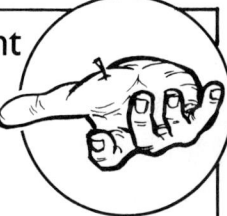

These things go straight
through my skin into
my bloodstream:

Here are some suggestions to help you

foods, drinks, medicines, powders, drugs, sunlight, ointment,
lotions, dust, germs, dirt, smoke, stings, diseases, injections,
splinters, pollution, cigarettes, solvents, alcohol, caffeine.

The World of Drugs

My name is ....

The persuaders

Look at the picture and talk about what you think is happening.

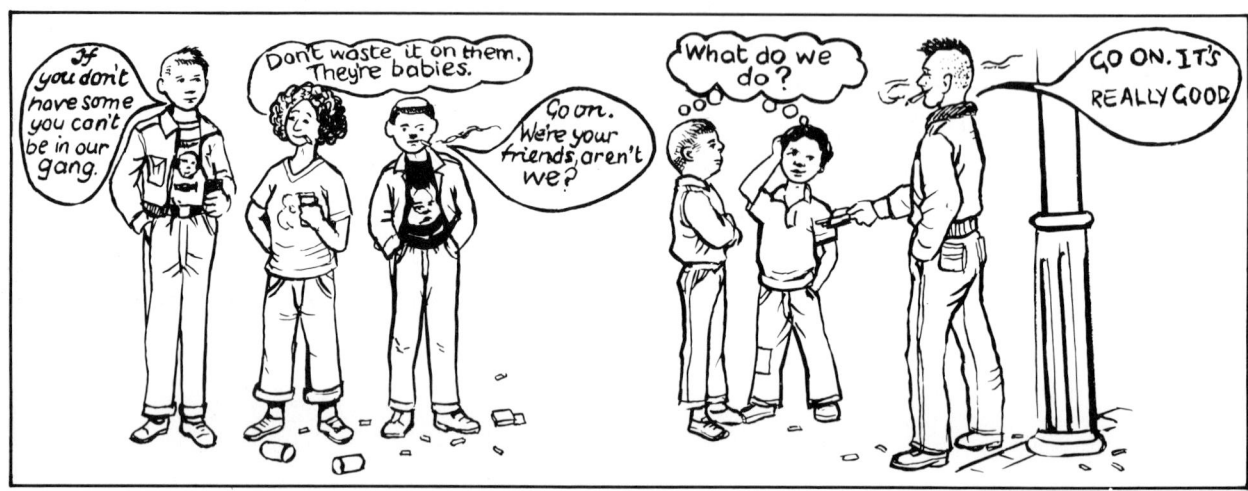

What are the older children trying to do?

_____

What do you think the two young children could do?

_____

Here are some ideas. What do you think of them?

_____

Can you think of some better ideas?

_____

– They could run away.

– They could cry.

– They could find someone to tell.

– They could have just a little taste.

Put a ring around the sensible
things to do.
Put a line under the risky things to do.
What do you think you would do?

I think they could:

_____

The World of Drugs

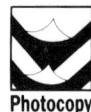

My name is ....

Where do we find medicines? 1

Talk about all the places where people can get medicines.

Write these places inside the rings. We have done one for you.

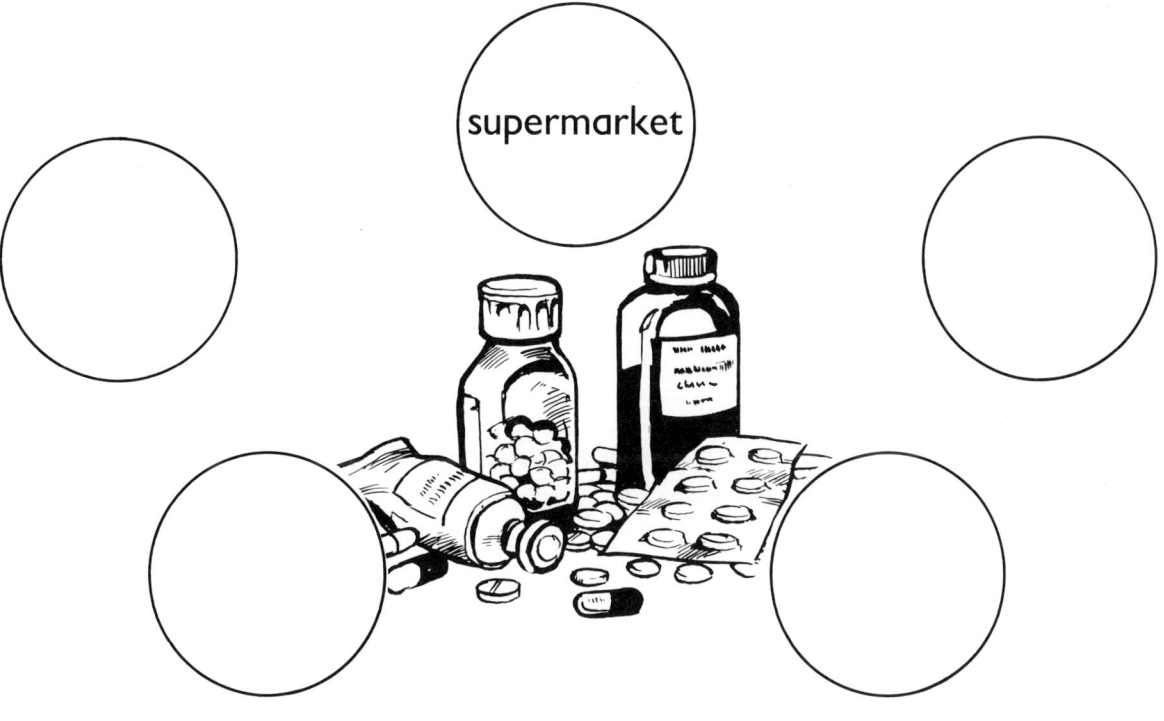

supermarket

aspirins – from the corner shop

Many medicines can be bought without prescription. You can even send away to newspapers and magazines for them. How many medicines of this kind can you think of? We have given you one.

_____

Photocopy

The World of Drugs

My name is ....

Learning to say 'No'

Most of the time our friends and other people only ask us to do things we know are safe and which we enjoy. Sometimes they can ask us to do things which are not safe and which are very risky or dangerous to our health.

One way to be prepared in case this happens is to practise asking yourself these questions:

– Am I sure it's safe?
– Is it risky? Is this a time to say 'No'?
– Who can I ask?

Talk about some safe things which people ask you to do. Write some of them here.

. . . .

. . . .

. . . .

Talk about the risky things which people ask you to do, write some of them here.

. . . .

. . . .

. . . .

Talk about times when it is difficult to say 'No', especially to friends. What can you do? What can you say? Write in the empty bubbles.

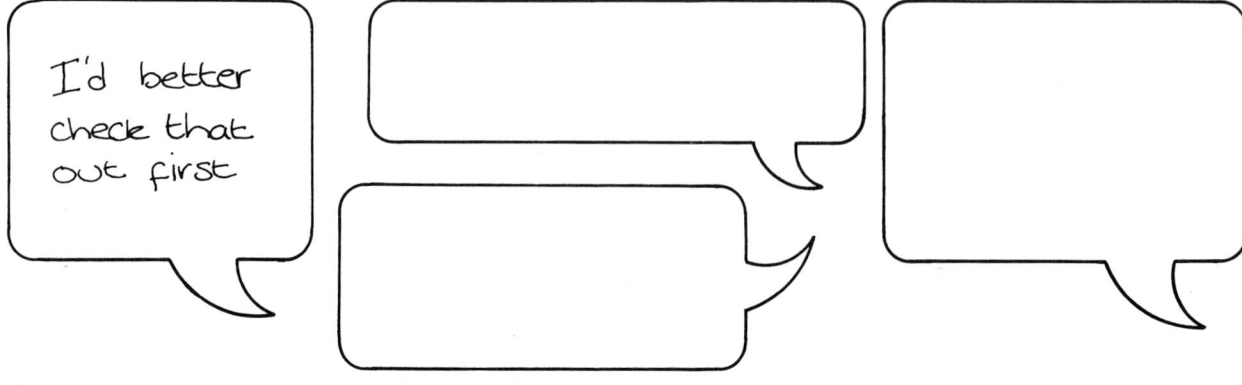

I'd better check that out first

The World of Drugs

 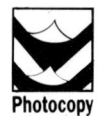
My name is ....

What do you do when you are ill?

Talk about what you would do. Draw lines to
show what you think you would do. We have
done one for you.

If I had:

a headache

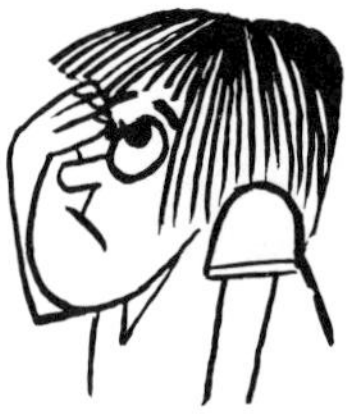

a stomach ache

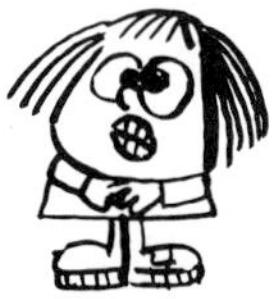

a cold

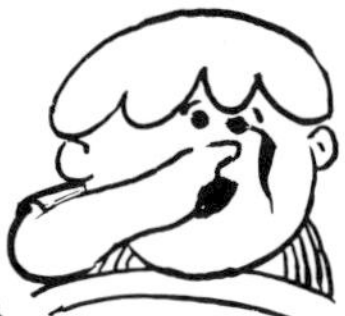

a cough

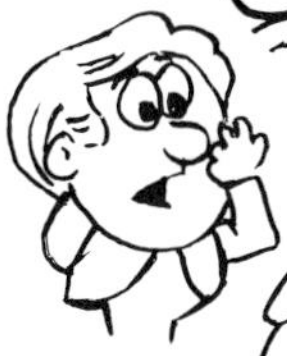

a sore throat

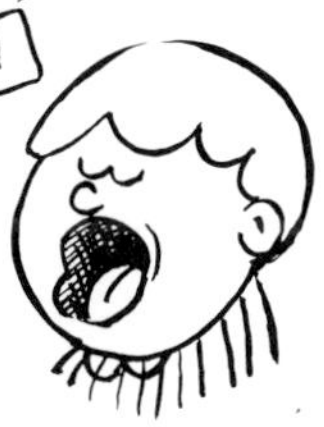

a splinter in my finger

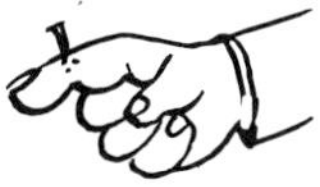

a cut hand

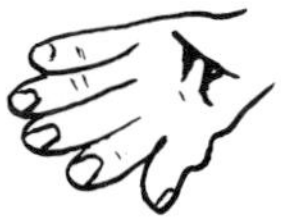

felt sick

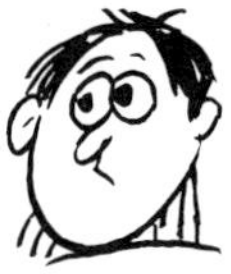

felt a bit low

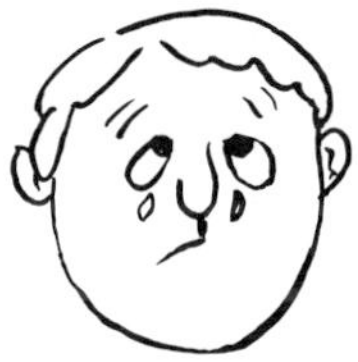

I would:

(tell a grown up)

(try not to pass on my germs)

(take my Mum's indigestion pills)

(wait and see if it got better)

(go out in the fresh air)

(look in the bathroom for something to make me better)

(take some of my sister's cough medicine)

(take a pill)

(dial 999)

(put a plaster on it)

(go to bed)

(go to the shop and buy some medicine)

(go to the doctor's surgery)

Talk about the things you think would be dangerous to do.
Put a star ★ by them.

The World of Drugs

My name is ....

Feeling low

Here is a circle of feelings about feeling low. Can you think of any more words to describe feeling low?

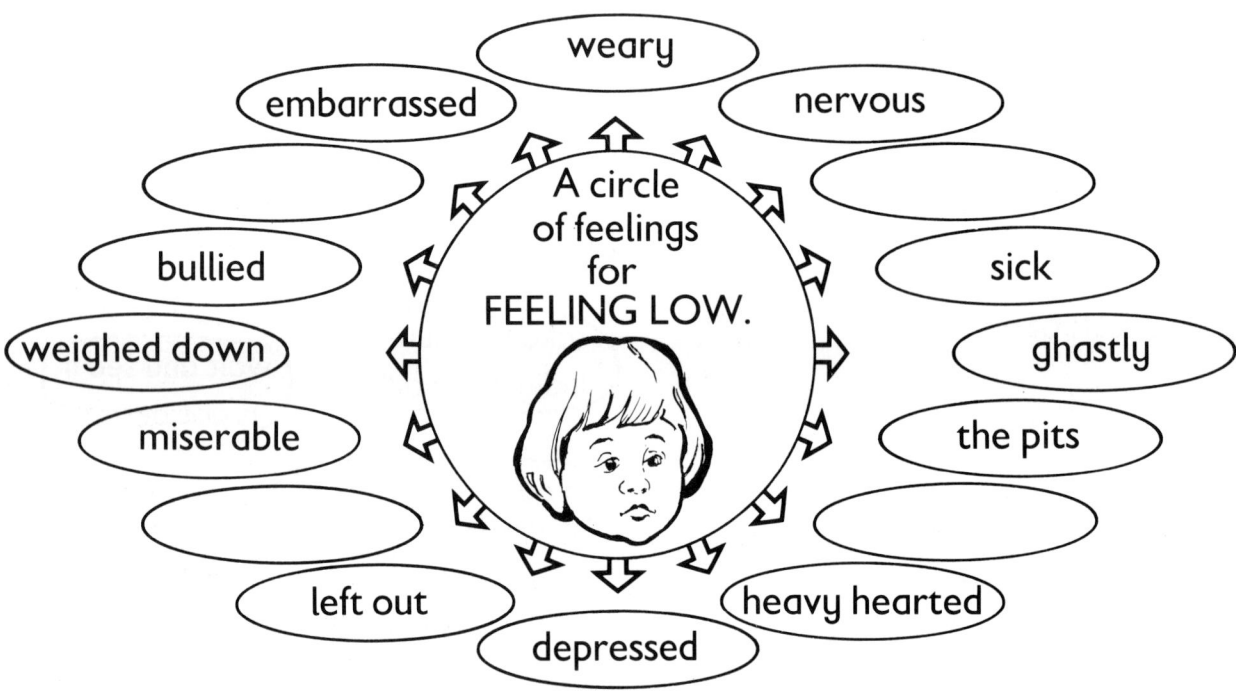

weary

embarrassed

nervous

A circle of feelings for FEELING LOW.

bullied

sick

weighed down

ghastly

miserable

the pits

left out

heavy hearted

depressed

Talk about what makes you feel low?
I feel low when

_____

What do other people do to make you feel low?
I feel low when other people

_____

What makes you feel better? What can you do to make yourself feel better?
I can

_____

The World of Drugs

 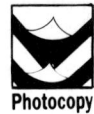

My name is ....

Feeling good

Class 3 have made a circle of feelings to describe feeling good.
Talk about the words they have used. Can you think of some more?
Think about the times when you are feeling good.

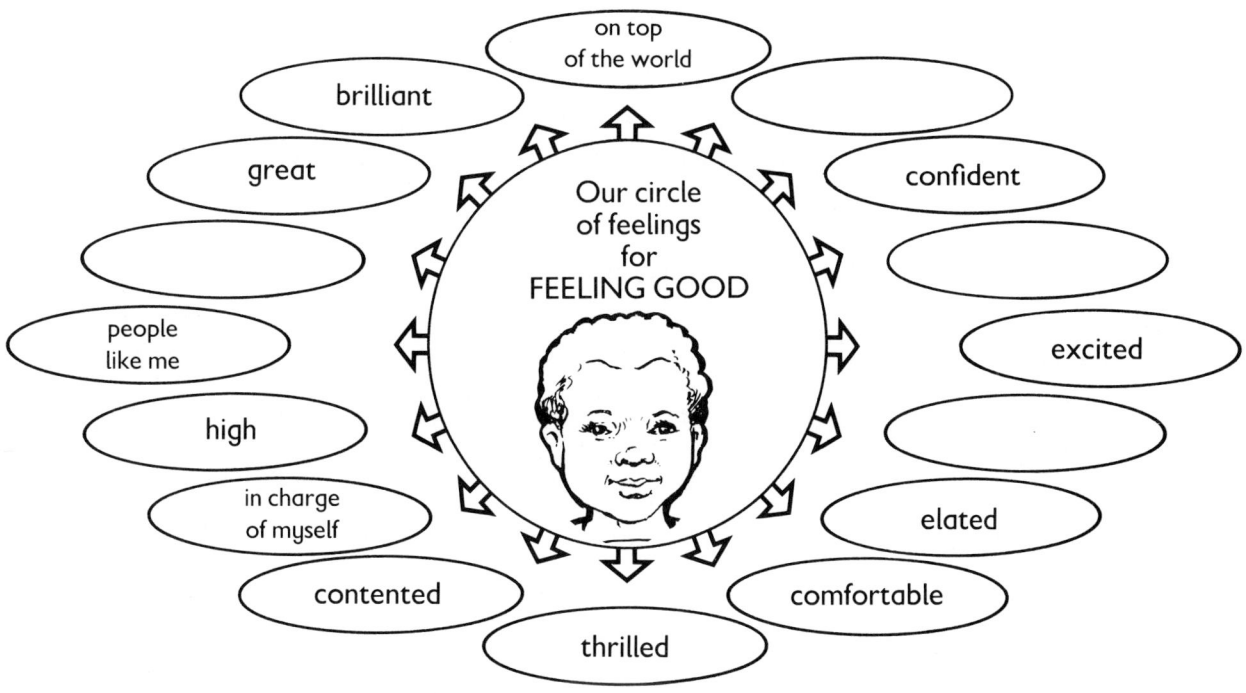

Talk about what makes you feel good.
I feel good when

_____

What do other people do to make you feel good?
When they

_____

What can you do to make yourself feel good?
I can

_____

The World of Drugs

My name is ....

Who needs medicine?

> **Health Education Notice Board**
> All medicines are drugs, but
> not all drugs are medicines.

Think and talk about people you know, or people you have heard of, who need drugs which are medicines. Who are they?

Write about some of these people who need drugs which are medicines. Draw some pictures, here are some ideas to help you:

disease	immunisation	illnesses	cure	get better
stay alive	normal life	problems	born too soon	accident
emergency	asthma	diabetes	epilepsy	

1. They are people who ....

_____

2. They are people who ....

_____

3. They are people who ....

_____

4. They are people who ....

_____

Where do they get their drugs?

_____

The World of Drugs

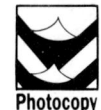

My name is ....

Where do we find medicines? 2

Think of some of the places where you could find drugs which are medicines.
We have written some for you. Can you think of any more?
Write them in the empty boxes.

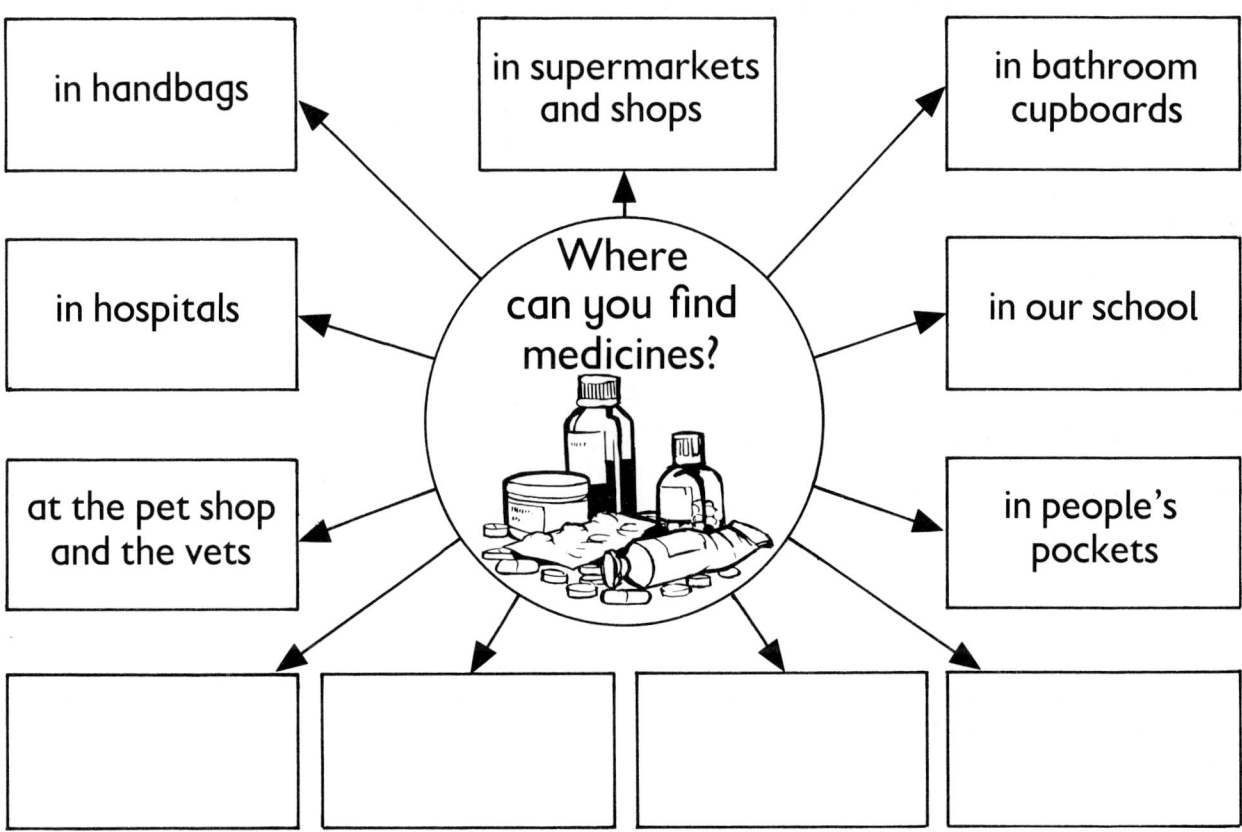

| in handbags | in supermarkets and shops | in bathroom cupboards |

Where can you find medicines?

| in hospitals | | in our school |

| at the pet shop and the vets | | in people's pockets |

Talk about the kinds of drugs you would find in each place.
Why are they there?

Do you have drugs which are medicines in your home?

_____

Where would you find them?

_____

Talk about what they are for.

Photocopy

The World of Drugs

My name is ....

Where do we find drugs which are not medicines?

Where can we find drugs which are NOT medicines? Write in the empty boxes. We have done one for you.

HEALTH EDUCATION NOTICE BOARD
REMEMBER
All medicines are DRUGS, but not all drugs are medicines.

Talk about the kinds of drugs that you find in these places? What are they there for?

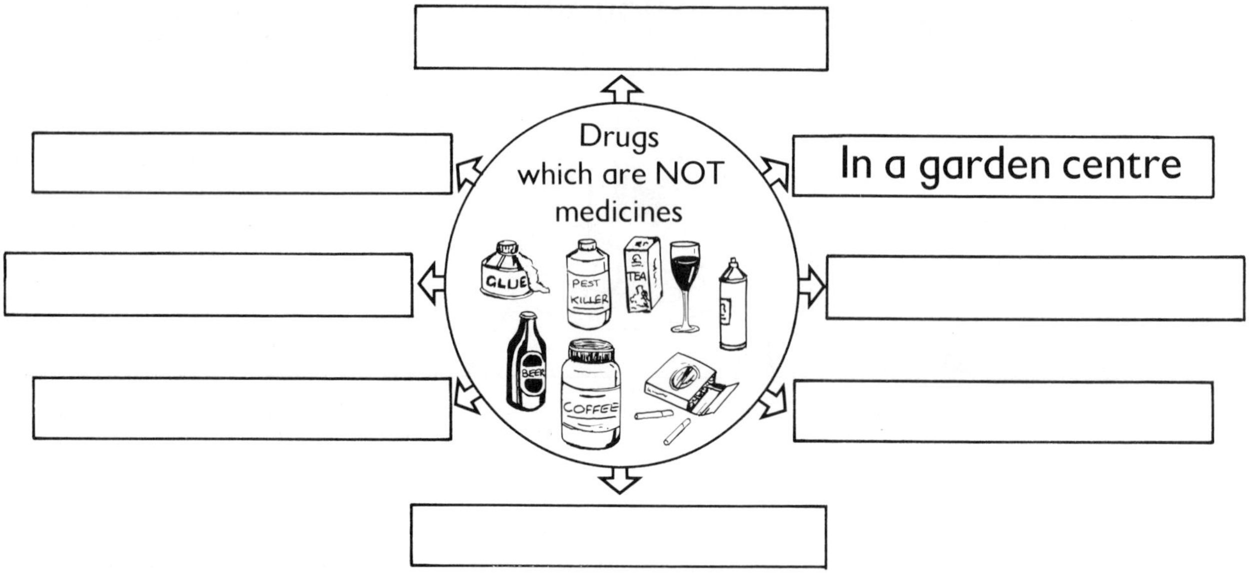

Drugs which are NOT medicines

In a garden centre

Talk about where you might find them. Who uses them and why?

_____

Can you think of any more drugs which are NOT medicines?

_____

Which of these drugs do you think are risky? When? Why?

_____

Which of these drugs are dangerous? Why?

_____

The World of Drugs

My name is ....

Why do people take drugs which are not medicines?

Here are some reasons why people take drugs which are not medicines. Can you think of some more. Here are some words to help you:

> performance   advertisement
> friends   addicted
> grown up   persuaded   weight

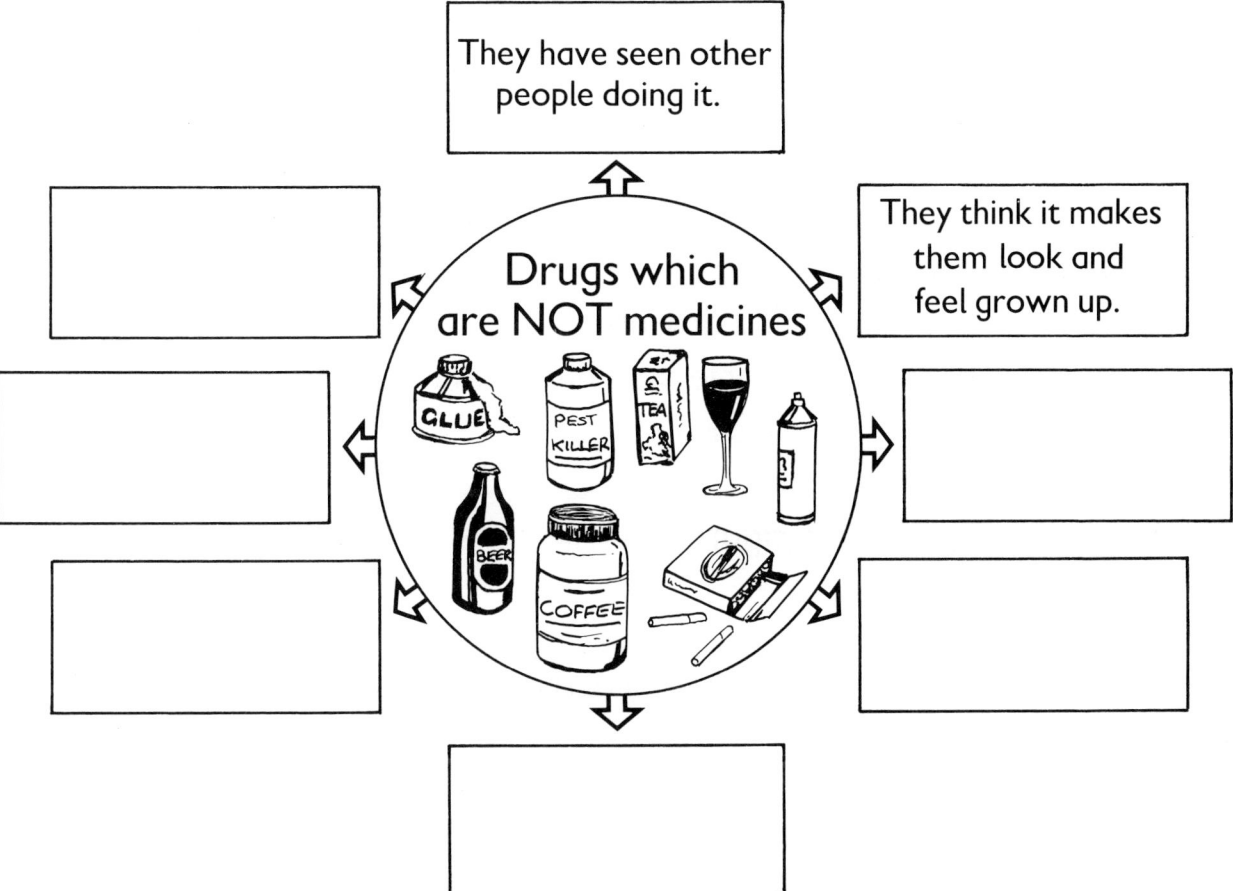

They have seen other people doing it.

Drugs which are NOT medicines

They think it makes them look and feel grown up.

Which of these reasons might tempt children?

_____

Talk about the risks involved in taking these drugs.

What do you think helps children to say 'No' to harmful drugs?

_____

The World of Drugs

My name is ....

Taking risks 1

Look at this page in a dictionary.

Risk: *possibility of something bad happening because a person decides to act in a certain way*

Now look at this list of things people can do.

  1 crossing the road
  2 swimming in the sea
  3 going off alone
  4 arguing with a bully
  5 going out late at night
  6 drinking alcohol
  7 rock climbing
  8 drinking and driving
  9 riding a bicycle on a busy road
10 using the subway
11 hitch hiking
12 smoking cigarettes
13 taking drugs
14 going off with a person you don't
      know or you know and don't trust

Can you sort out these things people do into 3 groups?

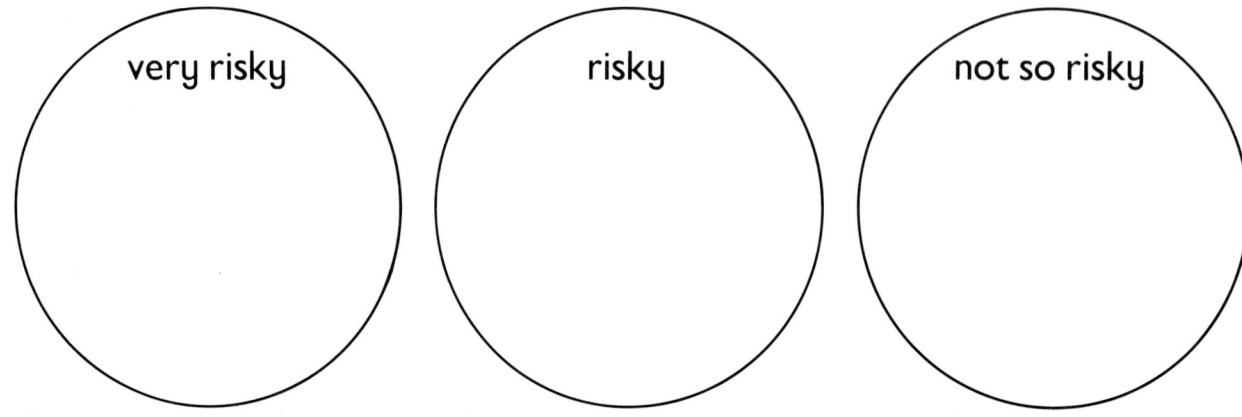

very risky   risky   not so risky

Can you give your reasons for the way you have grouped them?
Try explaining them to someone.

The World of Drugs

 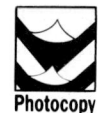

My name is ....

Taking risks 2

Look back at Worksheet 22 and the list of risky things which people sometimes do.
Talk about *why* people take risks.
Here are some ideas to help you. Can you think of some more?

- they think they can handle the risks
- their friends persuade them
- they have practised handling risks and feel confident
- they have learned about the dangers and made up their own minds
- they don't know how to say 'No'
- they believed what people said without finding out for themselves

Talk about some of the risks you think you face now and the risks you might have to face later on.

Which risks do you think you can handle now?

_____

What makes you think you can handle them?

_____

What skills do you need to learn and practise to make you more confident?

_____

Who can help you?

_____

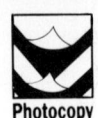

The World of Drugs

My name is ....

Warning signs

Here are some warnings you can see every day but perhaps you don't really notice them. Where are you likely to see them?

It is an offence to sell tobacco to children under the age of 16	You could see this notice _____
Warning: smoking can seriously damage your health	You can see this warning _____
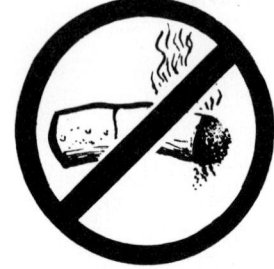	This notice means _____

Talk about why you think it is against the law to sell tobacco to children under 16?

I think it is because

_____

Talk about whether or not people keep the laws and take notice of the warnings.

_____

The World of Drugs

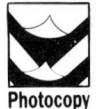

My name is ....

What do you know about smoking?

Try this quiz with your family.
Are these statements true or false?

	TRUE	FALSE
• Tobacco is made from the leaves of plants.	☐	☐
• Men smoke more than women.	☐	☐
• There are more people smoking now than there were five years ago.	☐	☐
• Smoking is the chief cause of fires in homes and hostels.	☐	☐
• Smoking is not allowed anywhere on the London Underground.	☐	☐
• Smoking can seriously damage your lungs.	☐	☐
• Smoking can seriously damage your heart.	☐	☐
• Smoking can damage an unborn baby.	☐	☐

Before cigarettes were invented tobacco was

☐ SMOKED IN PIPES   ☐ SMOKED IN CIGARS   ☐ SNIFFED AS A POWDER   ☐ CHEWED

Cigarettes were invented during the 17th century in

☐ GREECE   ☐ AFRICA   ☐ SPAIN   ☐ ENGLAND

Try explaining to a person from a non-smoking planet, what cigarettes are, and how and why people smoke them.

Part Two
Keeping Myself Safe

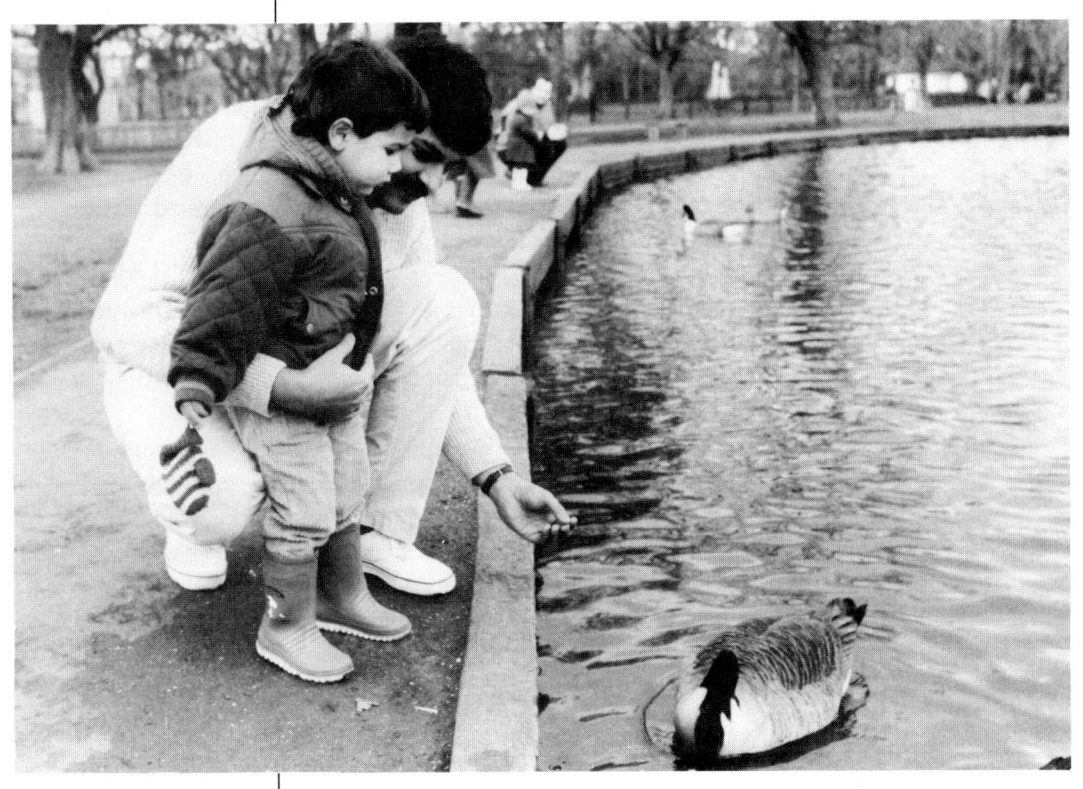

Introduction

Why we need safety education

The Health Education Primary School Project investigations revealed an overwhelming demand from parents and teachers for safety education in primary schools. Well over 90 per cent of those parents and teachers involved in the investigations (15,743 parents and 1,148 teachers) were unambiguous in placing safety education at the top of the list of health related topics they saw as important for primary schools. This is not surprising when we are reminded that accidents of one kind or another are by far the largest single cause of death, injury and permanent disability amongst primary school children.

That schools take safety education seriously is not in doubt, but unfortunately few develop a comprehensive and broadly-based plan which allows for the progressive acquisition and development of ideas, concepts and skills among successive age groups of children. The flexible curriculum offered here has grown out of a fusion of children's perceptions of 'keeping safe' with the messages and skills which we as adults know that children must understand and acquire in order to keep themselves safe.

The investigations, undertaken with 926 children aged 4–11, gave an understanding of what children felt they had to keep safe from, how they kept themselves safe and, particularly important, whose job it is to keep them safe. An insight into how children's perceptions change between the ages of 4 and 11 also emerged, and out of these perceptions themes have been developed for each of the age groups. It is upon these themes that the Scope and Sequence Chart, Classroom Strategies and Activities, and the Action Planners are based.

In response to the question, '*What are you keeping safe from?*' many children up to the age of 6 or 7 mentioned fantasy characters, many linked with television programmes. There was little mention of these imaginary characters and dangers after the age of eight, but this is not to say that they have ceased to exist.

Interwoven with the children's changing perceptions of what is dangerous or risky were several persistent themes: roads, strangers, bullies, stairs and adult (particularly parental) wrath or disapproval. Their view of 'getting told off', or 'getting into trouble' widened to include adults in authority or 'in charge' and was closely linked to specific strategies for avoidance, for example, keeping quiet, tidy, out of the way, playing in the bedroom and, most frequently quoted, watching TV.

The results showed that the older the children were, the wider their list of specific, hazardous objects and equipment. At first the focus was on the home, but this widened to include school and outdoors. At the earliest stages these objects were seen by the children as being there to harm them and being the cause of accidents. The awareness of their own role in this seemed slow to develop in some children and was linked with keeping safe strategies such as not touching and, not going near something.

The children's views of potentially dangerous people were given in very general terms as many were lacking in first hand experience. They were described as 'baddies', 'nasty men', 'strangers' and 'big boy bullies'. Their pictures showed that many saw, and persisted in seeing, such people in a very stereotyped way. Glue sniffers and drunks themselves were seen as dangerous before the children were really aware of sniffing glue, drinking alcohol or abusing other drugs.

Risky situations were described in generalised terms, with an early and persisting emphasis on 'going off' as a dangerous activity, and a widening awareness of the potential dangers of crowd behaviour, peer pressures, getting involved, dares or being dared, boasting, experimenting and 'messing about'.

When responding to the question, '*How are you keeping safe?*' children found it easier to describe and illustrate the hazards they perceived rather than their strategies for keeping safe. Many took refuge in a statement such as 'keep safe' without attempting to illustrate how they might do this. Between the ages of 4 and 11 there was a shift in the balance between 'do's and 'don'ts'. The youngest children saw running away, hiding, not looking and staying close to home, as positive keeping safe strategies. At 6 and 7 there was a shift of emphasis to 'don't' – 'don't touch', 'don't go near', 'don't go with', etc. Around the 8–9 year old stage there was a new emphasis on mastering the skills to handle potentially dangerous equipment, which was previously seen as something to keep away from. The children spoke of learning to handle things safely and using adults as instructors. Only towards the ages of 10–11 did the ability to evaluate risks emerge. This involved the awareness of the potential danger of people, places and, situations and strategies for resisting pressure and for thinking ahead.

The theme of adult disapproval as a hazard persisted and at the older age ranges showed an increasing awareness of parental concerns and fears, and the need to know the 'rules' connected with different places. Few children above the age of 5 saw 'telling', asking for support, discussion and sharing feelings as strategies for keeping safe.

In response to the question, '*Whose job is it to keep you safe wherever you are?*' there was a very slow but steady emergence of personal responsibility for personal safety. The view of responsibility which at the age of 4 was seen as belonging to Mum or Dad, widened to include a whole range of family, health, safety, education and government bodies and individuals. Only a small number of young children incorporated themselves into the list of those responsible for their safety.

Investigating children's perceptions of safety in the classroom

Before beginning work on **Keeping Myself Safe** activities, however, teachers might wish to use a Draw and Write Technique to discover the perceptions of the children in their class. This is the same investigation method adopted by the Project Team for their research. It is easy for the teacher to organise in the classroom and will reveal the children's knowledge of specific topics, and will provide a rich source of background knowledge from which starting points for the work will emerge. By using this technique before and after teaching the children, it will be possible to chart the children's progress.

The analysis of the children's work can be done quickly and simply to provide a quick overview of the children's perceptions, or extensively to provide a detailed picture of their thoughts and ideas. Full details of this technique, suggestions for its administration and analysis are given in Appendix 1 on page 410.

Coping with your pupils' safety problems

One of the most sensitive areas of children's safety concerns child abuse because it is likely to involve adults who are close to, and are known by, children. Often children are sworn to secrecy when they have been abused, so that a 'safety net' is necessary which allows them to relieve themselves of their burden. Regular opportunities for sharing experiences with teachers and other trusted adults are built into the materials and are clearly signalled, so that it is important for teachers to be aware of the procedures adopted by their LEA if a child reveals a possible incident of abuse.

In a more general sense it is particularly important that safety education is closely related to the local environment and local community. While national statistics relating to child accidents give an important context, close scrutiny of local figures will provide a more realistic guide. These local statistics can be readily obtained from the Safety Officers or from the Health Education Officer or Adviser and can provide teachers with an appropriate focus.

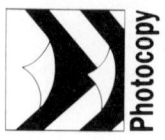

Keeping Myself Safe
Scope and Sequence Chart

Age	Children's changing perceptions of keeping safe	Suggested programme content	Suggested skills and strategies
4 & 5	We fear fantasy characters the most, traffic, things around the home, and bad boys or men. We think the best way to keep safe is to hide, run away, watch TV, stay with Mum, and lock the doors. It is Mum and Dad's job to keep us safe.	What is my name? Where do I live? Who is at home? Whose job is it to keep me safe? How can I help them? Where can I play safely? Which places are dangerous? Which people are safe? Should I keep all secrets? What is real and what is pretend? When should I ask for help? Why is getting told off different from being in danger? Why do accidents happen?	*Language skills:* Talking Listening Reading Writing Investigating Describing Recognising and naming Recording Categorising *General skills:* Illustration and presentation Observation Empathy Classroom play Decision making Keeping safe
6 & 7	We can list dangerous objects and places. We know we can cause accidents. Traffic and strangers are the greatest dangers. We know we should cross the road at a safe place.	Where do I live? What is my telephone number? Who knows where I am? Where am I going? How long does it take? Who can help me and how? Where are the safe and dangerous places?	*Language skills:* Talking Listening Reading Writing Investigating

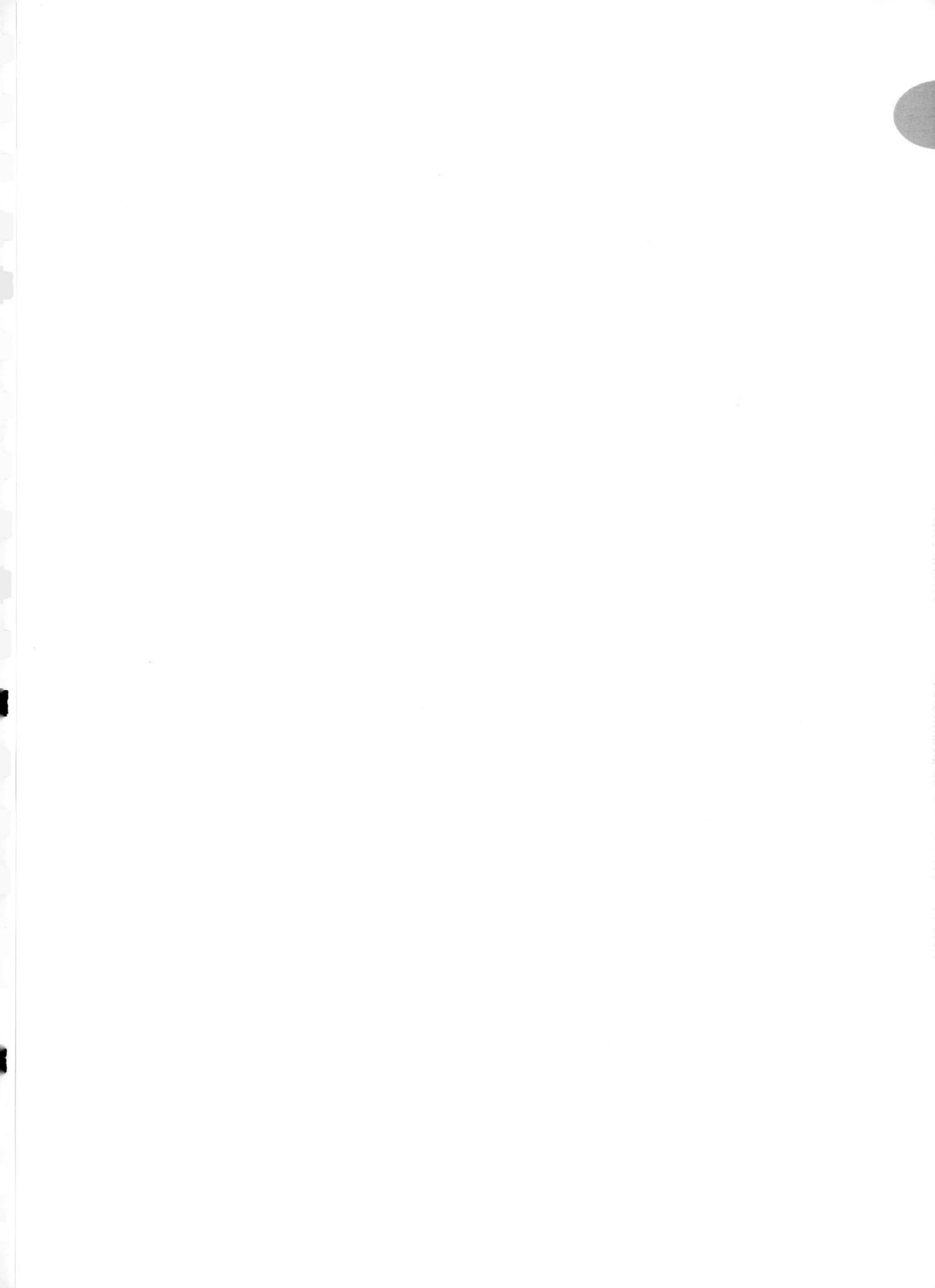

Classroom Strategies and Activities for Ages 4 – 11

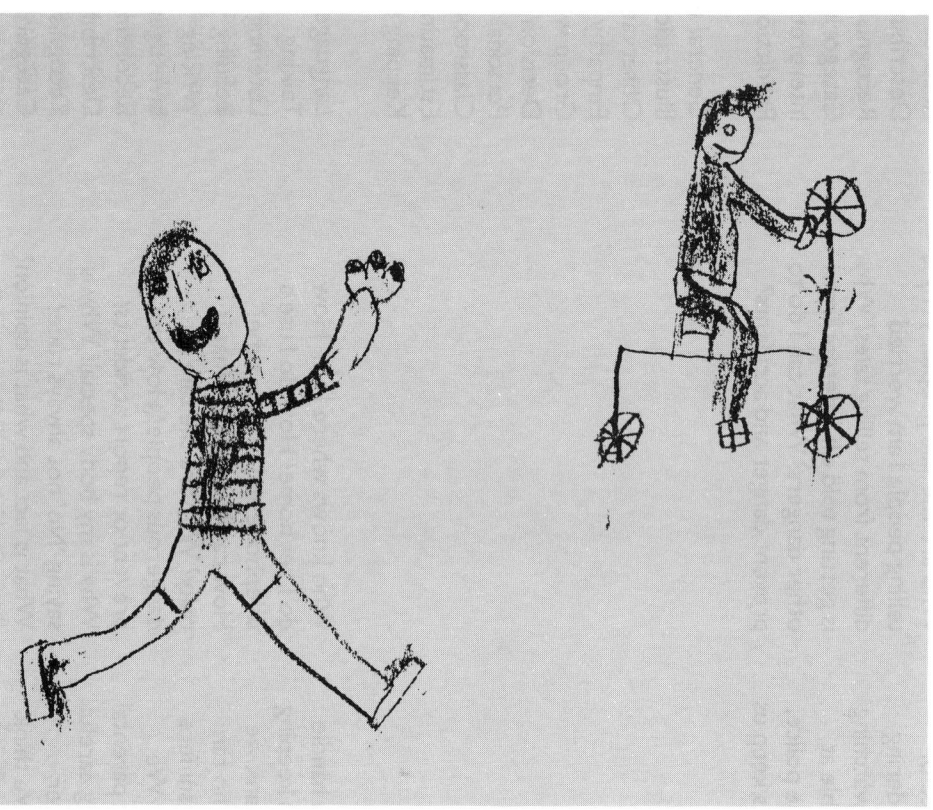

The activities in the following pages are based on the content boxes from the four Action Planners for ages 4 and 5, 6 and 7, 8 and 9 and 10 and 11. There are five content boxes on each Action Planner, each of which has a distinctive theme, providing five themes which run through the activities:

Content box 1: Focus on me

Content box 2: Focus on people

Content box 3: Focus on indoors

Content box 4: Focus on outdoors

Content box 5: Focus on feelings

The content boxes suggest questions which are explored in detail in the activities. All contain the important question: 'When am I most at risk?'

It is important that you select and modify these activities according to your needs. If you are devising your own keeping safe programme you may well be aware of the health education priorities of your school and may already have selected the key themes you wish to explore with your pupils. If this is the case, you may find that the following activities are useful as examples, alternatively, you may wish to incorporate them as they stand in your programme.

Action Planner
Keeping Myself Safe

4 & 5

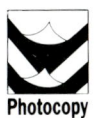

Photocopy

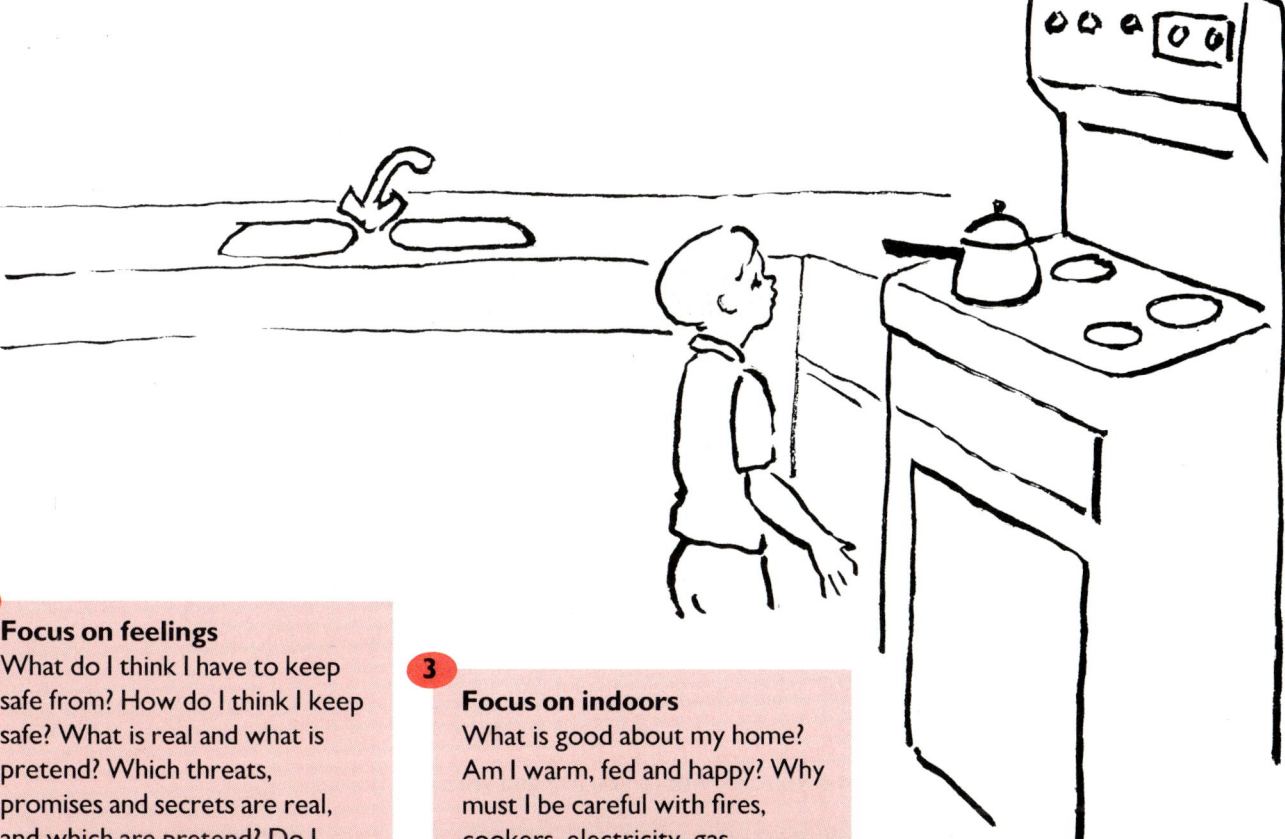

1
Focus on feelings
What do I think I have to keep safe from? How do I think I keep safe? What is real and what is pretend? Which threats, promises and secrets are real, and which are pretend? Do I always have to keep secrets? Which secrets are good and which are bad? Who can I ask for help? If I tell someone will I get into trouble?
When am I most at risk?

2
Focus on me
Who am I? Where am I? Where have I been? Who is (was) with me? Who is in charge of me? Where do I live? Who is there? How can I get there safely? What should I do when I am lost? What should I do to get help? What should I not do? How can I ask for help?
When am I most at risk?

3
Focus on indoors
What is good about my home? Am I warm, fed and happy? Why must I be careful with fires, cookers, electricity, gas, television, stairs, and medicines? How do accidents happen? What are the rules at home? How can I keep myself safe?
When am I most at risk?

4
Focus on outdoors
What is good about my outdoor world? Where do I play? Where do I go with my family and friends? What do I like about roads, cars, bikes, rivers etc? What do I need to practise? How do accidents happen? What is good about staying with what I know and where I am known?
When am I most at risk?

5
Focus on people
Who are my special people? How do I recognise them? What do my special people do to make me feel safe and happy? What do they do to make me upset, cross and worried? How do I make them happy, sad, cross and worried? What happens when I say: 'No', 'Please don't', 'I'll ask'? Which people make me feel unsafe? How do I say 'No' to them? How do I find someone safe to help me? Who has the job of keeping me safe? What is *my* job?
When am I most at risk?

Classroom Strategies and Activities for Ages 4 and 5

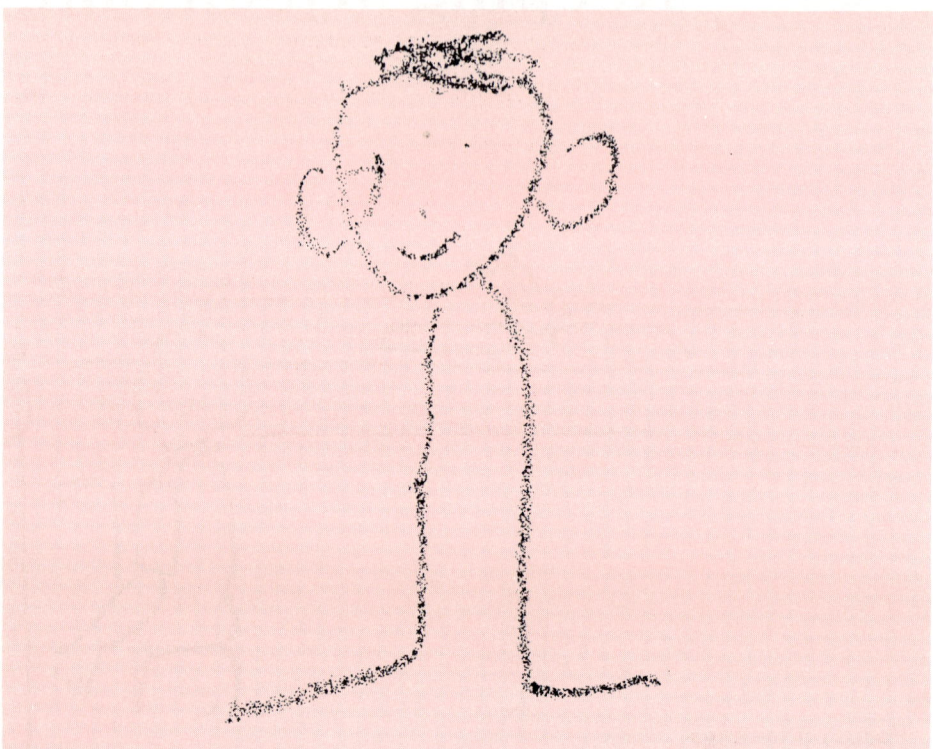

Key messages *Learn:*

- who you are, where you live and who is at home.

- where you are, who is with you and who is in charge of you.

- about some of the people whose job it is to help you keep safe and how you can help them.

- about the safe places to play, and how to play safely.

- about the dangerous places. What makes them dangerous?

- who are the safe people to be with?

- to stay close to what you know and what you are happiest with.

- to ask for help.

- to say 'No', 'Stop', 'I'll ask'.

- to tell people what happened and when and where it happened. Learn how to go on telling until someone listens.

Practise:

- the skills you need to do things, and to go to places, safely.

- the rules about people, places and things.

- playing safely, having fun, and feeling safe.

Understand:

- that you and your body are special, valuable and unique.

- that you don't cause all the adult problems around you.

- that it is good to keep some secrets, but bad to keep others.

- the difference between real and pretend?

- that asking and telling someone are the best things to do if you are worried, scared or unsure.

- that being told off is a different kind of thing from putting yourself in danger.

- that accidents are sometimes caused by what you do, sometimes caused by what others do, and sometimes no one is to blame.

Content box 1   Focus on feelings

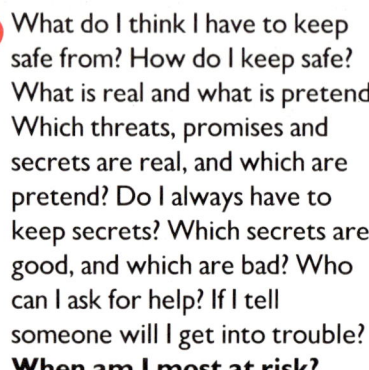

What do I think I have to keep
safe from? How do I keep safe?
What is real and what is pretend?
Which threats, promises and
secrets are real, and which are
pretend? Do I always have to
keep secrets? Which secrets are
good, and which are bad? Who
can I ask for help? If I tell
someone will I get into trouble?
When am I most at risk?

Activity 1

What do I think I have to keep safe from?

- Drawing and painting. Classroom play. Talking together.
- Class and group activities.

Invite the children to draw or paint pictures of themselves keeping safe, and things
they are keeping safe from. Explore their views of what the hazards are and how
they think they could deal with them. Although some imaginary dangers will seem
very real to some children, this could be a time to help them distinguish between
real and pretend dangers.

Bring their illustrations together to form a shared display or wall story. Write
captions for them. You can use this chart to prompt the children to talk about the
kinds of safety strategies they would use in different situations. Help the children
to practise these strategies through classroom play.

Activity 2

What is real and what is pretend?

- Talking together. Classroom play. Drawing and painting. Stories. Television.
- Class and group activities.

Many of the stories read to children at this age, and some television programmes
viewed both in and out of school, can provide starting points for distinguishing
between real and imaginary characters and situations. Children can look for stories
where solutions are reached by magic, where threats and promises can seem
impossible, unbelievable or dreadful. In other stories they can look for real
problems, threats and promises. Stories and programmes about real people who
have imaginary friends, pets or toys which come alive when adults are not there
make good starting points for exploring real and imaginary fears and secrets (an
important theme in later stages).

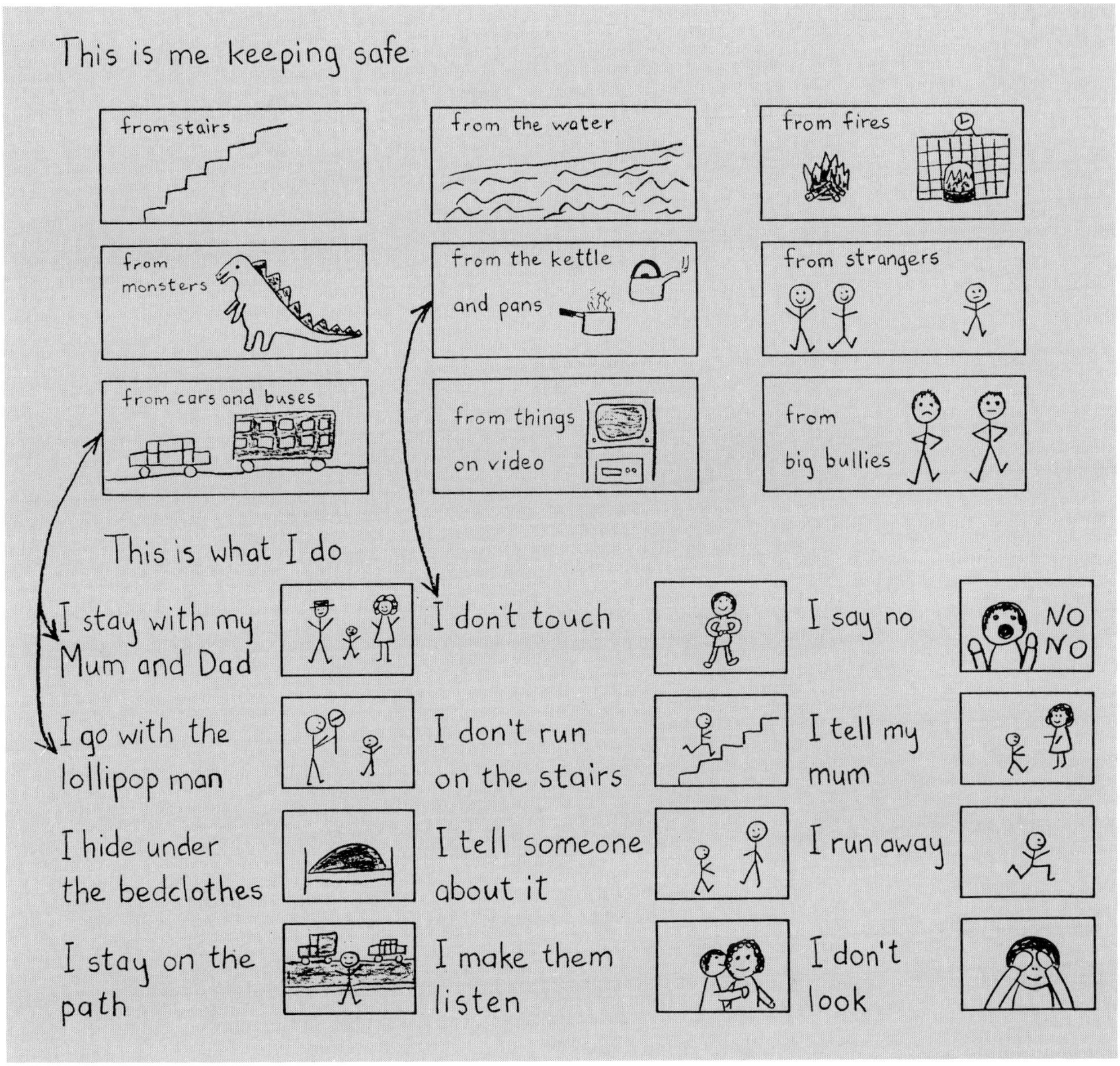

This is me keeping safe

from stairs	from the water	from fires
from monsters	from the kettle and pans	from strangers
from cars and buses	from things on video	from big bullies

This is what I do

I stay with my Mum and Dad

I go with the lollipop man

I hide under the bedclothes

I stay on the path

I don't touch

I don't run on the stairs

I tell someone about it

I make them listen

I say no   NO NO

I tell my mum

I run away

I don't look

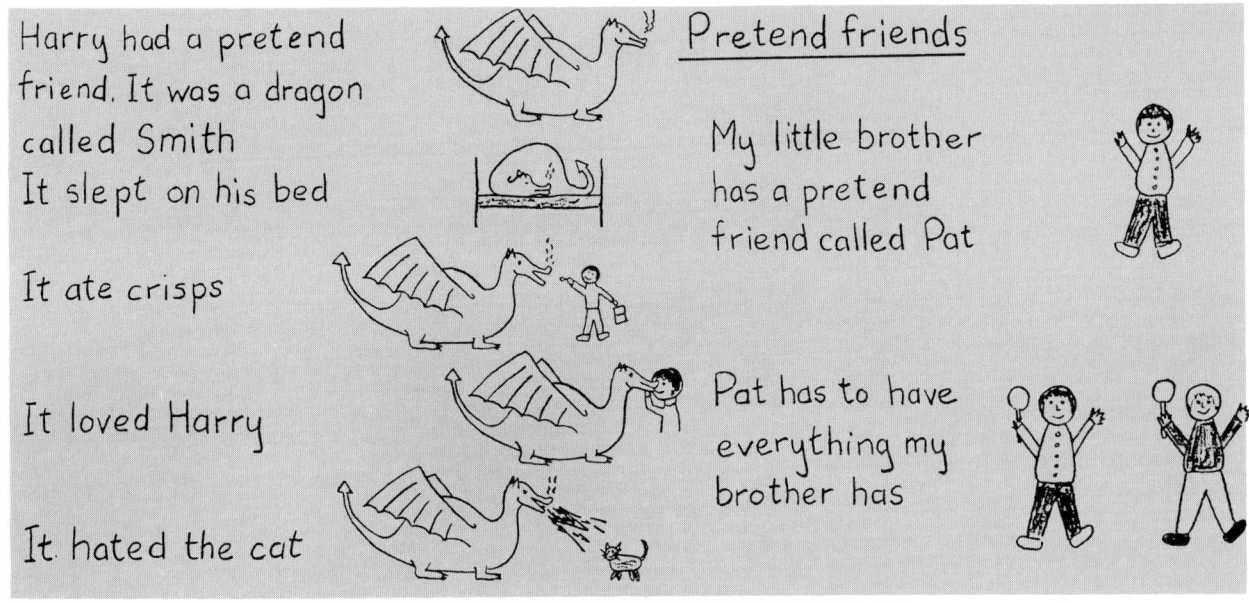

Harry had a pretend friend. It was a dragon called Smith
It slept on his bed

It ate crisps

It loved Harry

It hated the cat

Pretend friends

My little brother has a pretend friend called Pat

Pat has to have everything my brother has

Real friends

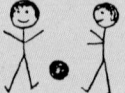

This is my friend at school

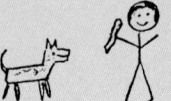

This is me playing with my dog. It's my friend

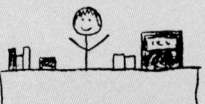

This is my grown up friend in the shop

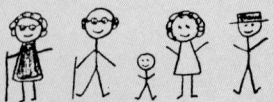

These are my family friends

Many of the children will have had experience of keeping secrets at home and school and these can be shared to emphasise the fun and caring aspect of good secrets.

I had a good secret. I didn't tell.

We hid my mum's present.
I didn't tell.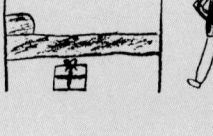

Benny cried at school.
I didn't tell.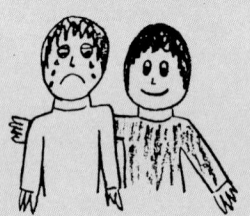

My teddy talks to me in bed.
I don't tell.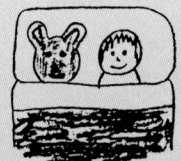

Our puppy wet the carpet.
We didn't tell.
He'd have got told off.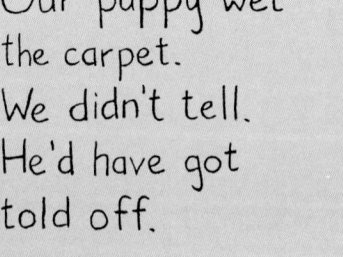

We're doing a concert for Christmas.
We aren't telling yet.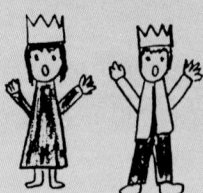

This is me keeping a good secret.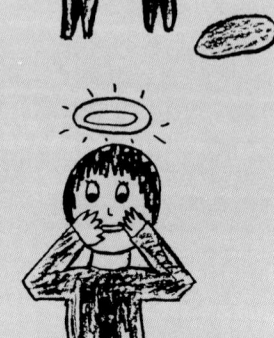

The children could then begin to distinguish between different kinds of secrets. Talk together about:

— secrets kept from them (and how they felt about this).

— secrets accompanied by some kind of threat or promise.

This will provide opportunities, where appropriate, for you to reinforce the difference between loving and non-loving secrets, and to emphasise the importance of telling someone and making someone listen when secrets are causing distress. Many of these experiences can be explored further in 'domestic' classroom play, drawing and painting.

Someone had a secret and didn't tell me.

My gran had a secret and she didn't tell me. It was a kitten. I was surprised.

My mum had a secret and she didn't tell me. It was a new baby.

I liked it

I cried. I didn't like it.

My friends had a secret and they wouldn't tell me.

I had a secret and I did tell

The video at Billie's house scared me. They said not to tell, but I told my mum

Some big boy bullies took my sweets. They said not to tell, but I told my teacher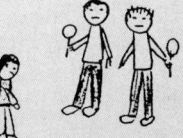

Someone tried to make me do things. They said they'd give me some sweets and not to tell—but I did tell

This is me with a bad secret.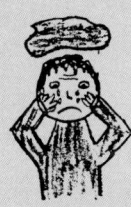

This is me feeling better when I told someone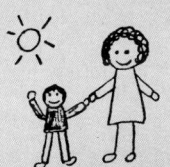

Content box 2   Focus on me

Who am I? Where am I? Where have I been? Who is (was) with me? Who is in charge of me? Where do I live? Who is there? Can I get there safely? What should I do when I am lost? What should I do to get help? What should I *not* do? How can I ask for help?
When am I most at risk?

Activity 1   *Who am I? Where do I live?*

- Classroom play. Drawing and painting. Number recognition. Stories and poems.

- Class and group activities.

Many different classroom activities can be used to help children practise saying who they are and where they live. In classroom play the theme of 'visitors' and 'visiting' can involve saying who you are, where you have come from and where you have been, other examples include going to the doctor's surgery and ordering things by telephone.

You could give the children stand up name cards with their names and addresses written on them. These cards could be used by the children in a variety of ways: to label their work, to be incorporated into displays and to be part of play activities.

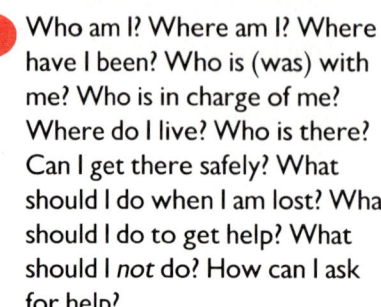

Invite the children to paint pictures of their front doors. Display them adding the number of the house for them in bold print. Play 'find your door', or 'find other people's doors'. There are many **cross-curricular links** with stories, poems and rhymes.

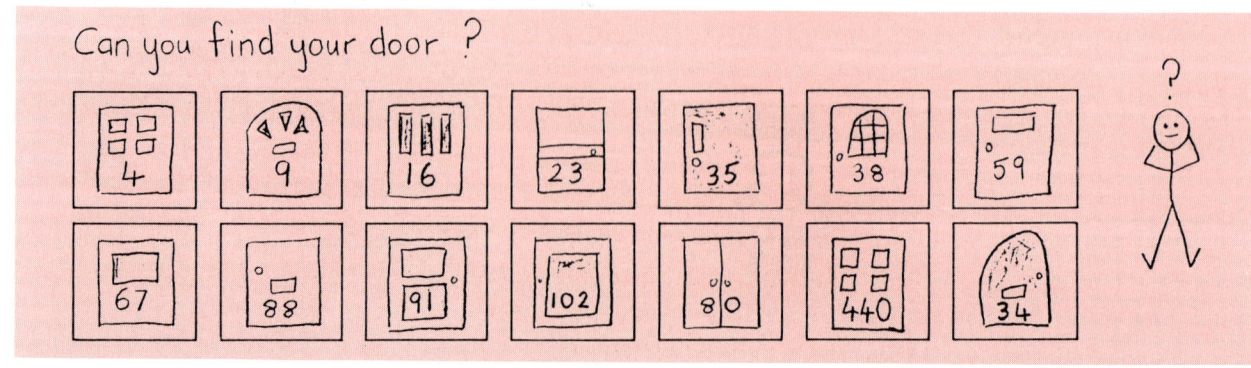

Ask the children what a character from a story would say if asked: 'Who are you? Where do you live?' For example, in *Jack and the Beanstalk*:

Jack: My name is Jack. I live in a cottage by a big tree.
Giant: I am the Giant. I live in a castle at the top of the tree.

Activity 2 ● *Where am I? Where am I going?*

- Drawing and painting. Talking together. Stories and poems

- Class or group work.

Invite the children to draw or paint pictures of themselves in different places, at different times of the day wearing different clothes and doing different things. Ask them to say where they are or where they are going and what they are doing. For example:

- I am at home in bed.

- I am going to the shops.

- I am at my Gran's house.

- I am at school, in the playground.

- I am going home.

Write the children's responses in 'speech bubbles' and add them to their drawings.

Talk with the children about how important it is to know where they are and where they are going, to ask for help; and not to go off alone, or with another person. These themes can be explored further and practised through classroom play.

Activity 3 ● *What should I do when I am lost?*

- Talking together. Drawing.

- Class or group activity.

Invite the children to talk about the times when they, or someone they know, lost something. Tell them a story of your own too. Talk about how they felt, who helped them, if and where they found the lost item and how they felt about its return. There are many stories and poems which use this theme which provide good starting points and children will enjoy hearing of other people's experiences.

Invite the children to talk about a time when they or someone they know was lost, or use a story or poem as a starting point for exploring the feeling of being lost.

Ask the children to describe or draw the place where they became lost. Encourage them to talk about what happened, and who, if anyone, helped. Was it someone they knew, or a stranger?

Explore with the children safe strategies for getting help, for example, in the street, in a store, in a car park or at a bus station.

We got lost

Sam got lost in the supermarket. The shop lady lifted him up to find his mum.

Anna got lost in the market. She asked a kind looking lady with some children

Joey got lost near his house. His big brother found him.

Benny got lost in the town. The policeman took her to the police station till her dad came

Tracy got lost at school. A dinner lady found her.

Opportunities will arise to:

— identify the 'safe' people in your community and talk about how we recognise them and ask for help.

— talk about safe people, how they help, and the limits of that help.

— talk about possible dangers from unknown people, or known people who cause unease or fear.

— warn children about people who use phrases such as: 'I am lost', or 'I've lost my dog' as a ruse for enticing a child away, and the importance of saying 'No, I can't help', 'I'll go and ask someone'.

Content box 3   Focus on indoors

What is good about my home?
Am I warm, fed and happy? Why
must I be careful with fires,
cookers, electricity, gas,
television, stairs and medicines?
How do accidents happen? What
are the rules at home? how can I
keep myself safe?
When am I most at risk?

Activity 1 *What is good about my home?*

- Talking together. Writing. Drawing and painting. Classroom play. Collecting and sorting magazine pictures.

- Class and group activities, with opportunities for individual work.

In order to look at some of the hazards in the home, it can be useful to look first at items of household equipment, first in terms of what is good and useful about them, and secondly, in terms of the possible dangers they present. Invite the children to think of the things in their house which keep them warm, comfortable, happy and safe.

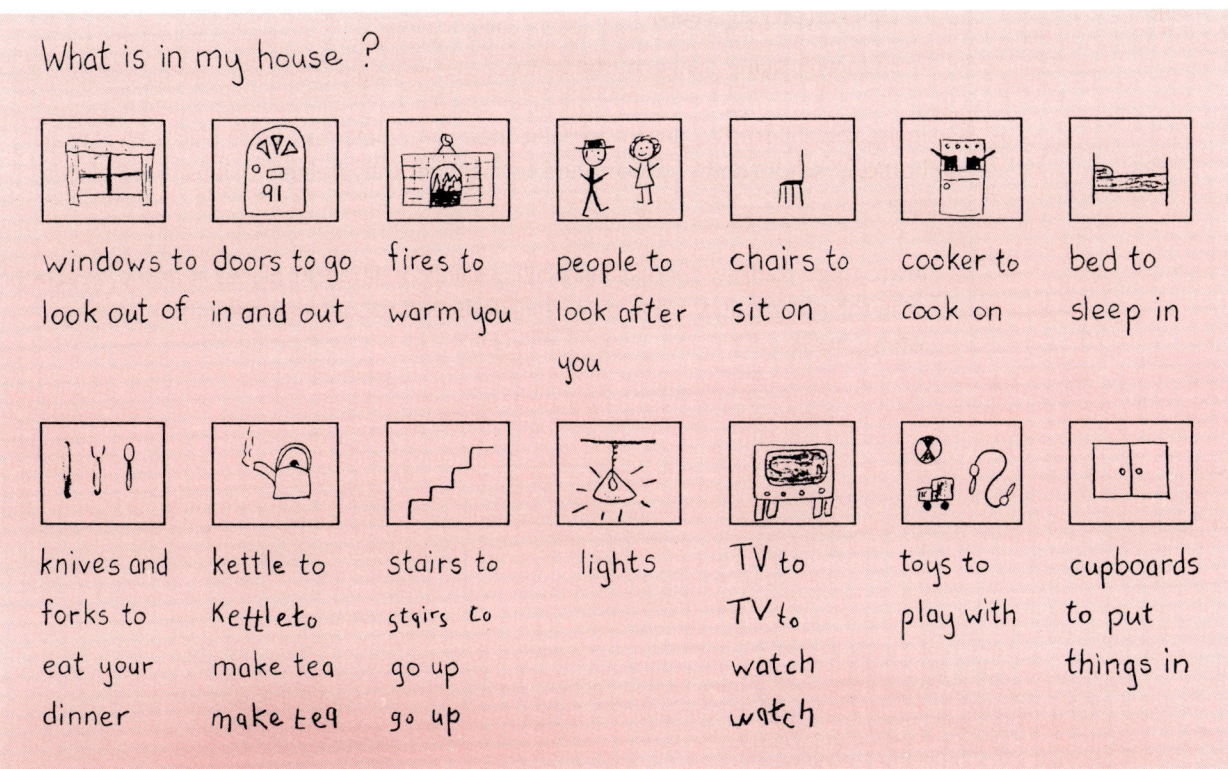

Talk with the children about what makes these things and people, good or useful. How would it be if there were no doors, windows, TV or people?

Ask the children to look again at these items and to say what could make each one unsafe. This could provide an opportunity for children to see the difference between what they might do which could cause accidents and what other people might do which could cause harm.

Look at strategies for keeping safe, for example, *not* touching, switching, opening, playing about, jumping or running. Talk about putting things away, listening to what people say, saying if you are worried or scared and telling someone you trust, especially if people's actions or demands are causing distress.

Use talking, writing, painting and classroom play to reinforce these safety strategies. Where appropriate, the children could begin to look at strategies they could use when they are alone, or with friends, or with family, or with other adults, or with strangers.

Invite the children to think and talk about the places in the home where accidents can happen, for example, on the stairs, in the kitchen, the bathroom and the living room. Look at 'do's' and 'dont's' in these places. Encourage the children to ask themselves: 'Is this a safe place to play?'

Ask the children to collect pictures from magazines of places to play, and children playing, and to sort out them into these categories:

— safe places to play.

— unsafe places to play.

— children playing safely.

— children playing dangerously.

Invite the children to draw and paint their own pictures of safe places to play at home, at school and outdoors, and to say what they believe makes these places safe.

Invite them to draw themselves playing safely in different places at home, at school or in the playground, alone or with friends, and to say what they think playing safely entails.

Content box 4   Focus on outdoors

What is good about my outdoor world? Where do I play? Where do I go with my family and friends? What do I like about roads, cars, bikes, rivers, etc? What do I need to practise? How do accidents happen? What is good about staying with what I know and where I am known? **When am I most at risk?**

Activity 1   ●   ***What is good about my outdoor world?***

- Talking together. Drawing and painting.
- Class and group activities.

Explore with the children all the places they go – to play, to visit and to use – in the outdoor world. Talk about where they go, who takes them, who goes with them, what they do, what they like and don't like about going out, what makes it fun, interesting, exciting, boring, worrying and frightening.

Invite the children to talk about and illustrate the theme: 'We are going out. What can we see?' For example,

- In the playground we can see the climbing frame, the fence, etc.
- In the garden we can see the gate, the shed, our toys, etc.
- In the country we can see water, bridges, trees, etc.
- In the street we can see cars, buses, people, shops, etc.
- In the park we can see the lake, the trees, the swings, etc.

Invite the children to think and talk about:

- the people they meet on their way to these places.
- the traffic and other hazards, for example, roads, water, lack of pavements, etc.

The children's responses and illustrations can be displayed as a focus for further activities on keeping safe.

Explore with the children the hazards or dangers they might meet during their outdoor activities and what they see as the best ways of keeping themselves safe. Invite the children to ask themselves the questions:

– 'Is this a safe place to go?'

– 'Should I go on my own or with someone I know?'

– 'Should I go with someone I don't know?'

– 'Is this a safe place to play or a dangerous place?'

Activity 2 ● *How do accidents happen?*

● Talking. Drawing. Writing

● Class and group activities, with opportunities for individual work.

Ask the children to talk, draw and write about, an everyday, minor accident, focusing on what caused it. Many young children believe that the cause of accidents lies in the object itself, rather than in the child's activity: 'Cars to run over you', 'bonfires to burn you', 'rough ground to make you fall over'. It is important at this early stage to help the children see that some accidents are caused by what they do, and others are caused by what other people do. Make a note of the children's responses. Note the number of times the children blame themselves, blame someone else, or put the blame on the object itself.

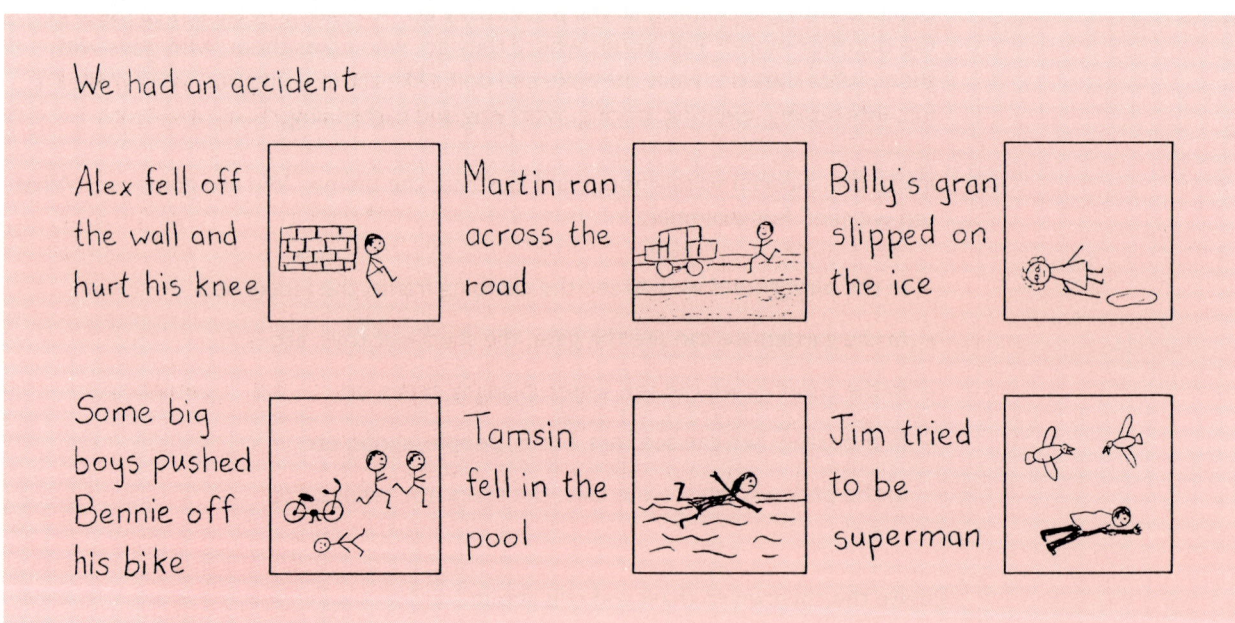

Use the children's illustrations and writing as a starting point for asking:

– 'What made this accident?'

– 'How did it happen?'

– 'Whose fault was it?'

– 'What could the people have done to stop the accident happening?'

This is a good time to remind children of the dangers of attempting to copy the actions of real or fantasy characters seen on television programmes.

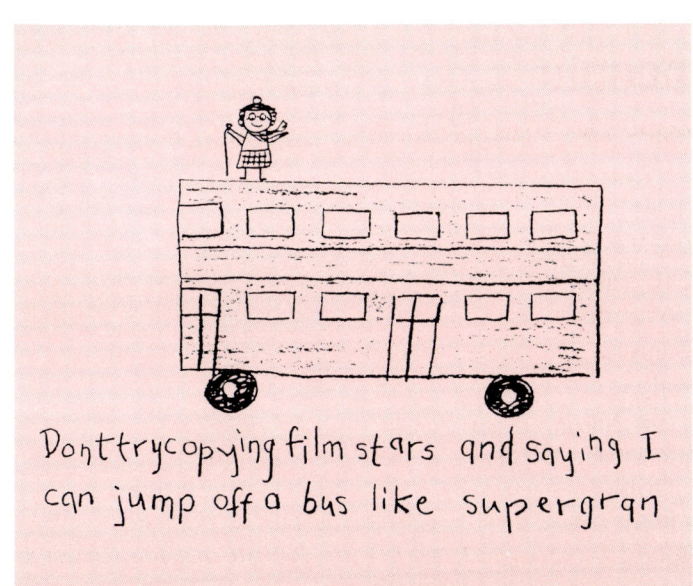

Donttrycopying film stars and saying I can jump off a bus like supergran

Look with the children at what they see as ways of keeping safe in different places. Invite them to illustrate themselves keeping safe in places such as:

— the playground.

— the shops or shopping centre.

— on the way to and from school.

— near the road or river.

— in a car, on the bus, at the station.

— alone, with others, with strangers.

The children's perceptions of how they keep themselves safe will be very illuminating and will provide a starting point for activities which develop safety skills, such as:

— knowing who they are, where they live, who is with them, or looking after them and what that person is called.

— being able to name and describe (or illustrate) a street, a path, a pavement, a bridge, a crossing, traffic lights, a drive, an entry, a car park, a parked car.

— being able to distinguish different kinds of vehicles.

— being able to understand and explain (or illustrate) what they mean by alone, with someone, a grown up, on, off, by, near, far, close, across the road, to cross the road, stop, wait.

— recognising people who control the traffic and how they do this.

— practical skills: walking purposefully, stopping, waiting, looking, listening, recognising and naming sounds.

— practical skills: handling large toys, such as tricycles.

144

Content box 5   Focus on people

Who are my special people?
How do I recognise them? What
do my special people do to make
me feel safe and happy? What do
they do to make me feel upset,
cross and worried? How do I
make them happy, sad, cross and
worried? What happens when I
say 'No', 'Please don't', 'I'll ask'?
Which people make me feel
unsafe? How do I say 'No' to
them? How do I find someone
safe to help me? Who has the job
of keeping me safe? How do I
recognise them? What is *my* job?
When am I most at risk?

Activity 1

Who are my special people?

- Talking. Drawing and painting. Classroom play. Writing. Sharing. Making books.

- Class, group and individual activities.

Invite the children to talk about, describe, illustrate and dress up as some of the people who are special to them. Most children will have people at home or at school who they trust or admire, with whom they feel safe and have a special relationship.

Exploring positive feelings of trust and safety, and what these involve (and don't involve) can be a good way of enabling young children to distinguish between safe and unsafe people. Ask the children to talk, illustrate and write (with your help) about:

- what their special people look like and how they pick them out in a crowd.

- what their special people do and say, or don't do and don't say.

The work resulting from these activities can be brought together to make individual, group or class books.

This basic work on what special people do and say, can provide a framework for children to talk about the different ways in which people show they love and care about others. Children who sometimes dislike being hugged, kissed or touched by some people, or who are afraid or abused, can be helped through these activities to talk about their feelings and concerns. The question of when it is important or appropriate to say 'No' in various forms such as: 'Please don't', 'I don't like that', 'I'd rather not' or 'I don't want to', is best approached in small group or one-to-one supportive situations. Parents and families will need to be aware of the reasons why children are exploring this topic.

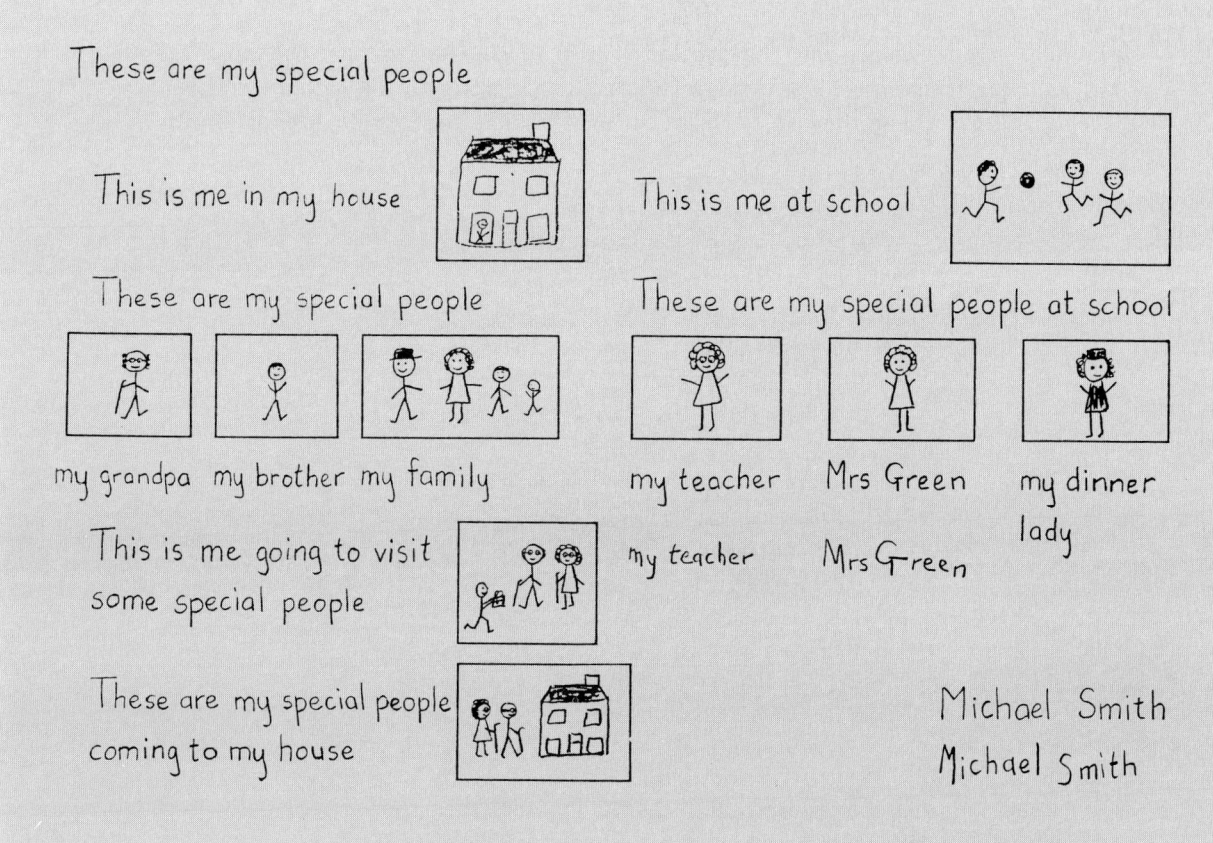

These are my special people

This is me in my house

This is me at school

These are my special people

my grandpa   my brother   my family

These are my special people at school

my teacher   Mrs Green   my dinner lady

my teacher   Mrs Green

This is me going to visit some special people

These are my special people coming to my house

Michael Smith

Michael Smith

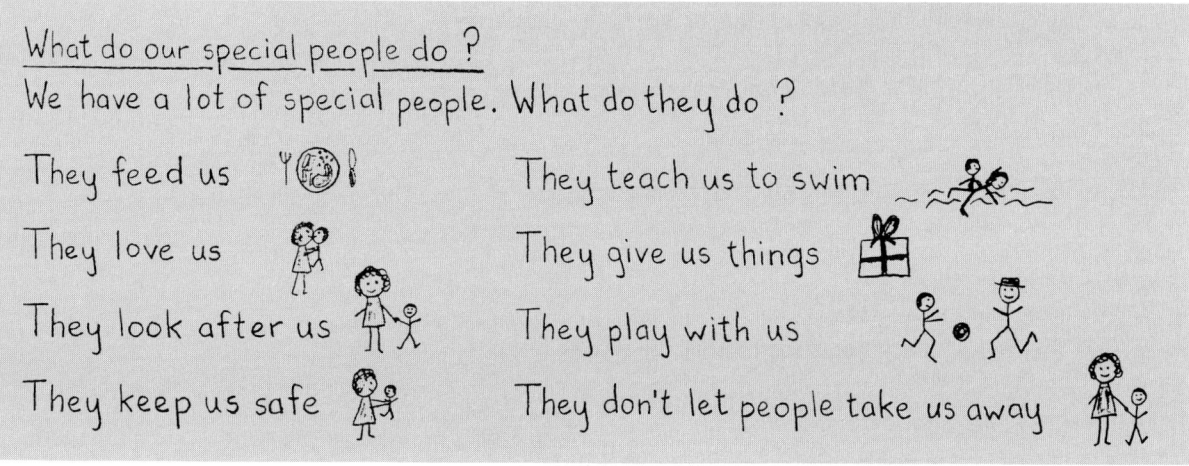

What do our special people do ?
We have a lot of special people. What do they do ?

They feed us

They love us

They look after us

They keep us safe

They teach us to swim

They give us things

They play with us

They don't let people take us away

The children could illustrate themselves saying 'Yes, please' and 'No, thank you' to people at home, at school and in the neighbourhood. Ask them to explain what it is they are accepting, refusing, or being asked to do. Opportunities may arise, or can be structured, to enable children to draw and talk about the more worrying aspects of saying 'Yes' and 'No', and to disclose pressures, fears, threats and abuse.

This work can provide a starting point for introducing other material relating to child abuse and personal safety. Its major purpose however, is to provide as many non-threatening, warm, sharing opportunities as possible, to encourage children to talk about things which bother them. It provides the first of a series of activities which enable the children to recognise risk and build up their own safety skills.

Explore with the children ways in which they can make the job of keeping themselves safe easier for their special people. Talk with the children about the things they do, or might do, which would worry their special people.

When do my special people worry about me ?

I ran off the pavement.
My mum was scared stiff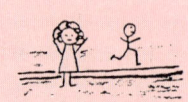

I went off and got lost.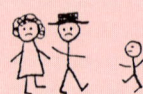
They were cross

I left toys on the stairs
and my grandpa fell.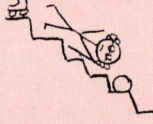
I cried

I went home from school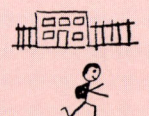
on my own.
My teacher was worried

I broke a window and
cut my hand

Ask the children about the things which their special people do which worry them, and make them feel unsafe. Responses might include:

Our special people worry us when they:

- leave us with babysitters.

- send us to bed.

- tell us off.

- tease us.

- scare us.

- cross the road at the wrong place.

- leave us alone in the car.

You can provide individual children with opportunities to reveal their own concerns, during small group activities when you can encourage a non-threatening sharing atmosphere.

Activity 2 ● *Who else has the job of keeping me safe?*

● Talking together. Visits and visitors. Topic work. Stories and poems. Classroom play.

● Class and group activities.

Beyond the children's special people are a wider group of people who share the responsibililty for keeping children safe, but at this stage the children's perceptions may not extend far beyond the family, the crossing patrol and the policeman.

Explore with them who it is they think keeps them safe wherever they are: indoors or outdoors. Make a note of children's responses, prompting them with questions such as: 'But what if you get lost?. . . if there is an accident . . . or a fire? . . . if you are at school?', etc.

Help the children to make a display of pictures and books which shows the range of people in the community who can and do help them. Invite the children to categorise these people using the question: 'How do I recognise them?' Look at the people who always wear a uniform, people who sometimes do or never do. What kinds of things do they tell the children to do or not to do?

This would be a good time to plan safety-related visits and visitors to increase the children's awareness of the role of those who keep them safe.

Follow up activities which focus on questions such as 'What do I do to help? . . . to make them pleased? . . . worried? . . . angry?' are particularly important in enabling children to begin to be aware of their own responsibility.

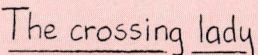

The crossing lady

This is our crossing lady   She came to talk to us today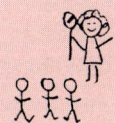

This is me making the crossing lady pleased

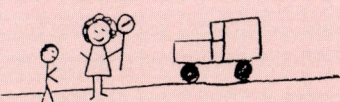

This is me making the crossing lady worried

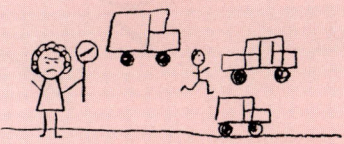

I am waiting till she says (NOW)

I am crossing in the wrong place

We are going to play crossing lady
We have got a coat and a lollipop stick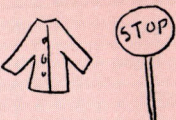

There are **cross-curricular links** here with

— topic work.

— the wider theme of people who help.

— stories, poems and rhymes.

— classroom play.

Action Planner
6 & 7

Photocopy

Keeping Myself Safe

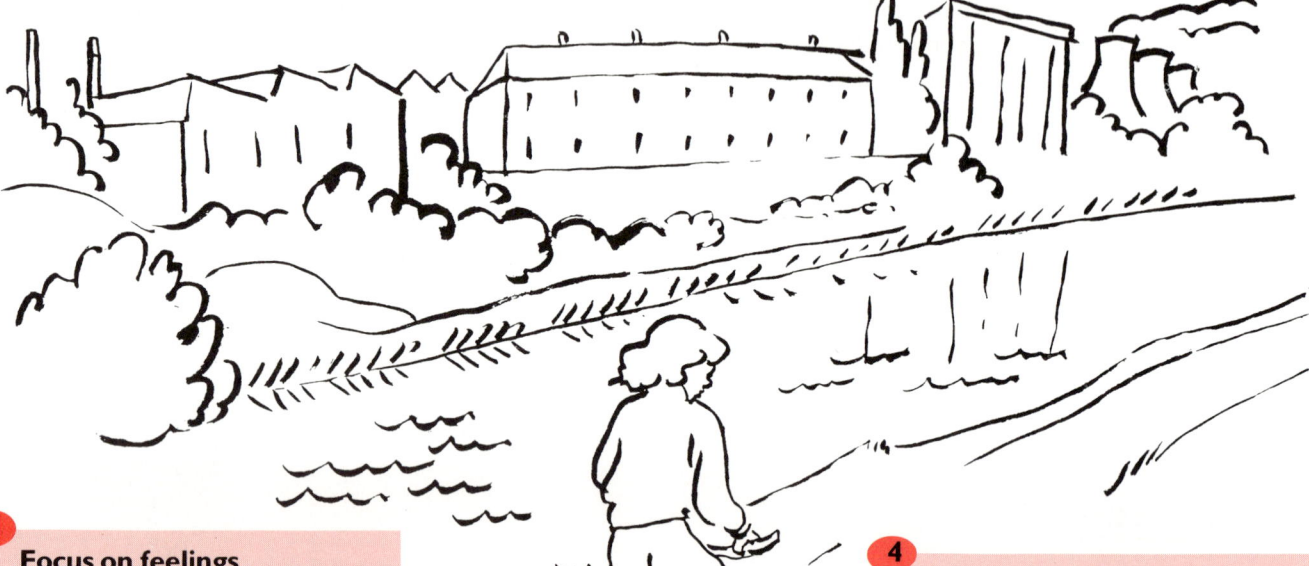

1

Focus on feelings

What do I feel I have to keep safe from? Are these real or pretend dangers? Which people and places are dangerous? Is it something I do that makes them dangerous? How do I keep myself safe? Do I have rules for different places? Is telling someone a good way of keeping safe? What makes me feel unsafe?

When am I most at risk?

4

Focus on outdoors

Where are the best places to play and explore? What makes these places safe, risky or dangerous? What makes them fun, exciting and interesting? What are the rules of these places? Can I remember them all? What am I getting better at? What can I learn to do so I'm safer in the street, by the water etc? How can I learn more about being a road user?

When am I most at risk?

2

Focus on me

Who am I? Where do I live? Where am I going? Where have I been? Who am I with? Who have I been with? Who is in charge? What time is it? How late is it? How do I get there? How do I ask the way, or ask for help? What does 'safe', 'dangerous', and 'risky' mean? What is good about being bigger and older? When is it risky? What can I do to help keep myself safe?

When am I most at risk?

3

Focus on indoors

What do I enjoy doing indoors? at home? at school? What can make play activities dangerous? What can make me safer? Is it something I can do? Who or what makes an accident happen? What are the rules indoors? Do the rules, and risks, depend on people and places? What am I getting better at? What would I like to be able to do? What does 'risky' mean?

When am I most at risk

5

Focus on people

Who will help me to keep safe? How do I recognise people whose job it is to keep me safe? What are they trying to teach us to do, or not to do? How can I help them? How do I know who to ask for help? Who are the people who threaten my safety? How do I recognise them? How can I keep myself safe?

When am I most at risk?

Classroom Strategies and Activities for Ages 6 and 7

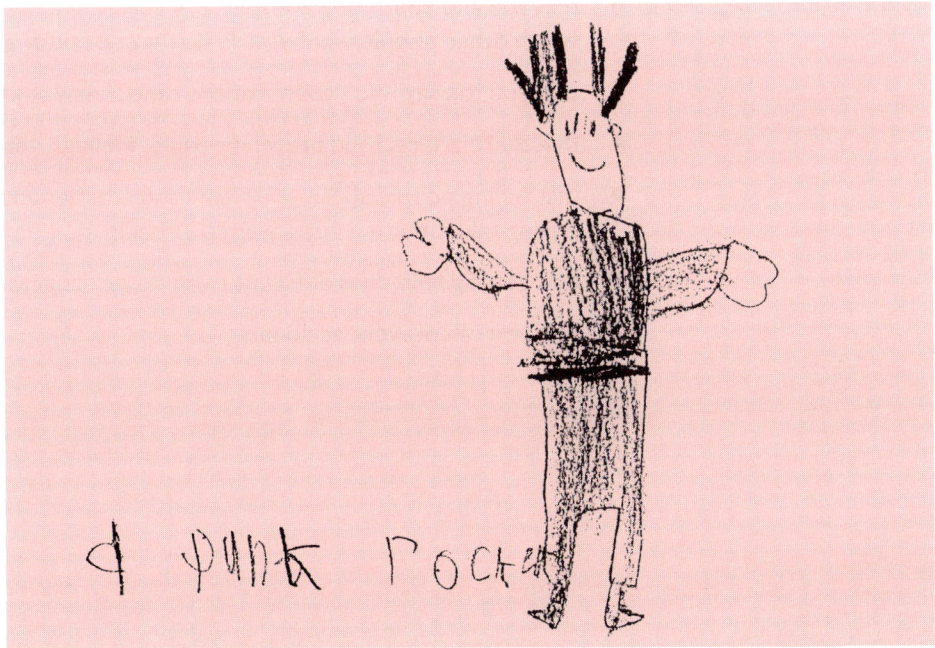

Key messages

Learn:

- who you are, where you live, who is at home, your telephone number, an alternative safe place to go.

- where you are, where you're supposed to be, who knows where you are, where you are going, where you've been, how to get out safely, the time, how long it takes to go from here to there.

- who can help you and what the limits of that help should be.

- about the day-to-day hazards where you live, play and go to school.

- about the safe places to play, how to play safely and the rules of different places.

- how to distinguish between the safe people, and the not so safe people.

- how accidents can happen.

Practise:

- the skills which help you to keep safe in traffic, near water, in and around the home, with people, and on your own.

- saying 'No', 'Stop', 'I'll ask'.

- asking for help, how to make people listen, how to describe exactly what happened.

- keeping family rules and the rules of different places.

- doing things for yourself.

- playing safely, having fun and feeling safe.

Understand:

- that you and your body are special, valuable and unique, and that some things which other people want you to do may not fit in with this.

- that you can say 'No', even if at the time it may seem rude or unkind.

- that there are real and pretend people, feelings, threats and promises.

- that telling people about your fears and worries and making them listen, is not 'telling tales', but is a good way to get help.

- that getting told off is different from other dangers.

- that you can prevent accidents.

Content box 1   Focus on feelings

 What do I feel I have to keep
safe from? Are these real or
pretend dangers? Which people
and places are dangerous? Is it
something I do that makes them
dangerous? How do I keep
myself safe? Do I have rules for
different places? Is telling
someone a good way of keeping
safe? What makes me feel
unsafe?
When am I most at risk?

Activity 1 ● *What do I feel I have to keep safe from?*

- Drawing. Writing. Talking together. Categorising.

- Class, group and individual activities.

Invite the children to think about the things they feel they have to keep safe from,
and, to draw and label as many of these as they can without discussion.

Ask them to pool their responses, and categorise them under the headings: 'real
things' and 'pretend things', or 'things', 'people' and 'places', which can then be
subdivided into 'real' and 'pretend'.

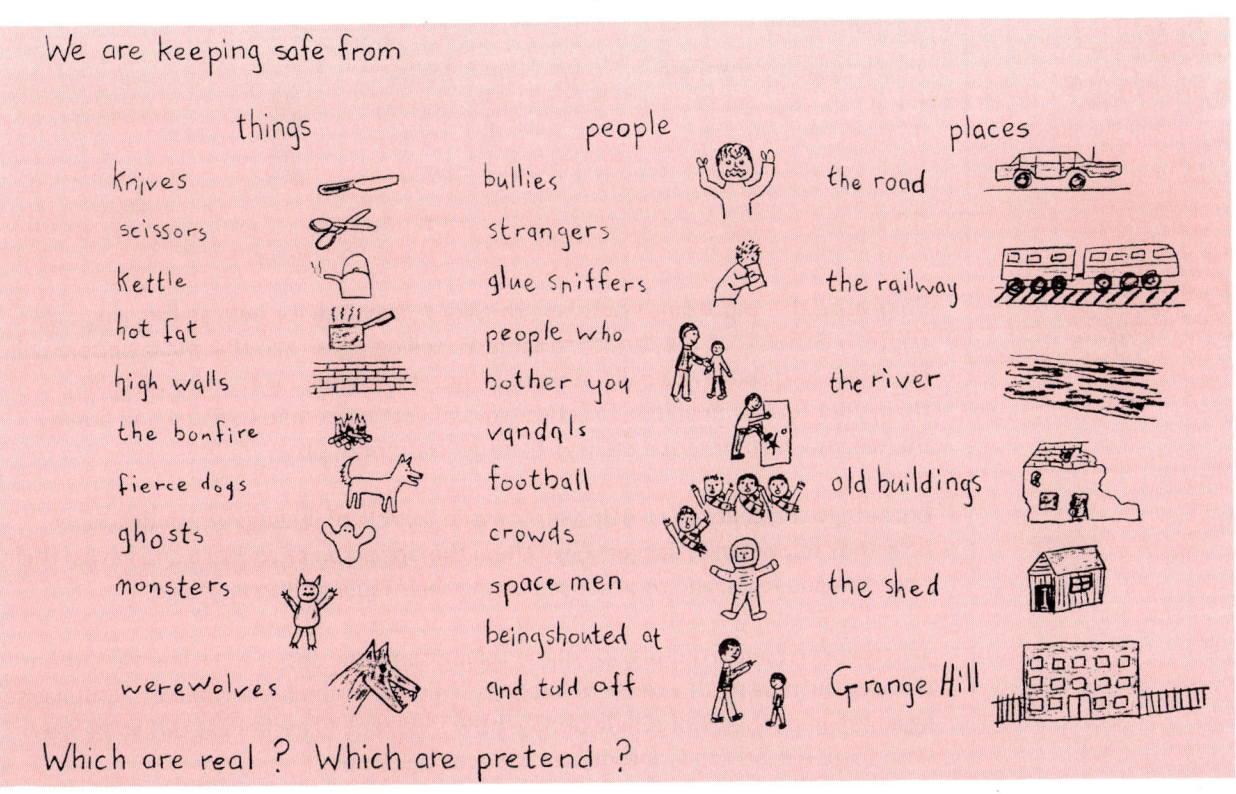

Explore with the children why they think these people, places and things are dangerous, asking the question: 'What can they do to hurt you?' Using this framework, children can begin to distinguish between hazards which they themselves can cause (for example, by being in an unsafe place, by playing with things not intended for play, or by taking risks) and hazards which are caused by other people not taking care, or other people who do things to them (for example, bullying or abuse).

Activity 2 ● *How do I keep myself safe?*

- Talking. Writing. Classroom play. Mime.

- Class or group activities.

Invite the children to review their list of things, people and places which they keep safe from. Ask them how they think they keep safe in different places and situations, and make a note of these.

Look at how many of the children's strategies are 'Do's' and how many are 'Don'ts'. They may include: 'Don't look', 'Hide yourself', 'Run away', 'Don't go with them', 'Say "No"', 'Keep away', 'Don't touch', 'Tell someone'. Help the children to distinguish between those which are specific to one kind of danger only, and those which can be used in different circumstances.

Invite the children to think of one or two safety rules, or reminders that could be used in any situation, for example,

– say 'No'.

– stop and think.

– ask someone for help.

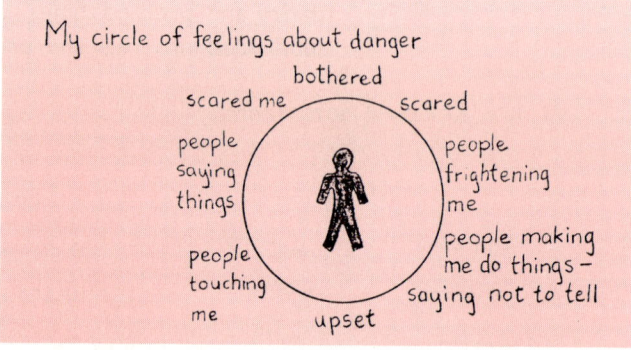

Emphasise the importance of telling or asking someone for help and sharing one's concern. Stress that this is not the same as 'telling tales', and that most people will not laugh or disbelieve a child in trouble, but it is important to keep on telling them your fear or problem. Practise ways of getting people to listen and finding the words which describe feelings through classroom play.

Encourage the children to help you compile a circle of feelings which describes how they felt when in danger. Give them the opportunity to share and reveal their concerns and fears, and to practise putting their feelings into language.

The children could role-play or mime telling someone about their fears and then share in the making of a circle of 'feelings which describe feeling better.' Emphasise again the importance of telling people how they feel. (Teachers at this stage may wish to go directly to Content box 5: Focus on people.)

Content box 2   Focus on me

Who am I? Where do I live?
Where am I going? Where have I
been? Who am I with? Who have
I been with? Who is in charge?
What time is it? How late is it?
How do I get there? How do I
ask the way, or ask for help?
What does 'safe', 'dangerous' or
'risky' mean? What is good about
being bigger and older? When is
it risky? What can I do to help
keep myself safe?
When am I most at risk?

Activity 1 ● *Who am I? Where do I live?*

- Classroom play. Mapwork. Stories. Talking together.
- Class and group activities.

The children can practise being able to say who they are and where they live
through activities centered around a topic such as the post office. You could set up
a post office and sorting office in the play corner and help the children to write and
sort letters and deliver cards and packages, which are addressed to themselves and
people within the school.

A map of the locality with the streets, houses, shops and blocks of flats clearly
labelled, can give the children additional practice, not only in knowing where they
live, but in working out safe ways to get from home to other places and back again.
This is a good time to ensure that they know their addresses and telephone
numbers.

Many traditional stories have characters who do not know who or what they really
are and where they come from, until a magical moment when all is revealed.
Children will enjoy talking about these characters, for example, the Ugly Duckling
who did not know it was a swan, the frog who was really a prince, the servant girl
who didn't know she was a princess. These stories can provide an opportunity to
remind the children of the importance of knowing who they are.

154

Activity 2 ● *Where are you going?*

- Talking together. Giving directions.

- Class and group work.

The ability to say where they are going and where they have been can be important safety skills for children. They can practise these skills during their everyday classroom activities and they can be reinforced when they make outside visits.

Ask the children, before they move to a different part of the school, to the hall, cloakroom, dining room or playground, to say where they are going, how they will get there and what they think they will see or pass as they go. Afterwards they can check if they were right. Before going on a visit away from the school, you can ask the children to describe the part of the route closest to the school, to practise saying who they are, the name of the school and their home or school address.

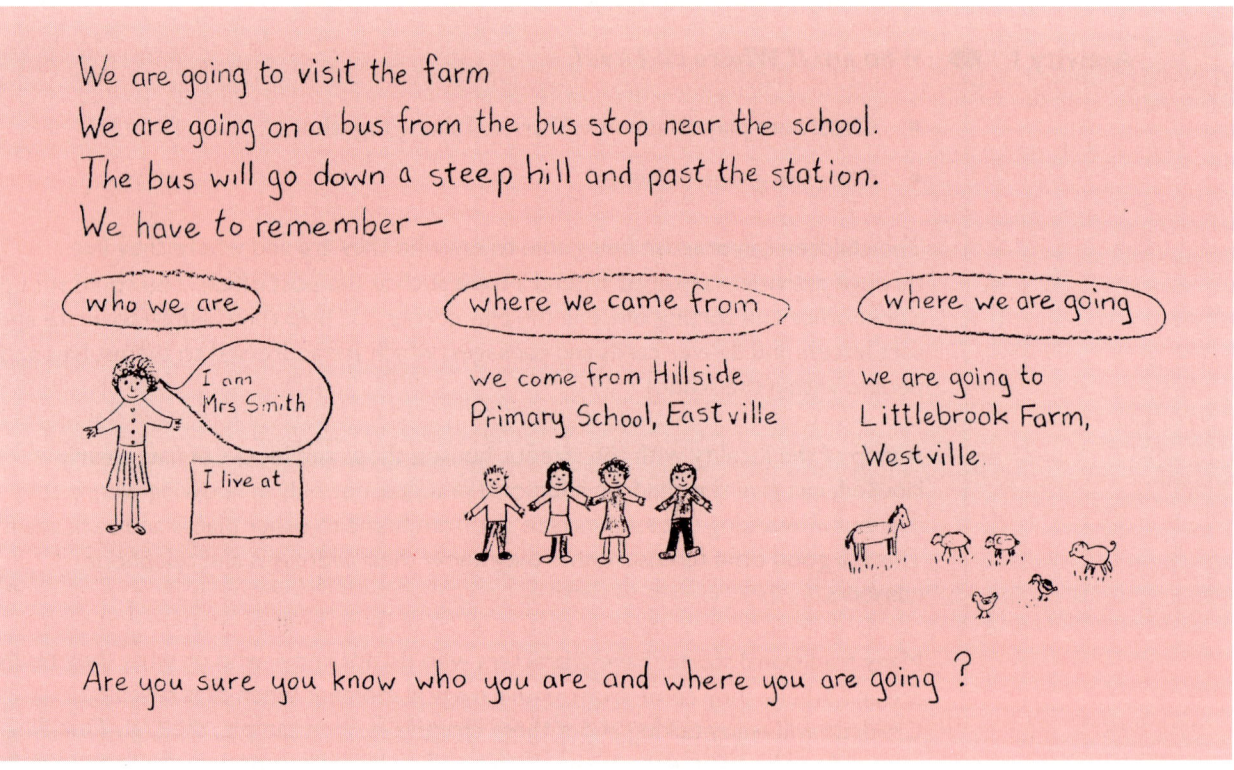

We are going to visit the farm
We are going on a bus from the bus stop near the school.
The bus will go down a steep hill and past the station.
We have to remember —

who we are

I am Mrs Smith

I live at

where we came from

we come from Hillside Primary School, Eastville

where we are going

we are going to Littlebrook Farm, Westville.

Are you sure you know who you are and where you are going?

Activity 3 ● *Who is with you? Who is in charge?*

- Talking together. Painting and drawing. Collecting and sorting pictures. Classroom play.

- Class and group activities.

Talk with the children about the importance of knowing who is with them, and who is in charge of them or the place where they find themselves. They could talk about the different places that they go to at different times of the day. This is a good opportunity to emphasise the dangers of going into places which are closed, fenced off etc.

Invite the children to collect, or make their own pictures of children in places such as: swimming pools, playgrounds, parks, river banks, beaches, shops, streets, classrooms and school visits. Display the pictures under a heading: 'Who is in charge here?'

Talk with the children about who might be in charge in each situation and how they could recognise that person. Ask the children to look at the possibility of no one being there to take charge. Who then would be in charge? This would be a good time to help them consider the importance of being in charge of themselves and their own behaviour, and look at the skills which they need to do this.

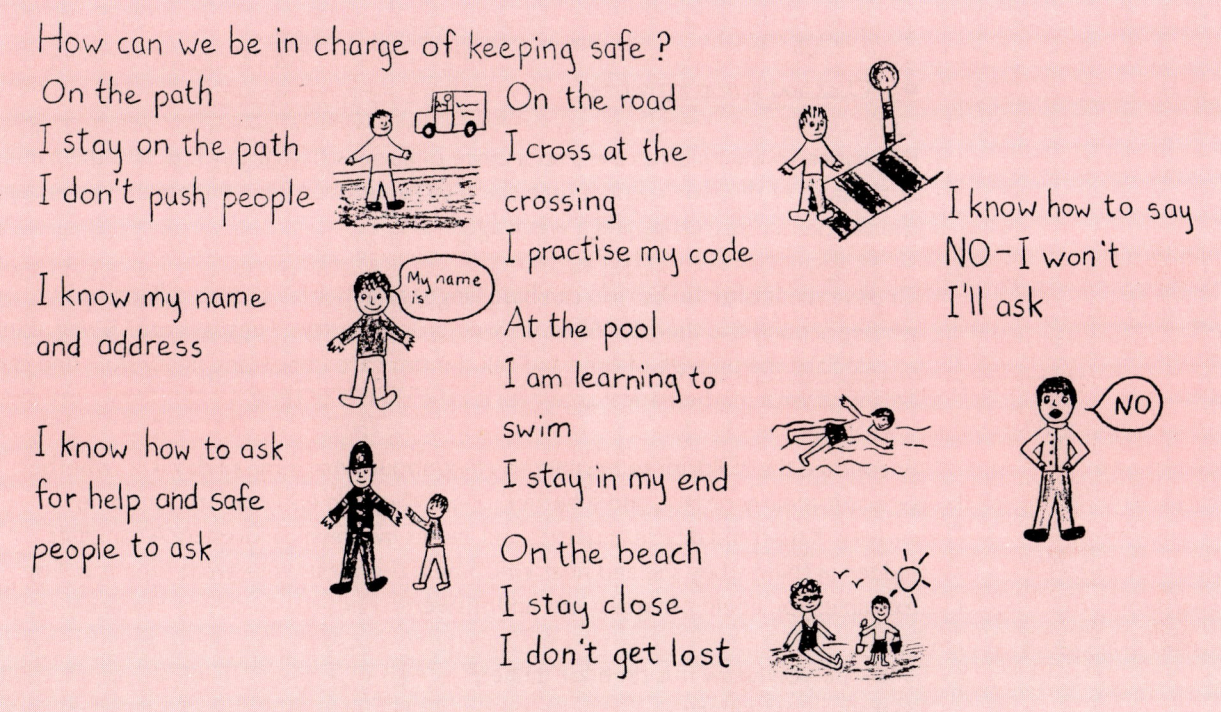

This activity provides an opportunity to look at safe people to ask for help, in school, in the neighbourhood, and in and around the home. You can use classroom play to share, practise and reinforce ways of approaching people to ask for help.

Activity 4 ● *Where have I been? How do I get home?*

- Describing. Observing. Drawing and painting.
- Class, small group and pair activities.

The skills of observing and describing sequentially where you have been can be of importance in the area of keeping safe. Young children sometimes find it difficult to describe the routes they have taken, the places they have visited, and the people they have encountered. Encourage the children, particularly when they are sharing their experiences with others in the class, to try to describe places, persons and routes so that others can 'see' them. Invite them to draw or paint pictures of places, events or class visits, arrange them sequentially and to try to recall exact details.

Invite the children to recall the routes they take from their homes to school, to the shops, to places where they play and to the other homes that they visit. Ask them to pick out the danger spots along the route, for example, heavy traffic, isolated or dark areas, or places where people congregate. Invite the children to work in pairs or small groups and to draw themselves on some of these routes illustrating some of the hazards (these illustrations are often very revealing). Ask the children what they would do if they needed help along the route. Where would they look? Whom would they ask? Ask them to illustrate their replies.

Activity 5 ● *What day is it? What time is it?*

- Talking together. Language activities. Telling the time.
- Class and group activities.

Emphasise to the children the importance of knowing what day it is, and the names of the days of the week. Encourage them to remember what happened yesterday, the day before yesterday and a week ago.

Cross-curricular links: you can base language activities such as talking and writing around the theme: 'What do we do on Mondays/Tuesdays etc.' Being able to calculate the passage of time and tell the time are important safety skills and can be linked with mathematical activities on the theme of time.

Encourage the children to be alert to clues about what time of day it is, whether or not it is early or late, and whether or not they are early or late for some activity. You could devise activities and games in which children look for clues hidden in things they see and hear which help them estimate what time it is. For example, you could use questions and answers:

'How do you know it is time for dinner?'
'Because I am hungry.'

Encourage the children to think of more clues provided by their own feelings, for example, hunger, tiredness and cold, and clues provided by their surroundings.

Activity 6 ● *What is good about being bigger and older?*

- PE. Talking. Writing.
- Class and group activities.

Cross-curricular links: explore through physical education activities the children's increasing ability to reach up, to span, to jump higher and further, to balance and to control small apparatus. In language activities you can help them to describe all the new things they can do, reach and control, now that they are bigger and more skilful, using talking and writing.

Talk with the children about 'looking after yourself'. Explore questions such as: Can they look after themselves all the time? Some of the time? When? Can they keep themselves safe? All the time? Some of the time? Which things are risky? What might happen? What can I do to keep myself safe?

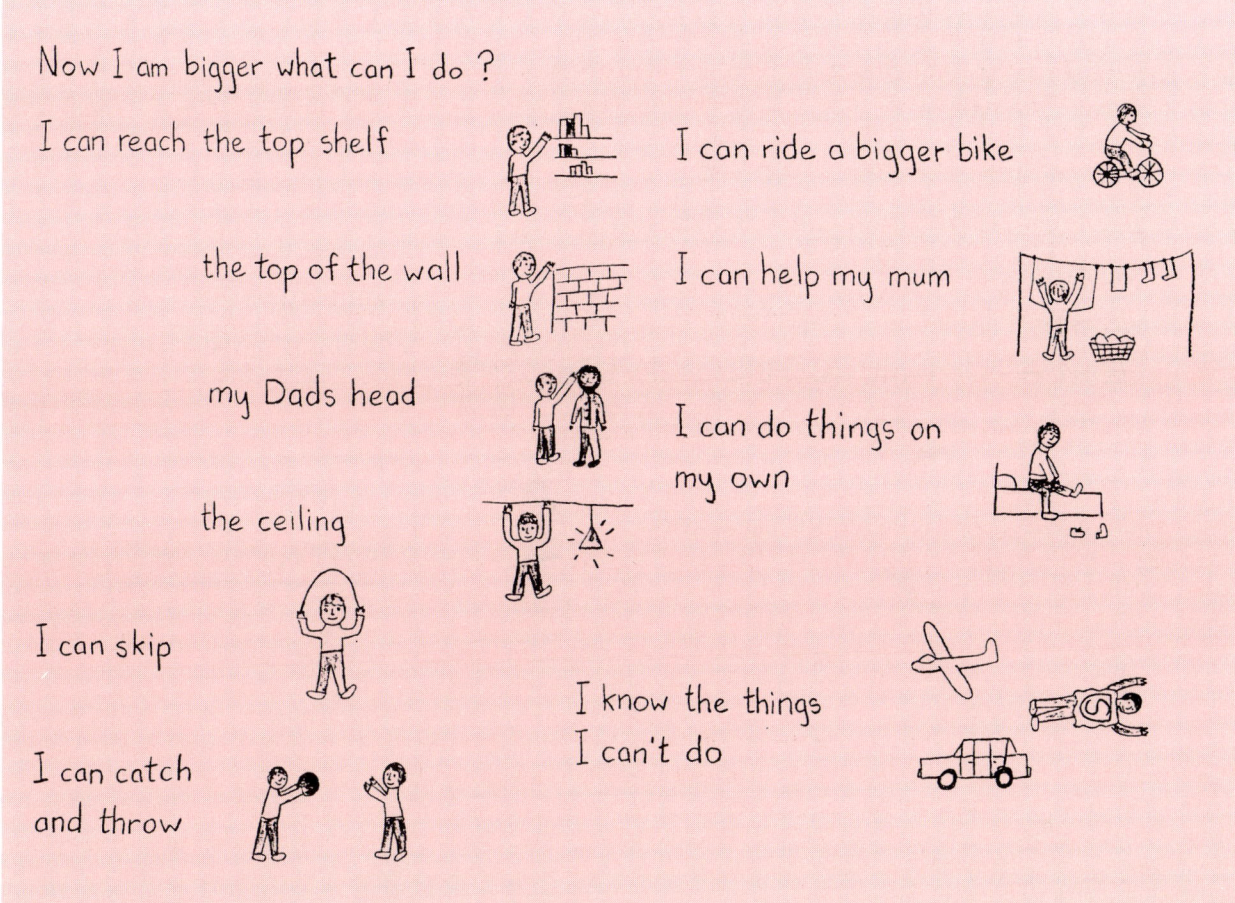

Now I am bigger what can I do ?

I can reach the top shelf

the top of the wall

my Dads head

the ceiling

I can skip

I can catch and throw

I can ride a bigger bike

I can help my mum

I can do things on my own

I know the things I can't do

Activity 7 ● *When am I most at risk?*

- Talking together. Describing situations and feelings.
- Class or group activity.

The concepts of 'taking risks' and 'being at risk' are not easy for children to grasp at this stage, but can best be explored through activities which focus on what other people do to make things risky for themselves and others. Children are made aware of the concept of risk more effectively by observing others in risky situations than by relating their own behaviour to risk taking.

Talk with the children about how they behave when they get excited, frightened, upset and angry. Ask them to think of ways in which this might affect their ability to keep themselves safe. Make a display on this theme. Remind them of the three main safety rules which they learnt earlier:

– say 'No'.

– stop and think.

– ask someone for help.

| Talk about the importance of keeping calm.

What do we do when we are excited ?
We jump up and down
We shout
We rush about

What do we do when we are scared ?
We run away
We don't look
We let people bully us, make us do things

What do we do when we are upset ?
We cry
We don't look where we're going
We run off

We forget our Keeping Safe Rules

We forget our Keeping Safe Rules

We forget our Keeping Safe Rules

Content box 3   Focus on indoors

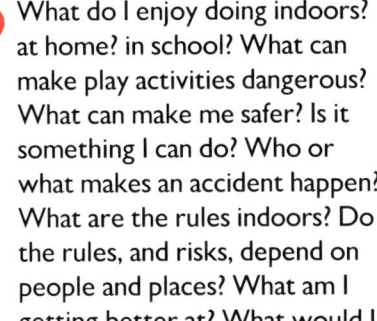

What do I enjoy doing indoors? at home? in school? What can make play activities dangerous? What can make me safer? Is it something I can do? Who or what makes an accident happen? What are the rules indoors? Do the rules, and risks, depend on people and places? What am I getting better at? What would I like to be able to do? What does 'risky' mean?
When am I most at risk?

Activity 1   *What do I enjoy doing indoors?*

- Talking and writing together. Describing situations, places and feelings. Making 'bendy books'. Drawing and painting. Model making.

- Class and group work.

Explore with the children the things they enjoy doing when they are indoors: at home, at other people's homes and places where they play.

Each child or group could make a 'bendy book', consisting of drawings and writing which show how they have fun and enjoy being indoors, and which says where they have fun, what they do, who is with them and what day and time it is.

Make a list with the children of all the places where they play that they have included in their work. Ask them to tell you which places, and ways of playing, are dangerous. Prompt them to include in their list: stairs, cupboards, balconies, the kitchen, bathroom, swimming pools, the classroom and any local danger spots. Ask the children to look through the 'bendy books' in groups, marking the dangerous places with a red danger sign.

Encourage them to talk about what could cause an accident in these places. Focus on:

— what the children might do;

— what others might do;

— or how others might persuade them to do something which could cause an accident.

Help the children to review each of these places in terms of how likely it is that accidents might happen there:

– at different times of the day;

– when they are alone;

– or when they are with other people;

to help them decide when they are most at risk.

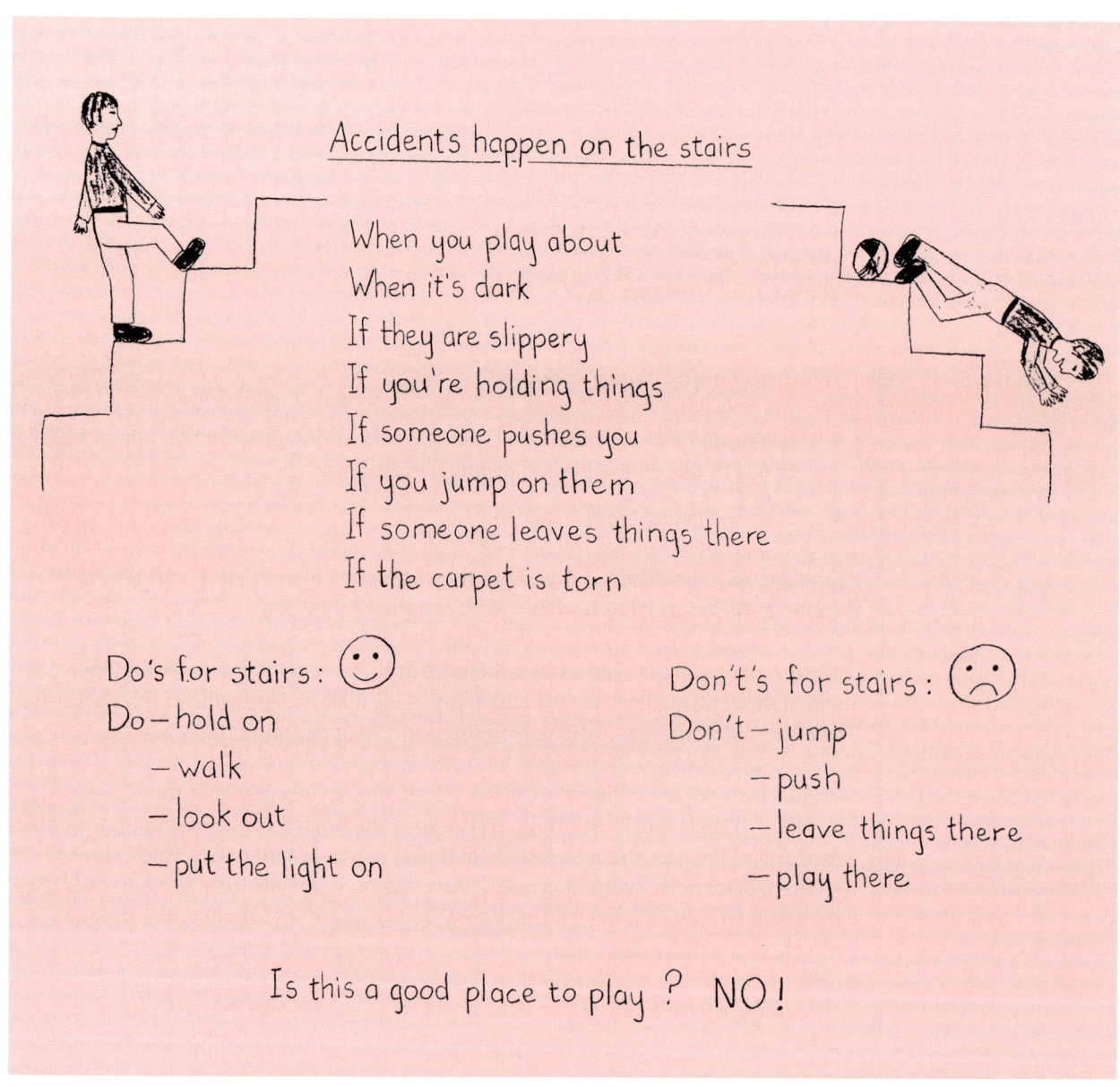

Accidents happen on the stairs

When you play about
When it's dark
If they are slippery
If you're holding things
If someone pushes you
If you jump on them
If someone leaves things there
If the carpet is torn

Do's for stairs : ☺
Do – hold on
  – walk
  – look out
  – put the light on

Don't's for stairs : ☹
Don't – jump
  – push
  – leave things there
  – play there

Is this a good place to play ? NO!

Through this kind of activity, children can learn to distinguish places which are safe to play in from those which are dangerous to play in. Invite them to make a set of Keeping Safe Rules for some of these places, for example: home, school, the swimming pool, etc. Ask them if their rules are different for each place and help them to look for general rules which can be applied to any place.

It is important that children now begin to think beyond things, people and places as hazards, to look at situations which are *potentially* dangerous, and at the impact that their own actions have in such situations.

It's safer in the classroom when:

- we keep ourselves safe

- teacher is there

- we walk and don't run

- we put things away

- we listen

- we point scissors down

Can you write some more DO'S for the classroom ?

Accidents happen in the classroom when:

- we play about, tease, dare

- we get upset, excited, silly

- we rush about, push

- we leave things on the floor

- we come in when there is no one

in to look after us

Can you write some more DON'TS for the classroom ?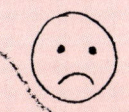

Talk with the children about some of the activities which are forbidden in their homes or in other people's homes which they might like to be able to do. Ask them to tell you about forbidden places which they would like to explore. Ask them what they think they would most enjoy about doing these things or going to these places? Is it the excitement? Or feeling grown-up?

Ask them to suggest the reasons people (adults?) give for not allowing them to do these things. Help them to categorise these reasons, for example:

- It belongs to someone else.

- They think I'll hurt myself.

- It's dangerous.

- It's risky.

- You have to be grown-up.

- They think I'll break it.

- I'm too small.

- They think I don't know how to do it.

- I don't know how to do it.

Talk with the children about the indoor things, places and activities which they think are *always* dangerous, for example, fires or electricity. Talk about the things which could be risky, but are less risky if they have the skills to cope with them.

Encourage the children to continue to explore their list of dangerous places, and think about the different times of the day, or days of the week, or seasons of the year, when these places may become more risky. Invite them to ask themselves the question 'Is this a good place to play?', and help them to look for a range of answers, such as:

- No, not ever.

- Only if/Only when . . .

- Yes, if you know the safety rules.

Explore with the children the outdoor places where they might find displayed safety rules which have been decided on by other people, for example:

- in the park (no cycling).

- by lakes, rivers and canals (no swimming, paddling).

- on electricity pylons and sub stations.

- in escalators or lifts.

- on railway crossings and pelican crossings.

- on building sites.

- in playgrounds.

Talk about the reasons for keeping the rules and the risks involved in not keeping them.

This could provide a starting point for exploring the locality of the school, for making visits and inviting safety officers to come and talk with the children.

The children could illustrate different aspects of these rules and warnings through drawing, painting or model making.

Activity 2 ● ***What am I getting better at?***

- Talking together. Drawing and painting.
- Class, group and individual activities.

Talk with the children about the things that they (and you) are learning to do, and getting better at: at home, at school and in other places. For example, swimming, using scissors, doing PE, throwing and catching. Invite them to say whether these activities are risky, and what makes them so. (This can reveal a great deal about young children's perceptions of risk.)

Invite the children to illustrate this list of activities and to say what might make them risky, completing sentences as follows:

'Swimming can be risky if . . .'
'Cooking can be risky when . . .'

Explore with the children how they are getting better at these things. Is it just that they are older, or bigger? Help them to think about generalisations like the ones below.

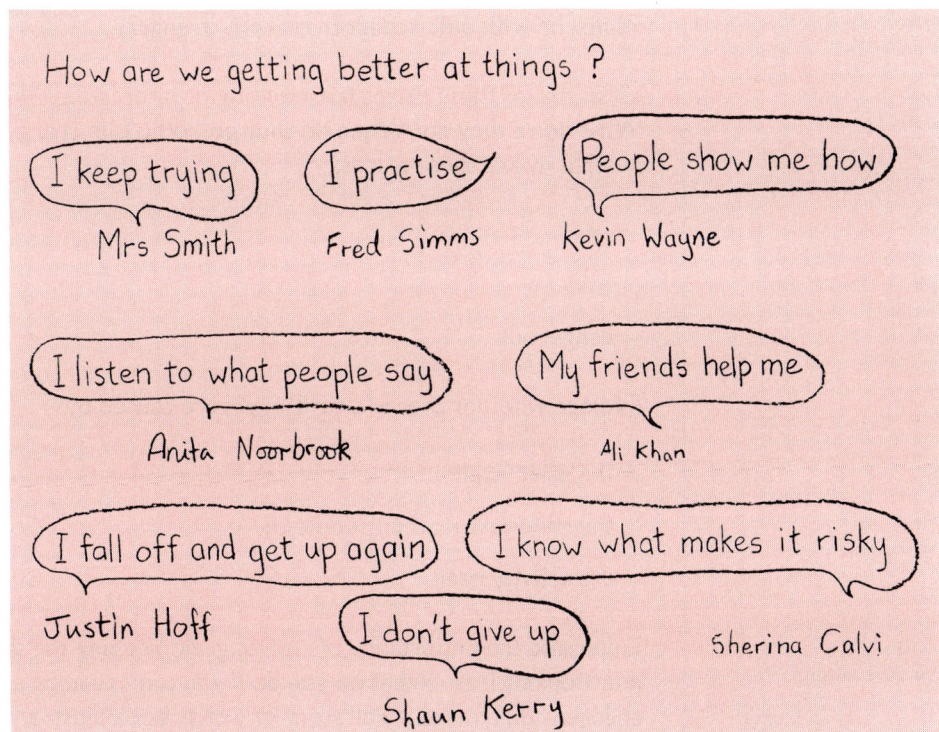

Invite the children to pick out one skill which they think they could improve and to think how they could do this and who could help them. Encourage them to set themselves a target and to ask for support from friends and family to reach that target.

Content box 4 Focus on outdoors

Where are the best places to play and explore? What makes these places safe, risky and dangerous? What makes them fun, exciting and interesting? What are the rules of these places? Can I remember them all? What am I getting better at? What can I learn to do so I am safer in the street, by the water etc? How can I learn more about being a road user? **When am I most at risk?**

Activity 1

Where are the best places to play and explore?

- Talking and writing together. Drawing and painting. Making books.

- Class, group and individual activities.

Invite the children to describe, draw and paint places in the locality where they go, or have been, with the class, or alone, or with friends, or with family, or with other adults, or with older children or with strangers.

What makes these places fun, exciting or interesting? What do they do there? What don't they do? When do they go? Who is in charge? Look with the children at what makes these places;

– safe.

– risky.

– dangerous.

Explore whether the risks or dangers are caused by:

– the place itself.

– the children or other people there.

– the activity itself.

Emphasise the importance of knowing and keeping the safety rules. Ask them questions such as: 'What do you do if you can't read or understand them? The children could make a wall story or a class book illustrating these places, with the rules boldly printed.

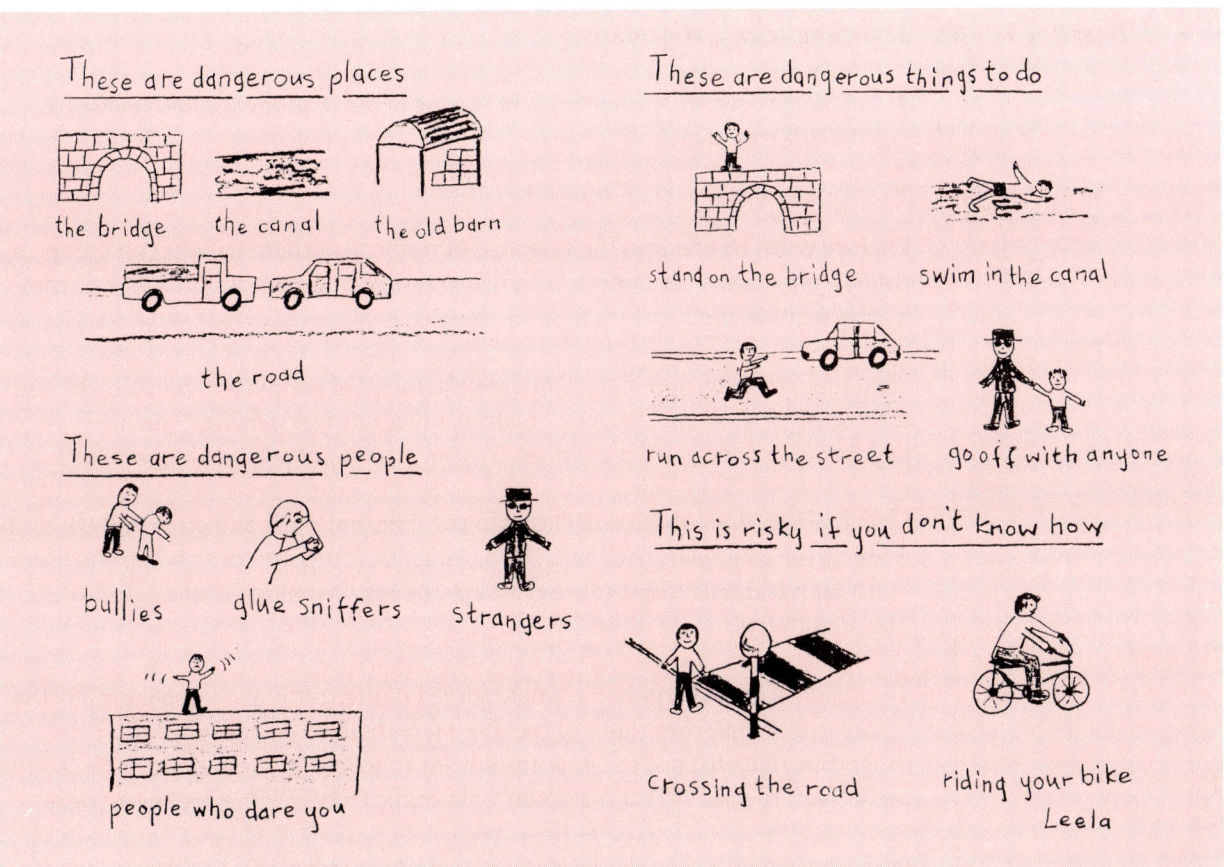

Invite the children to make an individual book with pictures showing themselves in some of these places keeping the rules. They could add to these with pictures from magazines, photographs, and leaflets from safety organisations. You could suggest that the children ask their families to share in this activity, and extend the range of the books.

The children could also look at those places where there are no safety rules displayed, for example: in the school playground, at zebra crossings, near the school crossing patrol, on pavements, on roads, at traffic lights, in the garden, derelict or abandoned buildings, railways and subways. (This will provide you with opportunities to focus on specific hazards in the locality.)

The children could work together, in small groups, to illustrate some of these places and to decide what the rules of these places should be. They could then compare the different sets of rules. Ask them whether or not it is possible to remember all these rules all the time.

Review the sets of rules and check how many are 'Do's' and how many are 'Don'ts'. Identify the rules which are repeated. Encourage the children to try to condense the rules into one or two which can be remembered all the time. These can be added to the children's individual books, and to the wall stories or class books.

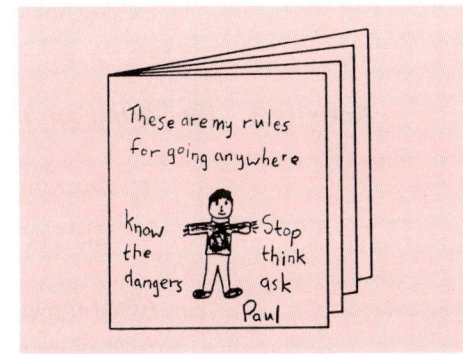

Activity 2 ● *Learning to use the roads*

- Talking together. Collecting and sorting pictures. Drawing. Survey work. Talking together.

- Class or group and individual activities.

Explore with the children the language of traffic. Ask them to collect pictures of traffic from magazines, and sort them into categories, such as: lorries, vans, cars, tractors, buses, etc.

Help them to think about and illustrate the range of people and animals who use the roads, for example, families, children, horses, drivers, delivery men, pedestrians, traffic wardens, police, crossing patrol people, building workers.

Help them to think about and illustrate the different areas and places where traffic is found, for example, roads, streets, pavements, footpaths, driveways, entrances, exits, car parks, bus stops, zebra crossings, pelican crossings, traffic lights, traffic islands, subways.

The children could carry out a simple survey of the traffic and people passing the school gate at different times of the day. Help them to decide when it is most dangerous and what are the important rules to follow at these times. You can give them clues, such as: 'What makes being in traffic risky?', 'What makes it safer?'

Invite the children to look at the skills for dealing with traffic which they can practise, for example, stopping, moving, listening and looking. Talk about how they can recognise danger:

– as they go out of the school gate;

– on the pavement;

– when getting ready to cross the road;

– when crossing the road;

– when alone;

– with friends;

– with adults;

– when going out to play.

A similar approach could be used in order to focus on other areas of risk in the locality, for example, railway lines, bridges and canals.

Activity 3 ● *What am I getting better at?*

- Drawing. Writing. Mathematical representation. Talking together.

- Class or group and individual activities.

Adapt the Draw and Write Technique (see Appendix 1, page 410) to investigate what the children think they are getting better at doing outdoors.

Without any prior discussion or sharing of ideas, ask them to draw themselves outdoors, doing some of the things they are becoming better at. Ask them to label their pictures, starting with these words: 'I am getting better at . . .'

There is a **cross-curricular link** with mathematical representation here: you could either analyse their replies and present your analysis to them, or you could help them to present the investigation results themselves. Use bar charts, graphs or any other methods of mathematical representation you think are appropriate.

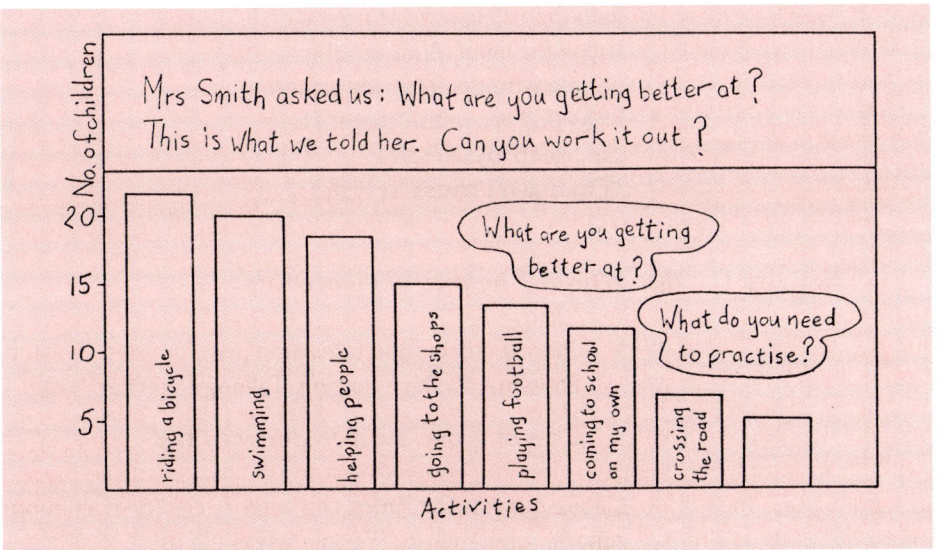

The children could then identify those skills which they as individuals think they most need to improve or extend.

They could make contracts with themselves and pinpoint ways in which they might best succeed, for example:

— by practising.

— asking for help.

— observing others.

— learning the rules.

— remembering the risks.

— identifying people at home, in school and in the local community who could help them fulfil their contracts.

Content box 5   Focus on people

 Who will help me to keep safe?
How do I recognise people
whose job it is to keep me safe?
What are they trying to teach us
to do, or not to do? How can I
help them? How do I know who
to ask for help? Who are the
people who threaten my safety?
How do I recognise them? How
can I keep myself safe?
When am I most at risk?

Activity I   ● *Who will help to keep me safe?*

- Sharing stories and television programmes. Collecting and sorting pictures. Drawing. Collage making. Talking together. Visits. Classroom play.

- Class or group and individual activities.

Cross-curricular links: this activity can form an important strand in a more general topic such as: 'People who help us'.

Explore with the children what they would do if they lost something, or became lost themselves. Use their experiences, a story, or a television programme as a starting point. This could be an opportunity to reinforce the work on the theme 'Who am I? Where do I live?' from Content box 2. It might also be prudent to remind children about the dangers of agreeing to strangers' requests for help in searching for lost things.

Invite the children to help you to collect pictures from magazines, photographs and posters. Combine these with their own drawings and paintings of people who help to keep them safe, and arrange them in a collage. Encourage them to include pictures of family, friends, teachers and members of the community. Ask each child to add a picture of herself or himself as a very important part of this team.

Who helps to keep us safe?

The keeping safe team

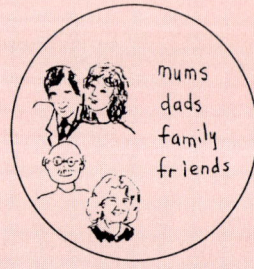
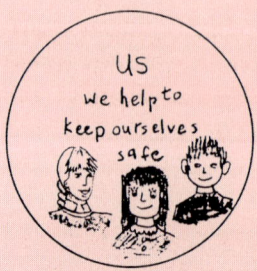
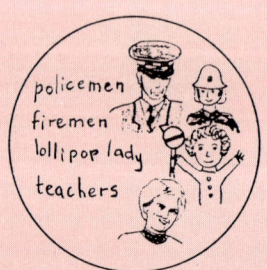

Explore with the children the roles of some of these helpers by asking these questions:

– Do they wear uniforms? Can they describe them?

– How do we recognise helpers if they do not have uniforms?

– What kind of job is it? Is it risky? What makes it risky?

– What do they have to do so it's not so risky?

– What do they do every day?

– What do they do in emergencies?

– What do they do to stop people getting hurt?

– What do they try to teach us?

– What are their messages to grown-ups and children?

You could use visits, visitors, recall, observation, role-play and creative activities to help the children find the answers to these questions. You could display safety messages from different helpers as reminders and reinforcement.

Ask the children to reflect on what they can do to help these people and to take on their share of the job. Help them to consider:

– learning the messages and keeping the rules.

– being aware of what makes the helpers' jobs difficult.

– practising getting better at doing things.

– being aware of the risks.

– setting a good example and passing on the messages.

Ask the children if it is possible to take all these people with them wherever they go. Is it possible to remember all their messages? What can they do if it isn't possible? Would it be helpful to reduce all the messages to one or two important ones which could help them in any situation?

Activity 2 ● *Who are the people who threaten my safety?*

● Drawing. Writing. Talking together.

● Class or group and individual activities.

It is important to tap the children's perceptions of people who they see as threatening, and to explore with them how they think these people can, or do, harm them, and how they can be recognised. Many children have a very stereotyped picture of people with whom they could be at risk, and this is based almost completely on appearance.

It would be valuable to use the Draw and Write Technique at this point (see Appendix 1, page 410 for more information). Invite the children, without discussion, to draw themselves keeping safe from dangerous people, and to label or describe the person, the danger and their method for keeping safe.

Children may name specific people in their replies or respond in more general terms, such as: strangers or people who tease, dare, threaten, vandalise, bully, sniff glue, touch, scare and abuse. You will undoubtedly uncover aspects of the children's perceptions, fears or misunderstandings which are not covered here, but which need to be followed up.

Explore this question with the children: 'How can we tell this is a dangerous person?' Help them to focus less on appearance and more on the kinds of things these people might say, or do.

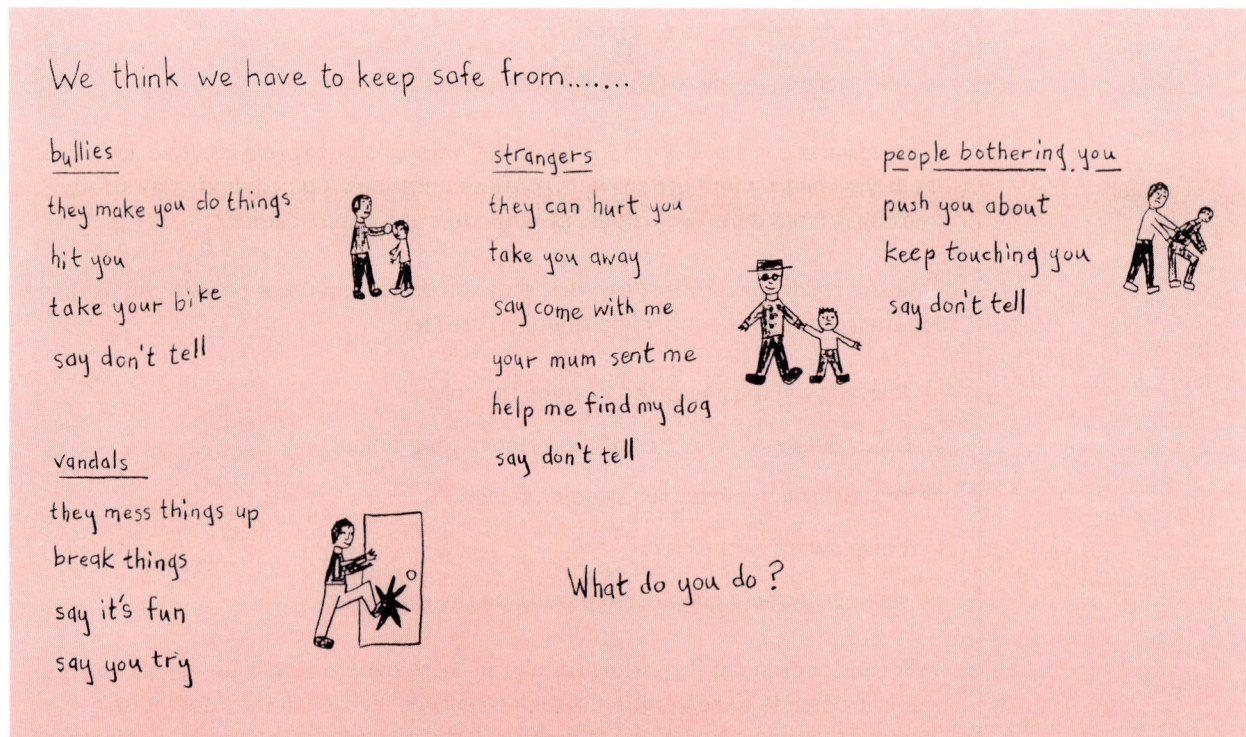

We think we have to keep safe from.......

bullies
they make you do things
hit you
take your bike
say don't tell

strangers
they can hurt you
take you away
say come with me
your mum sent me
help me find my dog
say don't tell

people bothering you
push you about
keep touching you
say don't tell

vandals
they mess things up
break things
say it's fun
say you try

What do you do?

Explore with the children some of the best strategies for dealing with these situations, for example

– stay with people you know, like and trust.

– don't join other groups, or follow older children.

– get help from people you can trust.

– tell other people about what happened, where it happened and how you felt.

– say 'No, don't', 'I'll ask someone' etc.

Provide opportunities for the children to practise these strategies using role-play.

Cross-curricular link: use stories and poems to illustrate how to deal with threatening people. Contact your children's librarian for help or compile your own list of relevant material.

Action Planner
Keeping Myself Safe

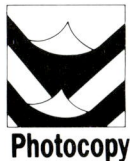

Photocopy

1

Focus on feelings

What is it like to feel safe? Is feeling safe different for other people? How does it feel to be uncertain or unsafe? What is it like to feel high or feel low? How do my feelings affect my safety? What do we have to keep safe from? Do people keep safe in different ways?

When am I most at risk?

2

Focus on me

Who am I? How do I describe myself and other people? Where am I? Who is in charge? Where am I going? Where is home? Who is there? How do I get home? What would I do in a dangerous situation? Are the rules and the risks different in different situations? How can I keep safe in any situation? Whose rules are the most important?

When am I most at risk?

3

Focus on indoors

What makes indoor places fun and exciting? What new places am I going to? What new things am I learning to do? What makes these places risky or dangerous? How can I make things less risky? Who is responsible for me indoors? How can I learn to be responsible for myself? What is an accident? How do accidents happen? Is being told off a danger?

When am I most at risk?

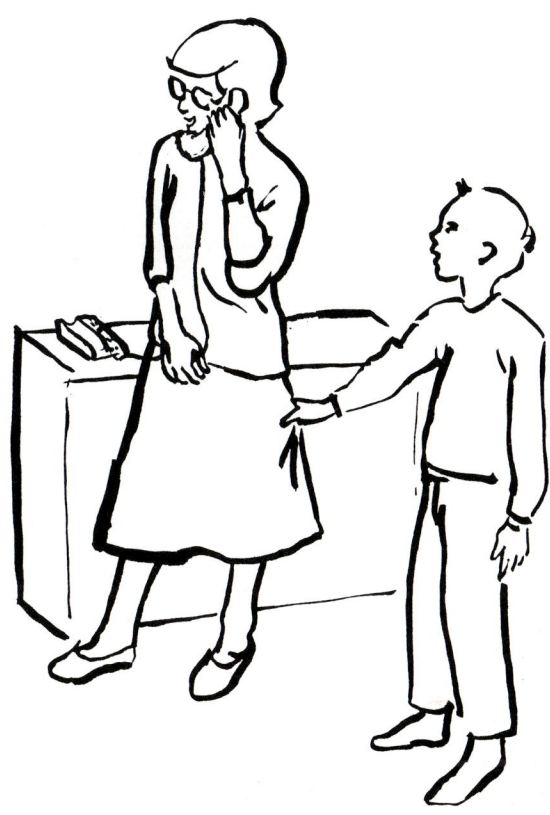

4

Focus on outdoors

Where are my favourite outdoor places? What makes them special? What do we do there? What are the rules? Do the rules and risks change with the place? What would I do if something dangerous or frightening happened? What can I practise so I am ready to cope? Who can help me? How do I get to these places and back again? What are the risks on my journey? Where are the safe people and places? What kinds of accidents happen to children of my age?

When am I most at risk?

5

Focus on people

Who do I see when I am out and about? Who has the job of keeping me safe? What can we do to make their jobs easier? What does being responsible mean for me? Who can I trust? How can I tell what kind of a person someone is? How can I learn to keep safe from, and cope with, threatening people?

When am I most at risk?

Classroom Strategies and Activities for Ages 8 and 9

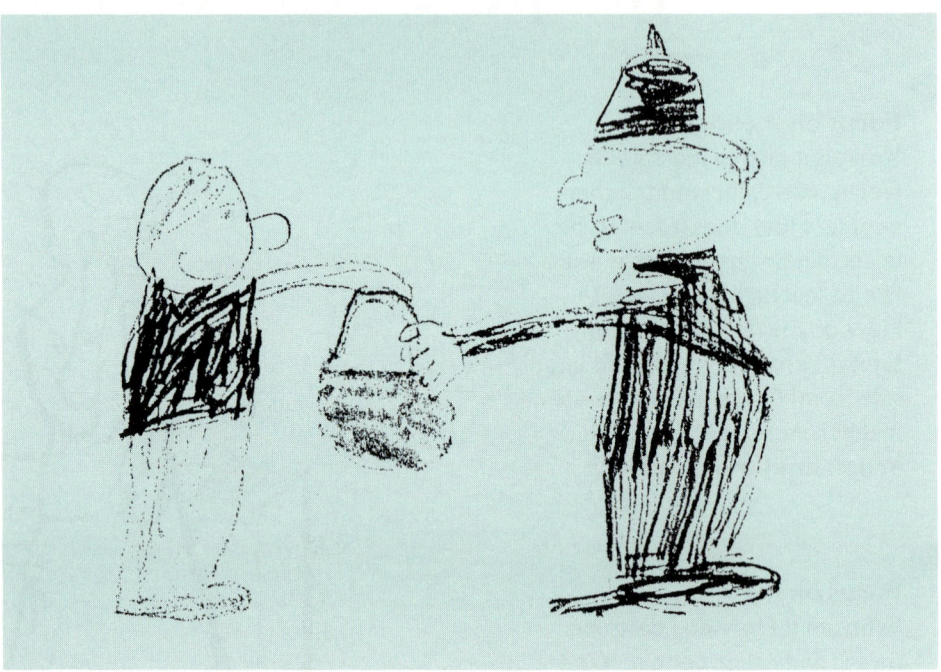

Key messages

Learn:

- who you are, where you are, where you're supposed to be, who is in charge, who knows where you are.

- the way out, the way home, how to contact home, about an alternative safe place, how to tell the time, use a telephone, judge time and distance.

- how to get help in time of need.

- about the hazards and risks, especially when you are away from adult supervision or help.

- about safe people and not so safe people, and how they can be recognised.

- how accidents can happen, when and where children are likely to have accidents, how to report an accident or incident.

- all the skills which keep you safe in traffic, in and on water, at home, away from home, alone and in groups.

- to resist pressure from your own age group, and older children, who want you to take risks or experiment.

- to say 'No', 'I won't take that risk', 'I'll ask', 'I'll check that out first'.

- to tell people, how to make them listen, how to explain and describe what happened and how you felt.

- to keep the rules designed for different places.

- some simple lifesaving skills.

Practise:

- sharing things and feelings with your friends and family.

- playing safely and using things safely.

- having fun, feeling good, and feeling safe.

- the skills you need to keep safe.

Understand:

- that your growing body is yours and is special, and that you can keep it, and the space around it, free from interference.

- that saying 'No', even if it seems to cause problems or threats, is not rude, thoughtless or unkind if what you are saying 'No' to is frightening or upsetting you.

- that what people tell you could be true, but could also be an opinion or 'pretend', and that some secrets need to be told.

- that telling people you are worried, and continuing to tell them, is not telling tales, but is a good way of getting help.

- that 'getting told off' is a different kind of worry from other dangers and may be something to do with grown-up worries.

- that although lots of people can and do help you to keep safe, it has to be your job too.

- that younger children will copy you and copy the way you keep safe or take risks.

Content box 1   Focus on feelings

What is it like to feel safe? Is feeling safe different for other people? How does it feel to be uncertain or unsafe? What is it like to feel high or feel low? How do my feelings affect my safety? What do we have to keep safe from? Do people keep safe in different ways? **When am I most at risk?**

Activity I   *What is it like to feel safe?*

- Talking together. Describing feelings and experiences. Painting. Role-play.

- Class or group and individual activities.

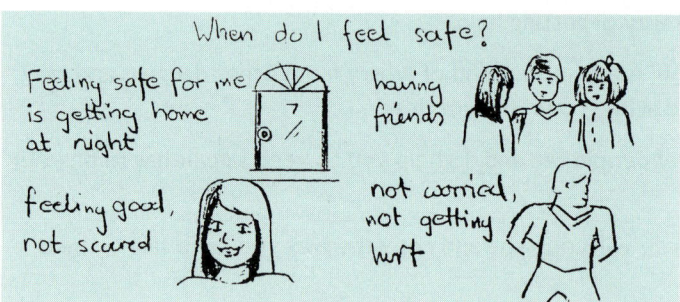

Ask the children to try and capture the feeling of being safe in words, in pictures or through movement and mime. Help them to extend their vocabulary, and explore their personal experience. Draw on relevant current, local or national events, and the experiences of characters in stories and television programmes.

Invite the children to think about what feeling safe means to different members of their families, and explore the idea that different people will have different views of keeping safe. Look at the physical aspects of safety: being warm, being fed and having a home, and look at people who do not have these things. Look at other aspects of safety, for example, feeling protected, cared for, having friends, being free from fear, and having someone to trust and tell.

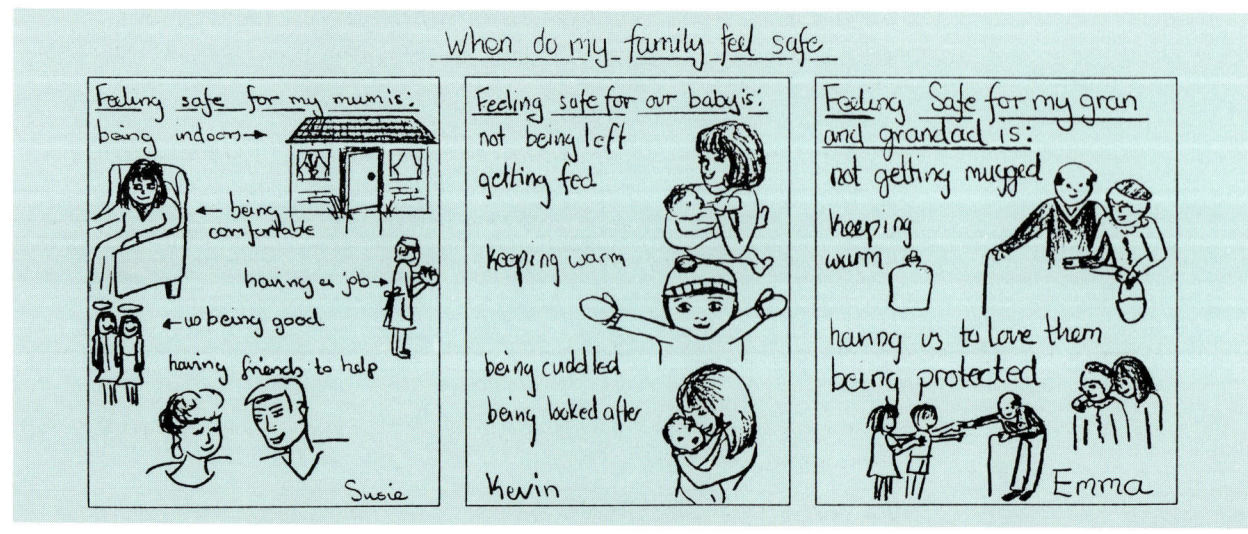

Activity 2 ● *How does it feel to be unsafe or uncertain?*

- Talking together. Describing feelings. Drawing and painting. Role-play. Family work.

- Class or group and individual activity.

Explore different feelings of unease with the children using movement and mime, drawing, painting and discussion. Ask them to consider what it is like not being safe, being uncertain about people, places and situations, or being uncertain about what to do or say.

Tie in examples from current local or national events, from children's literature and television programmes.

Explore and extend the vocabulary the children use to describe these feelings and look for new shades of meaning. Encourage the children to suggest examples of situations where they, or others, may have felt unsure or unsafe. How did they react? What were the outcomes?

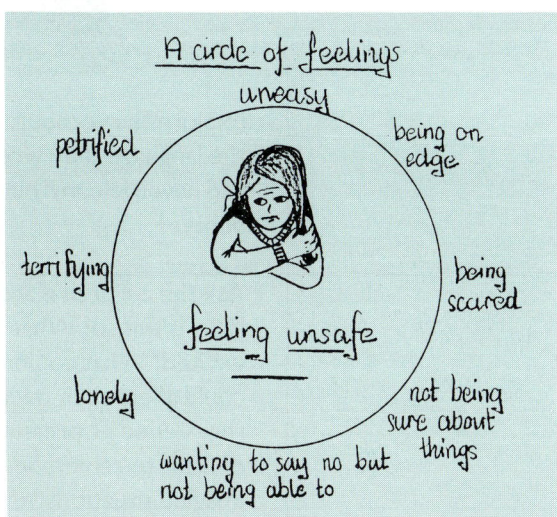

Talk with the children about coping with some of these situations, the importance of recognising feelings of uncertainty and fear, and of finding a trusted person to tell, or ask, before the fear becomes a reality.

Encourage them to practise saying: 'No, I won't', 'I don't want to', 'I'll ask'.

This activity will provide opportunities for children to share their personal concerns, real fears about what might happen, imaginary fears, and personal unease or abuse.

The work on feeling safe and unsafe could be carried over into **family work**. As well as involving the family in the children's safety education, this could provide a starting point for negotiating and planning a shared school and family programme to approach the problem of child abuse.

Activity 3 ● *What is it like to feel high or feel low?*

- Talking together. Describing feelings and situations. Drawing and painting. Mime. Role-play.

- Class or group and individual activities.

Invite the children to describe times when they have been excited using talking, drawing, writing, painting, mime or role-play.

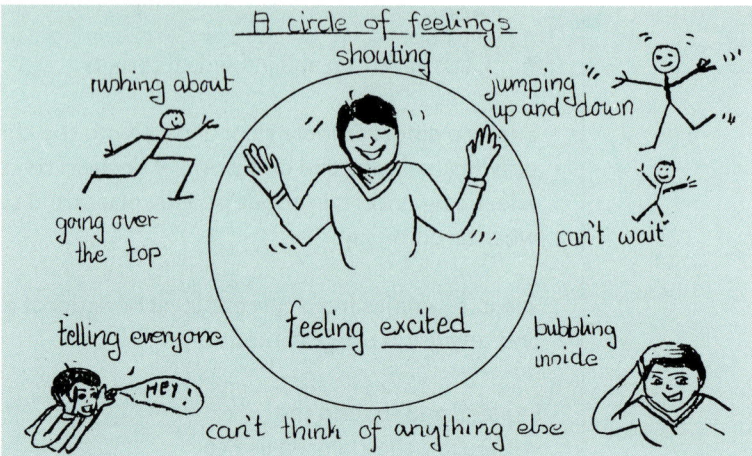

Explore the vocabulary which describes feeling excited. Ask them to write down the language they would use if they had to explain being excited to a robot who had never felt anything. How would they explain the way excited people look and behave?

Ask the children if accidents are more likely to happen when people get excited. Why is this so? What happens to all the keeping safe rules when people get excited? What could happen? Ask the children to explore other feelings which could affect their awareness of risk, for example, feeling upset, frightened, bullied, threatened or pressured by friends. Do these feelings make it easier or more difficult to remember the keeping safe rules? Invite the children to recall or imagine situations when their feelings made them forget the keeping safe rules and accidents occurred.

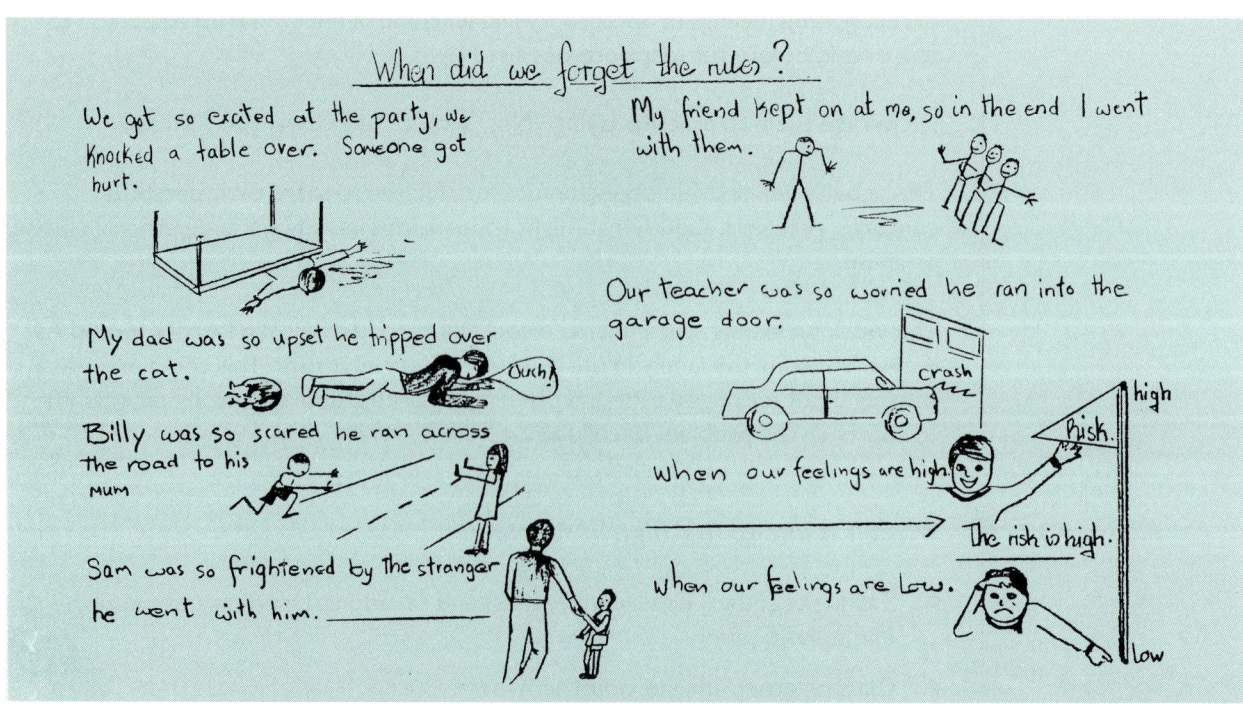

Some groups of children could write and perform their own role-plays to illustrate this connection between the emotions and risks.

Ask the children to think about their own feelings. Do they get upset or angry quickly? When does this happen? What does it make them do? When and where is it most risky to get upset, angry or frightened? What is the best thing to do? This could be a good time to talk about peer pressures and the influences of older children.

Activity 4 ● ***What do we think we have to keep safe from?***

- Drawing. Writing. Survey work. Talking together. Problem solving. Categorising.
- Class or group activity.

Use the Draw and Write Technique (see Appendix 1, page 410) as the basis of a survey. Ask the children to make and illustrate a list of all the things they think they have to keep safe from.

Talk with the children about the ways in which they might sort their responses. Ask them to work in groups to produce a shared solution to this problem. You could use categories such as people, places, real things, imaginary things or things that might happen. It is possible that the children will include categories such as: getting into trouble, being told off, being in disgrace, losing friends or family, separation and bereavement.

Ask the children to analyse the responses to the survey in groups. Then ask them to come together to collate their findings, and decide how these might be presented.

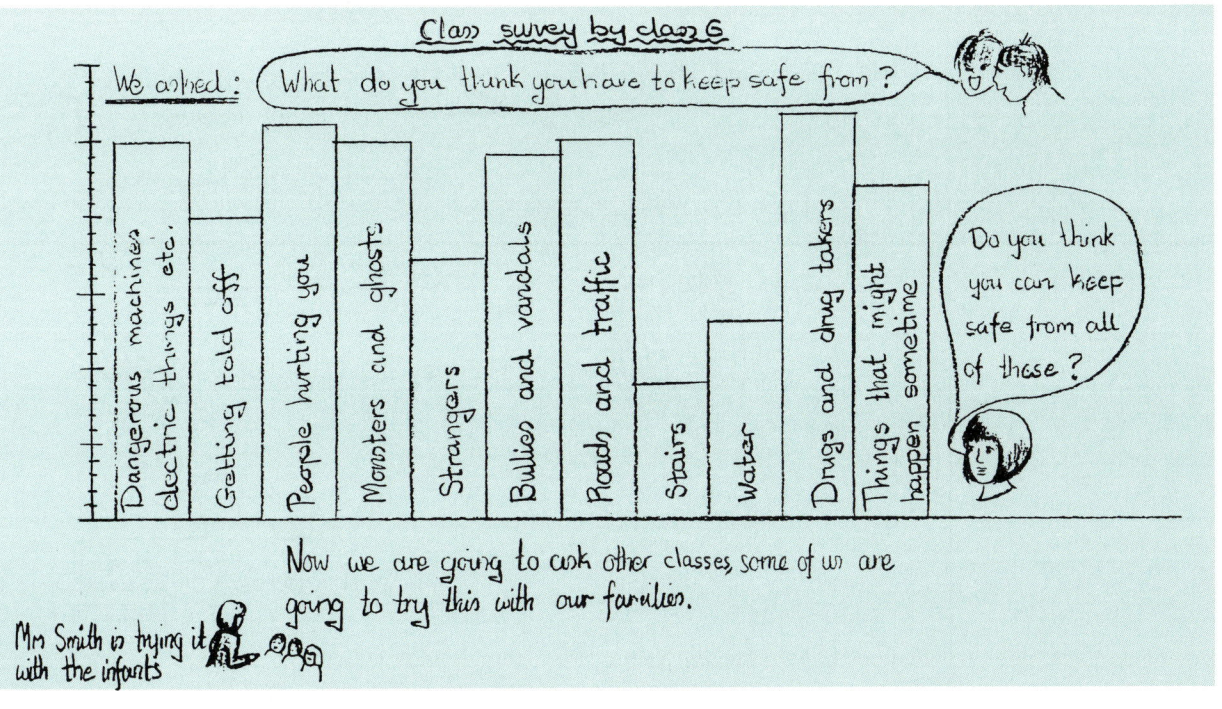

The children and their families (if they become involved) may be surprised to see the range of fears revealed by the survey, and the way danger is seen from different perspectives. In group and class discussions opportunities will arise for children to ask questions and talk about this wide range of perceived hazards. This could be the time to give them appropriate information and clarify the things which they have heard but only partly understood. This may include questions about child abuse, divorce, drugs, substance abuse (including tobacco, alcohol and solvents), death, disease, sexuality and AIDS. They may want information, reassurance or positive help. You will need to be prepared for this and to have, as a school, consulted with families about what to do when these topics arise.

The children could repeat the survey with children of a different age group particularly children in the infant age range. They could compare the results, and try to explain any differences. Alternatively you could present them with the results of such a survey. Ask them what they have learned which the younger children did not know or understand, and what surprised them about the younger children's responses.

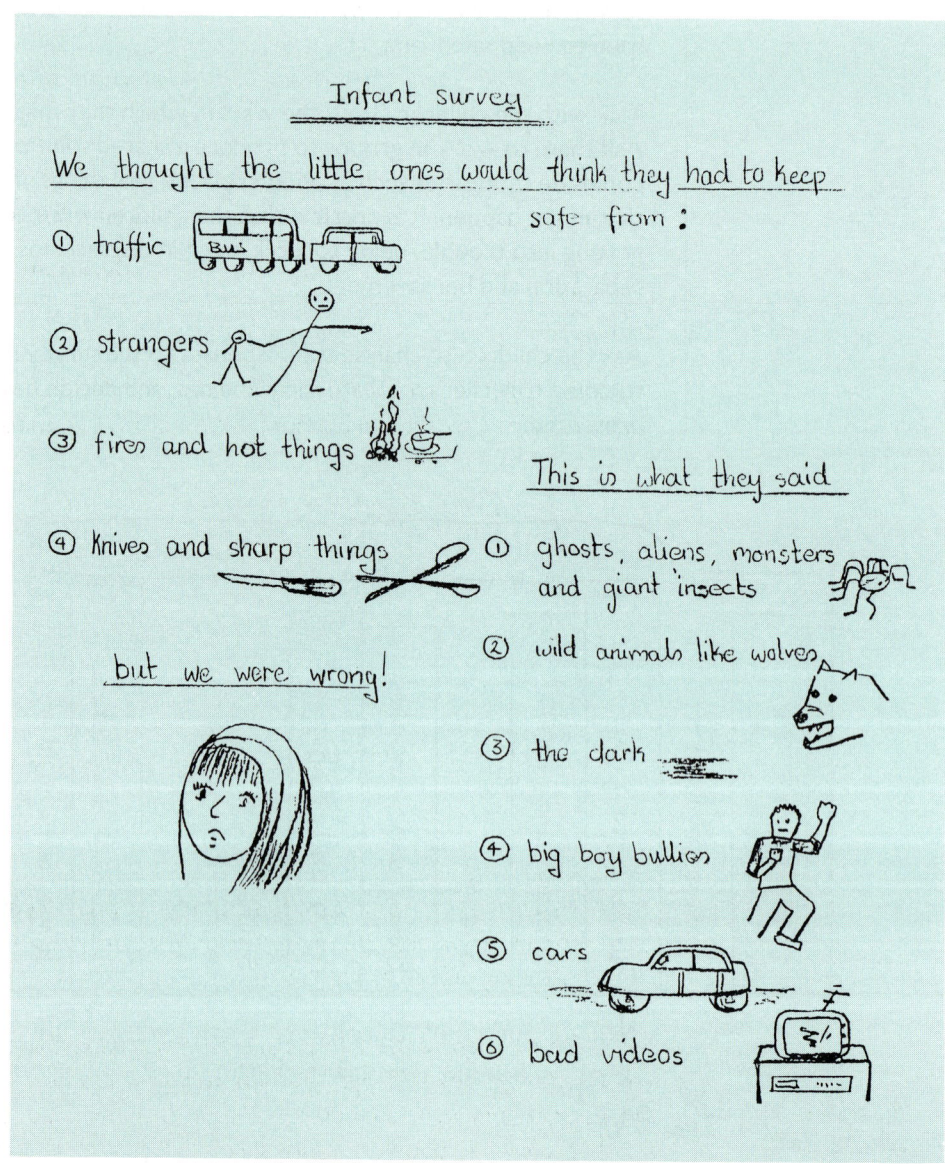

Activity 5 ● ***How do we keep safe?***

- Brainstorming. Talking together. Categorising.

- Class or group activity.

Ask the class to review the results of their class survey from Activity 4. Hold a brainstorming session to encourage them to think of all the possible ways they can keep themselves safe. Help them to categorise their replies under these two headings:

The things we say we *wouldn't do:*	**The things we say we *would do:***
– we wouldn't let people persuade us to do things.	– we would read the instructions.
– we wouldn't play in dangerous places.	– we would be aware of the risk.
– we wouldn't dare each other or boast.	– we would ask someone how to do it properly.
– we wouldn't go off without telling someone.	– we would use things properly.
– we wouldn't fool about on bikes, in buses or cars.	– we would practise.
– we wouldn't do things just because our friends do.	– we would learn the difference between real and pretend.
	– we would look after the little ones.
	– we would learn to say 'No'.
	– we would learn how to get help.

Invite the children to guess the type of answers 5 year olds would give to the question: 'How do you keep yourself safe?' Show them the results of such a survey, or a list of typical responses. For example:

– hide under the bed or the bed clothes.

– don't look.

– run away.

– cry and shout.

– stay with Mum.

– don't touch.

– hold on.

Invite the children to look at these responses and ask them: Are these sensible or risky ways for 5 year olds to keep themselves safe? How and why are their answers to this question different from ours?'

Invite the children to think through their day, at home and at school. It could be a weekday or a weekend day. Ask them to pick out times when they think they are most at risk, and what they do to keep the level of risk down. For example: 'I am most at risk when people dare me to do things. I can say that doing dares is daft.'

Content box 2   Focus on me

Who am I? How do I describe myself and other people? Where am I? Who is in charge? Where am I going? Where is home? Who is there? How do I get home? What would I do in a dangerous situation? Are the rules, and risks, different in different situations? How can I keep safe in any situation? Whose rules are the most important?
When am I most at risk?

Activity I ● *How do I describe myself and other people?*

- Drawing and painting. Talking together. Writing stories and poems.
- Class or group activity.

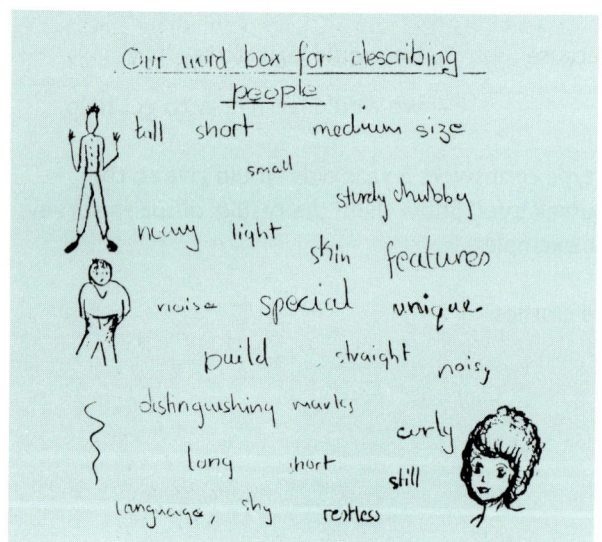

Ask the children to draw or paint a portrait of themselves, or to bring a photograph of themselves to school. Invite them to write a description of themselves to accompany the portrait. Can they estimate their height and weight? Can they describe their size, build, colouring and voice? Can they think of some unique way of identifying themselves?

Draw a word box of useful words for describing people. Encourage the children to add to this with more words and pictures cut from magazines to illustrate the many different characteristics which people have.

Give the children a set of descriptions and set of pictures and ask them to match them in pairs.

You can use this activity to give the children practice in oral and written work by asking them to describe accurately the people that they see in and around the school. Encourage them to look beyond what the people wear, especially if this is a uniform, and concentrate on their characteristics as individuals. Emphasise to the children how important it is to be able to tell people about those who cause them alarm or unease, and therefore, how necessary it is to be able to describe people accurately.

There is a **cross-curricular link** with children's literature here. Select your own examples of descriptions, or word pictures of characters, read them to the children and ask them to illustrate them.

Activity 2 ● ***Who am I? Where am I going? Who am I with?***

- Talking and writing together. Describing situations and feelings. Drawing. Stories.

- Class or group and individual activity.

Emphasise the importance of being able to say, and/or write:

– who we are.

– where we live.

– who is at home.

– where we are going.

– where we have been.

– who is with us.

– how long we have been out.

– who is in charge.

Encourage the children to develop this into a personal file, with photographs and illustrations, and details of their height, weight, accomplishments etc.

Cross-curricular links with literature: take a story which the children have heard or read, and look at the different characters' knowledge of who they are, where they are, where they are going and where they have been.

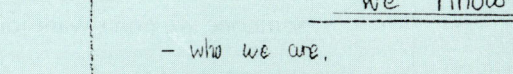

Where am I going? Who am I with?

In the story:

- Richard knew his name, but not where he lived.

- He didn't know how old he was, but he knew he had a sister.

- He was in a car with a family who had rescued him.

- He knew the old grandmother was in charge.

He didn't feel very safe.

We know:

- who we are,
- where we live,
- who is at home,
- where we are going,
- where we have been,
- who is with us,
- how long we have been out,
- who is in charge,
- how to use a telephone,
- how to ask for help safely,
- how to say 'NO'.

This helps us to keep safe.

Invite the children to recall, by drawing a comic strip illustration, a time when they went out with their families, or other adults. Ask them to represent where they went and what they did by answering these questions:

– Where are we?

– What are we doing?

– Who is in charge?

– How did we get here?

Invite the children to explore unforeseen situations which might have happened on their outings, such as, getting left behind, left out, scared, worried, told off, etc. How would they cope safely?

Suggest they illustrate two different ways in which they might cope, leading to two different outcomes.

The activity could be repeated. Invite the children to recall, again using comic strip illustration, times when they went out in a group of children without adult company. Ask them to answer these questions:

– Where are we?

– What are we doing?

– Whose idea was it?

– Who is in charge?

– How did we get here?

– How will we get home?

– What if . . .

   . . . someone we don't want joins the group?

   . . . the group splits up?

   . . . someone wants to play in a dangerous way or in a dangerous place?

   . . . someone threatens, bullies, or tries to persuade us?

   . . . someone we don't know or aren't sure about tries to take charge?

Repeat the activity again. This time ask the children to recall a time when they went somewhere alone. Ask them to answer the question 'What do I have to remember when I'm alone?'

Encourage the children to pinpoint the risks in these different situations and say how and why they differ. Ask them to say what kinds of rules would apply to all of the situations, and what kinds of rules would only apply to some of the situations.

Invite the children to think about how best to cope with these situations. Ask them to suggest ways in which they can practise or rehearse these skills, for example, through role-play and writing role-play scenes for others to enact.

This is a time when peer interests and rules are becoming more important to children, and their safety can be strongly influenced by these pressures. Children need to become aware of who is with them, who is at the centre of the group, who is on the edge, who is the leader and who are the followers. This can be done by inviting them to talk about friendship groups portrayed in stories and television programmes, before asking them to be more analytical about their own. Some children may be finding that some of the group secrets which they are being asked to keep are worrying or frightening. Talking with them about this in a general way will provide them with the opportunity to express their personal concerns.

Content box 3   Focus on indoors

What makes indoor places fun and exciting? What new places am I going to? What new things am I learning to do? What makes these places risky or dangerous? How can I make things less risky? Who is responsible for me indoors? How can I learn to be responsible for myself? What is an accident? How do accidents happen? Is being told off a danger?
When am I most at risk?

Activity 1

What makes indoor places fun and exciting?

- Talking and writing together. Describing. Evaluating. Drawing.
- Class or group activity.

Look with the children at the new activities they have been involved in at school, for example, learning to handle new equipment or material, taking on new responsibilities, working in new ways, studying new areas, visiting new places, etc.

Record these activities and include the children's views (expressed in writing and illustration) on what has made the activity new, interesting, exciting or difficult.

Now turn the children's attention to things which they have been learning to do in other indoor places, such as: the home, other people's homes, the swimming pool, clubs, church, classrooms, and other places where they meet and pursue interests.

Ask the children to work in groups and to choose two or three of these places, and explore:

- the things they have had to learn.

- the problems they have had to overcome.

- the things which might make some of the activities risky or dangerous.

- how the risks have been cut down.

Ask the children to evaluate the places they have talked about using a 'high-low' risk scale, and to identify the high risks at specific places.

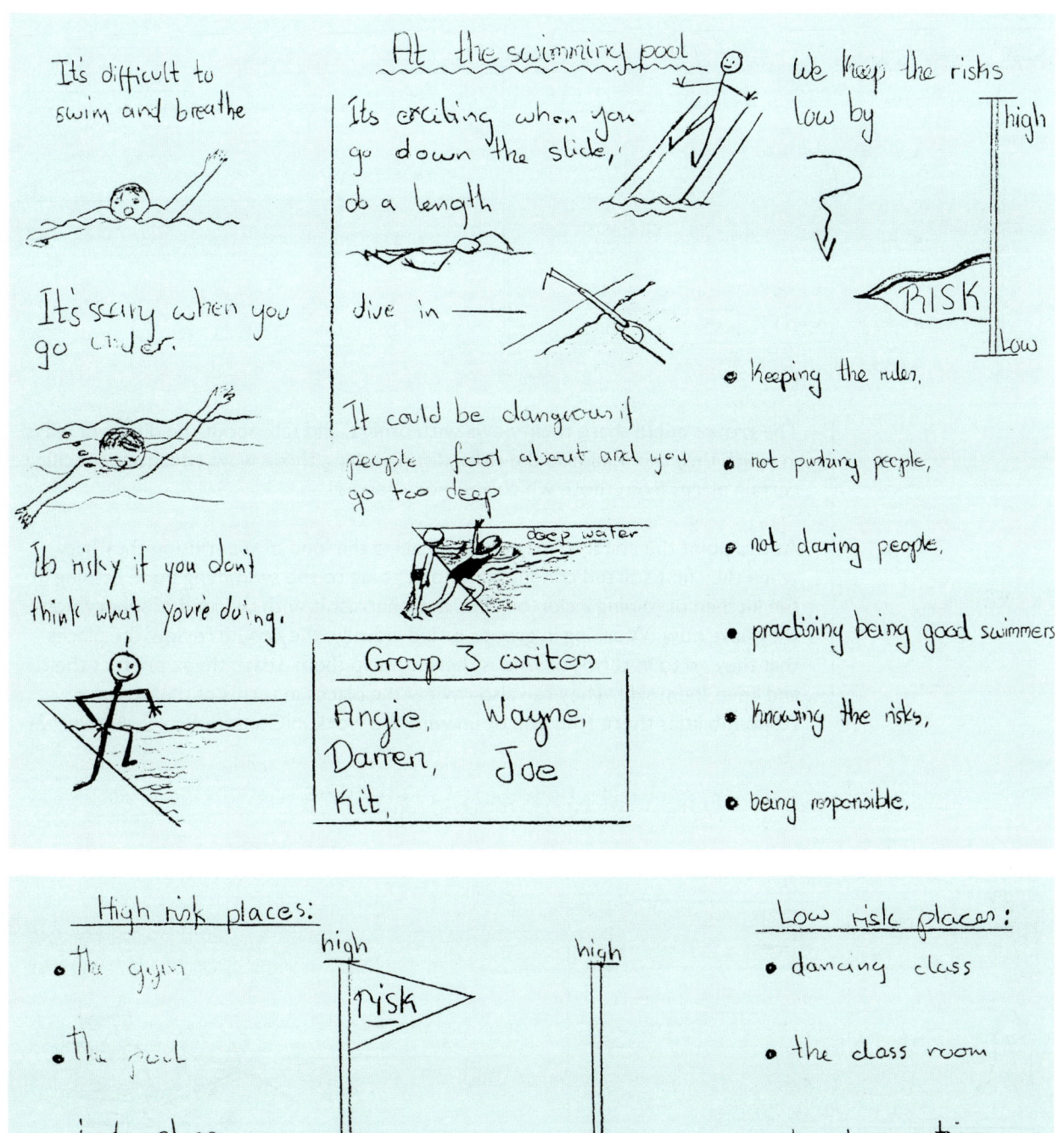

It's difficult to swim and breathe

It's scary when you go under.

It's risky if you don't think what you're doing.

At the swimming pool

It's exciting when you go down the slide, do a length

dive in ———

It could be dangerous if people fool about and you go too deep

deep water

Group 3 writers

Angie,	Wayne,
Darren,	Joe
Kit,	

We keep the risks low by

high

RISK

low

- keeping the rules,
- not pushing people,
- not daring people,
- practising being good swimmers
- knowing the risks,
- being responsible.

High risk places:
- the gym
- the pool
- judo class
- my friends house when no one is in

high

risk

low

high

risk

low

Low risk places:
- dancing class
- the class room
- band practice
- scouts
- my home

How can I keep the risk down?

This activity, especially when done in small groups, can provide opportunities for children to communicate, or hint at, a range of concerns and fears. Children can explore the idea of high risk and how it can vary in different situations, for example, when they are alone, with friends, in a group they don't know well, or with known adults or strangers.

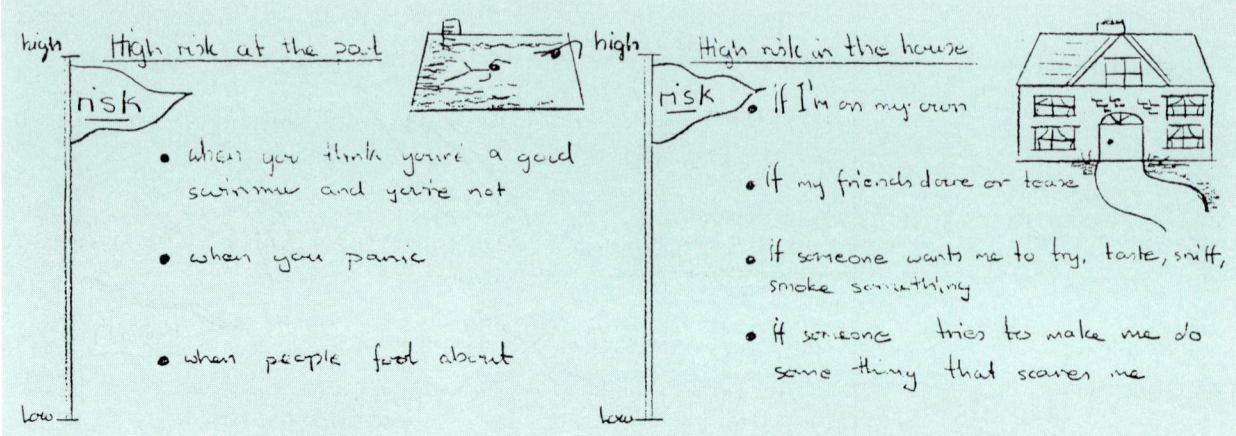

The groups could share their views with others, and talk about the different ways in which they can minimise the risks, distinguishing those ways which are specific to certain places from those which are more general.

At this point the children may enjoy recalling the kind of supervision they had when they first started coming to school, going to the swimming pool, helping in the kitchen or joining a club or class, and contrast it with the kind of supervision they have now. Working in groups or individually, they could review the places that they go to in terms of who is there to help them, teach them, protect them and keep them safe. They can also review the places in terms of their own responsibilities there (this will tie-in with the work in Content Box 2, Activity 2).

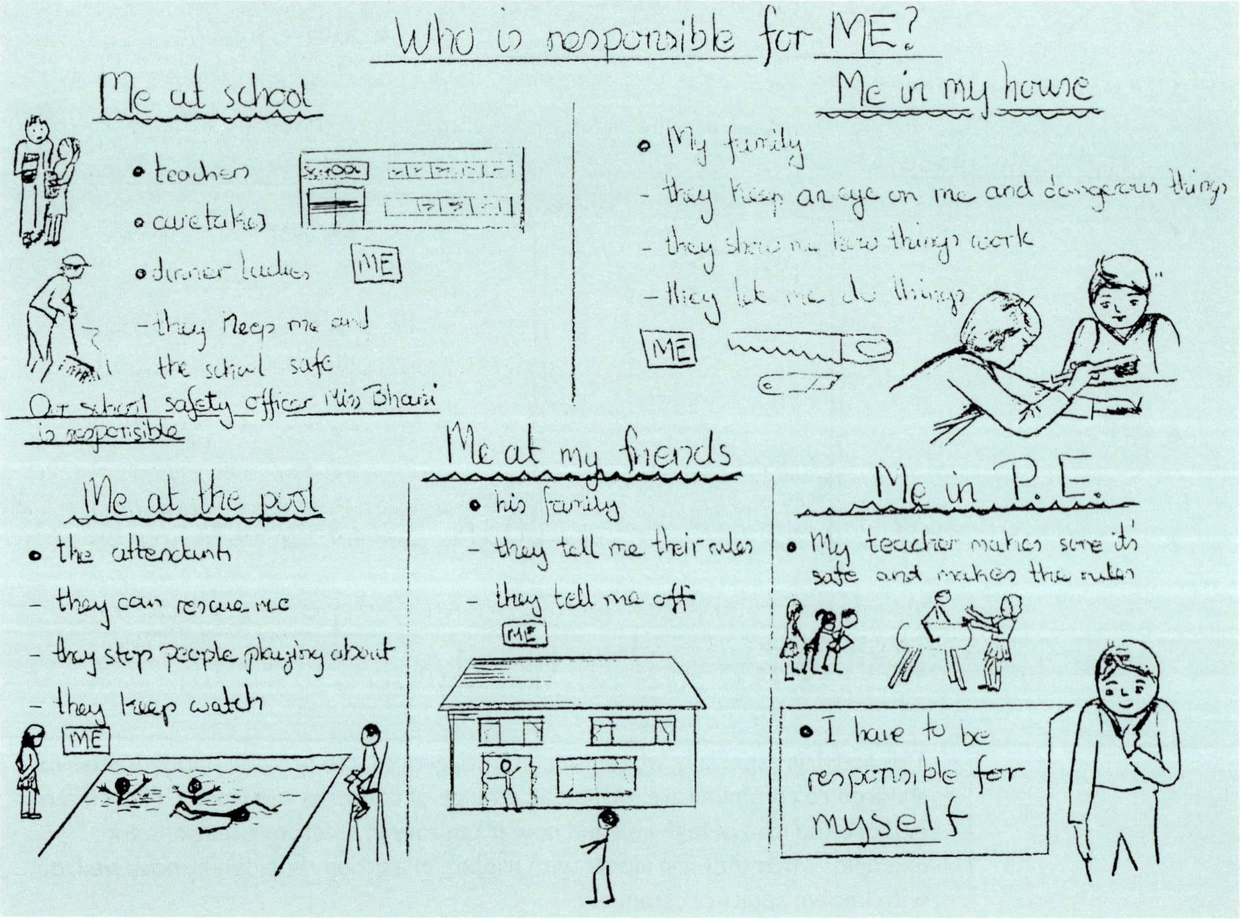

Activity 2 ● *What is an accident?*

- Talking together. Vocabulary work. Survey work. Writing. Drawing.

- Class or group activity.

Explore with the children the meanings of the words 'accident' and 'accidental'. Talk about the meanings of phrases such as:

– 'We met them by accident'	– 'Accidental death'
– 'A terrible accident'	– 'It was accidental'
– 'The accident ward'	– 'He is accident prone'
– 'I had an accident'	– 'This colour paint happened by accident'
– 'It was just an accident'	

Which phrases have these meanings?

– by chance	– not deliberate
– not planned	– something good
– a disaster	– unexpected
– a mishap	– careless
– a misfortune	– something bad
– not on purpose	– a calamity

Invite the children to recall occasions when they or someone they know:

- was involved in an accident.

- caused, or nearly caused, an accident.

- was able to avoid an accident.

Look at how these situations happened. Which risks or skills were forgotten or remembered?

Invite the children to take part in a class survey. You could organise it in a similar way to the Draw and Write Technique, outlined in Appendix 1 on page 410. Ask them: 'Which are the places where children are most likely to have accidents?'

Cross-curricular link: analyse and present the results using some form of mathematical representation.

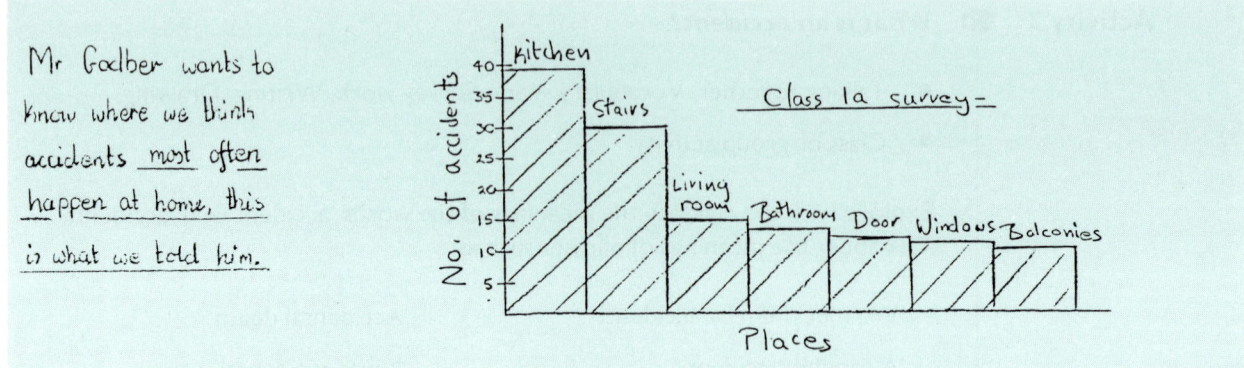

Mr Godber wants to know where we think accidents _most_ often happen at home, this is what we told him.

Class 1a survey

Ask the children to explain:

— why they see these places as dangerous,

— what kind of activity or behaviour is likely to cause accidents.

It would be interesting to ask the children to compare their opinions with some of the statistics on home accidents to children which are currently available. (See Appendix 2, page 426.)

Ask them to look around the school, evaluate different areas and decide which ones are potentially hazardous. They could work with the schools own appointed safety officer and other members of the staff.

You could reinforce all that the children have learnt in this activity by asking them to suggest generalised explanations of how accidents can happen inside buildings of all kinds, including derelict or dangerous buildings in the localilty. Help them to consider:

— entering dangerous or illegal places.

— ignoring the rules and the risks.

— taking part in activities for which they lack the necessary skills.

— being led into a difficult situation.

— being overwhelmed by feelings of excitement, fear or panic.

Ask them to suggest positive ways of minimising the risks.

This could be a good time to explore the notion held by many children that avoiding adult (especially family) disapproval is to avoid danger. Discuss how disapproval differs from other hazards.

Invite the children to explain the difference between:

— causing an accident by breaking the rules, or ignoring the risks, and

— causing an accident unintentionally.

This could provide you with an opportunity to explore adult reactions to these situations. Ask them to describe their experiences in writing and drawing.

<u>'We got into trouble ~ we got told off'</u>

- I ran across the road and nearly got run over.
  My mum was so scared she smacked me.

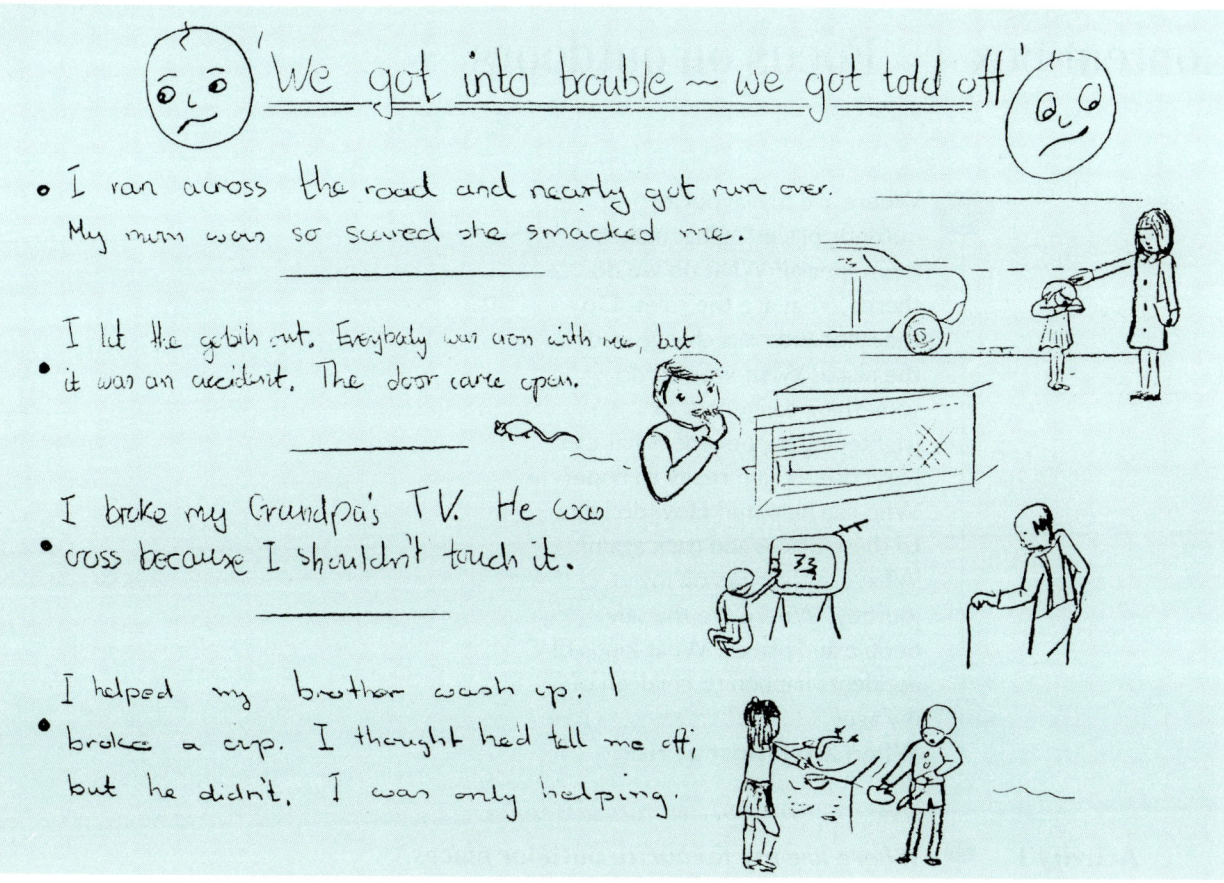

- I let the gerbils out. Everybody was cross with me, but it was an accident. The door came open.

- I broke my Grandpa's TV. He was cross because I shouldn't touch it.

- I helped my brother wash up. I broke a cup. I thought he'd tell me off, but he didn't. I was only helping.

190

Content box 4   Focus on outdoors

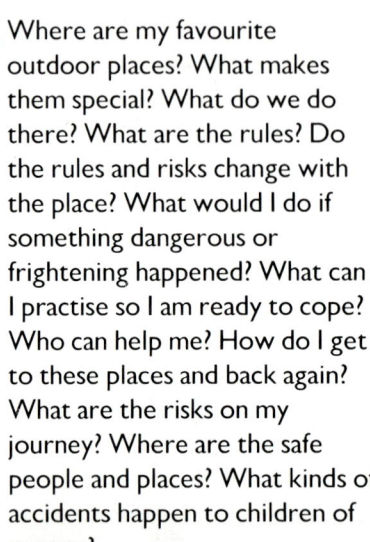

Where are my favourite outdoor places? What makes them special? What do we do there? What are the rules? Do the rules and risks change with the place? What would I do if something dangerous or frightening happened? What can I practise so I am ready to cope? Who can help me? How do I get to these places and back again? What are the risks on my journey? Where are the safe people and places? What kinds of accidents happen to children of my age? **When am I most at risk?**

Activity 1

Where are my favourite outdoor places?

- Survey work. Writing. Drawing. Talking together. Describing. Evaluating. Painting. Collage making.

- Class or group and individual activity.

Invite the children to set up, analyse and present the results of a survey of their favourite outdoor places, using this question as the starting point: 'If I could choose where I'd like to go this Saturday, I would choose . . .'

Invite each child to illustrate the chosen place and to answer these questions:

— Where is the place?

— Who would be with them?

— What would they be doing there?

— How would they get there?

— Is it a place they often go to, or is it a new place?

The children could work in groups or as a class to collect and present the information.

Ask the children to indicate how many of them have chosen places they visit frequently and how many have chosen new places. Ask them to record this. Explore with them what makes 'old' favourite places fun and exciting, and what they enjoy most about new places.

We analysed the results:

⑥ chose new places to go

㉒ chose old favourites

③ said they would go alone

⑬ said they would go with friends

⑫ said they would go with one of the family

⑤ said they would walk home

⑩ said they would go on bikes

④ said they would get a lift

⑨ said they would go on the bus

What are the risks?

Invite the children to think about who would be with them at these places. Did any child suggest going alone? How many would be with friends? How many would be with members of the family?

Ask the children to say how they would get to these places, and to describe what they would do there. Invite them to work in small groups to make a shared painting or collage to illustrate this.

Activity 2 ● *Rules and risks*

- Talking together. Writing. Drawing. Describing. Evaluating.
- Class or group and individual activities.

Invite the children to look at the survey work which shows their favourite outdoor places and, working in groups or as a class, to pick the places where the risk to their personal safety is highest. They could devise a 'riskometer' or 'risk scale' to illustrate this.

Ask them to consider whether the risk factor is higher or lower if they are:

– in new places;

– alone;

– with friends;

– walking;

– on bicycles;

– or taking a lift;

and to give their reasons.

The children could choose one popular place in the locality and explore how the risks might differ for children who go there:

– with family members;

– with friends;

– alone.

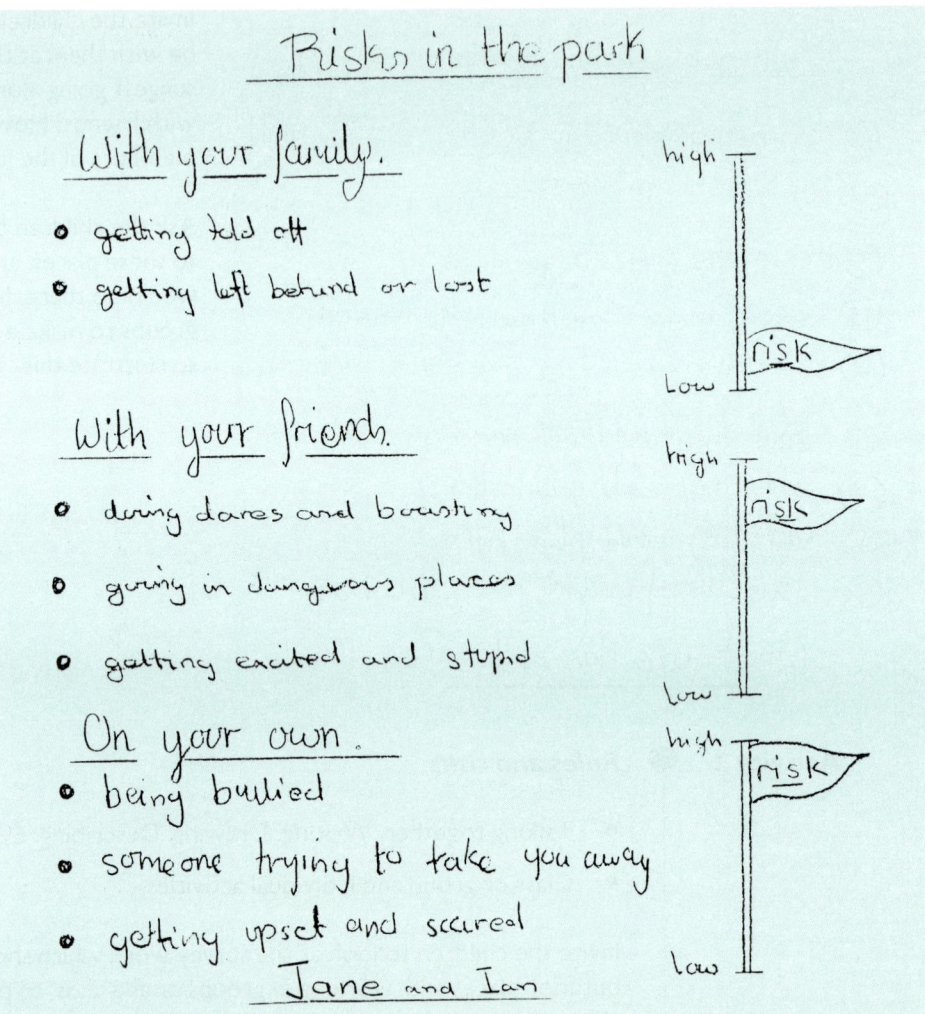

Ask the children to work in groups and suggest risks which are common to many places. Ask them to devise a set of rules for children on their own or in groups (with friends). Ask the children to look for general rules which can apply to all places at all times, and to pinpoint rules for particular times, places and circumstances.

Activity 3 ● ***What would I do if something dangerous or frightening happened?***

- Talking together. Describing. Generalising. Summarising. Drawing. Writing. Role-play. Family work.

- Class or group and individual activities.

Explore with your class what they think they might do in certain potentially dangerous or difficult situations. This might be a good time to discover any misconceptions which they may have. Use questions such as:

What would you do if . . .

– a group of older children dared you to sniff, smoke, drink, taste or try something?

- someone tried to persuade you to take part in something dangerous, stupid, risky, destructive or unkind?

- someone tried to persuade you to go to a locked, forbidden or dangerous place, such as a railway track, river or canal?

- someone you didn't know (or knew and felt uneasy with) asked you to go with them or help them, or said they had been sent by someone to collect you?

- someone bullied or threatened you?

- one of these things happened to a friend while you were there?

- a friend had an accident?

- you broke the rules and were found out?

Ask the children to work in groups, or individually, to express in drawing, writing or role-play, how they think they would react to these situations. They could then come together to share their ideas and decide which skills they need to learn, practise and revise.

This activity provides a useful opportunity for involving **families**, and the local community safety and environmental health personnel and resources.

The children can be asked to pick out those rules which apply when they are with friends, or when they are alone, and at different times of the day. They could:

- look at, and talk with, people who are in charge at specific places and find out what being in charge involves.

- look for rules on display in these places, make a collection of them and note which of them people tend to keep or ignore.

- devise rules for places where rules are not or cannot be displayed.

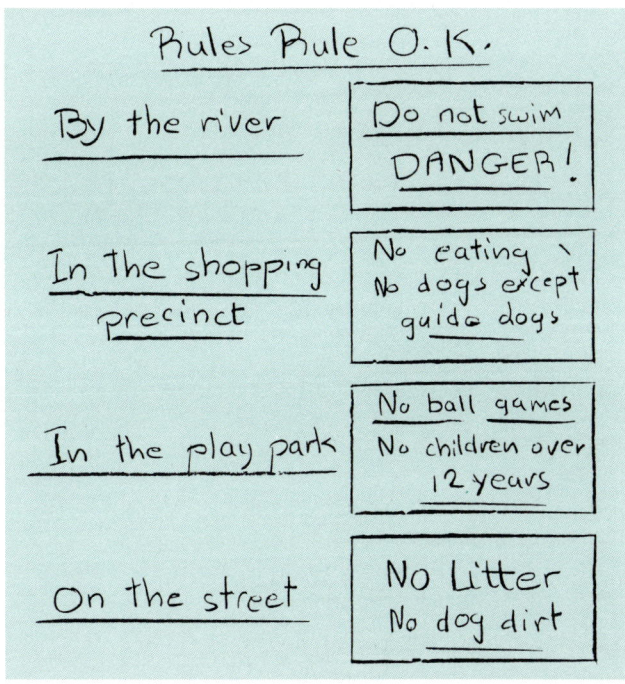

194

Activity 4 ● *How do I get there and back again?*

- Drawing. Map-making. Writing. Talking together. Describing. Evaluating. Visits. Family work.

- Class or group, pair and individual activities.

Ask the children to choose one of their favourite places in the locality and to make a picture map or plan which charts the route from school to that place. There is a **cross-curricular link** with geography here.

Invite the children to include:
— the hazards of the journey if they were to make it as a class, including such places as dangerous road junctions, crossings, exits, entrances, narrow or non-existent footpaths, railway crossings, rivers, canals, derelict sites, short cuts, places where people congregate, heavy traffic, parked cars.

— safe routes, crossings, safe shelters, refuges, safe people they can ask for directions, help or refuge.

— ways of behaving, thinking and skills which can minimise the risks.

The children could make their maps from memory and then check them by making a class visit. Display the map or plan, add to it the children's own illustrations, newspaper cuttings, photographs and leaflets. This activity could provide a useful starting point for work on specific aspects of keeping safe outdoors, such as roads and water. At the same time it offers opportunities to reinforce keeping safe strategies appropriate to the locality and to current concerns, and gives children a framework for looking at journeys they make or plan to make.

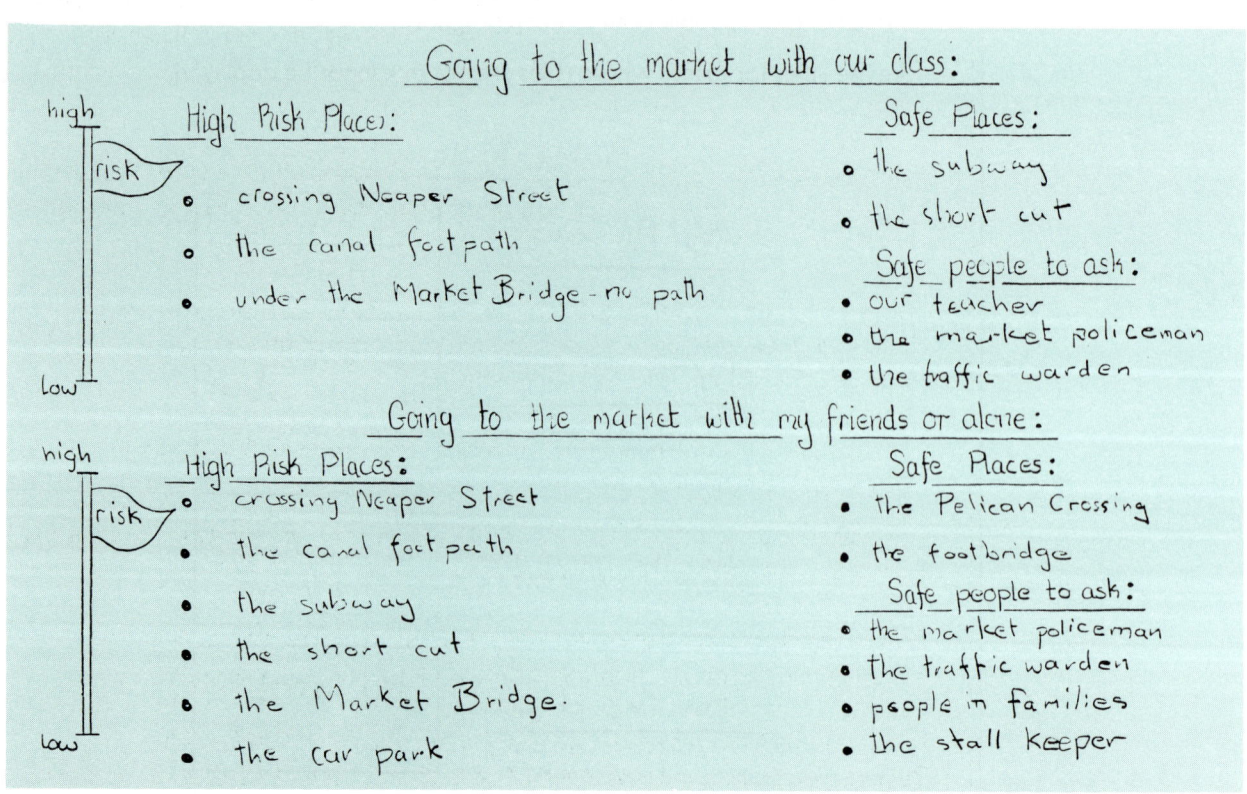

The activity could be extended by asking the children to review the hazards, risks, skills and refuges of the journey and to say how these might differ if they were to make the same journey, not as a class, but with one or two friends, or on their own.

Ask the children to talk about the different risks, refuges and skills needed on different days of the week and at different times of the day.

The children could work in pairs or small groups and use this framework to chart and illustrate the routes from their homes to their favourite places. You could ask their **families** to join in this activity. The work could be reinforced by asking the children to:

— pick out those skills which help them to keep safe as they go to and from places.

— pinpoint skills which they think they need to practise.

— set their own targets for improving these skills, inviting family and friends to help.

— revise the work of Content boxes 1, 2 and 3.

Activity 5 ● *Using the roads*

- Talking together. Survey work. Writing. Presentation. Evaluating. Drawing and painting.

- Class and group activities.

Children of this age are regular road users, as pedestrians, cyclists and passengers in motor vehicles. Many of them own bicycles and are allowed to use these alone and with friends. Some children are allowed considerable independence and freedom of movement to go to and from school, the shops, their friends homes and playgrounds without constant adult supervision.

You could use the earlier activities in this Content box which explored hazards in the locality as starting points for focusing on road user awareness and skills, and on road accidents and the causes of these.

Ask the children to take part in a class survey of their views on accidents to children of their age outdoors. Ask them to write down their responses to questions such as:

— What accident is most likely to happen outdoors to someone your age? to a boy your age? to a girl your age?

— Where are accidents most likely to happen? At what time of day? On what day of the week? At which time of year?

Invite the children to suggest ways of presenting their results, and ways of checking them against available statistics. (See Appendix 2, page 426.)

Invite the children to devise road safety rules, to cover the times when they are pedestrians, cyclists and passengers. Ask them to review their rules to cover the times when they are with adults, with friends or on their own. (You could mention courses for cycling proficiency here.) This would be a good time to revise the work done on feelings (Content box 1, page 174) and the way these can affect safe behaviour

This work can be reinforced by inviting the children, their families, friends, members of the community and safety officers to contribute to the making of a Keeping Safe on the Roads poster. The children could add to this with their own illustrations, photographs, pictures from magazines, leaflets or advertisements.

The children will be able to compare their views with statistics, and the recommendations of road safety officers. Ask them to say where and why these may differ. This will help them to learn what causes road accidents, and motivate them to learn the skills and safety precautions they need.

This could also be a good time to explore what makes an accident (see Content box 3, page 184). Give the children a story line which describes an accident, and ask them to analyse it and find possible causes by answering questions. For example, Sam had an accident on the road. Was it because:

— Sam did something?

— Sam forgot to do something?

— someone else forgot, or failed, to do something?

— someone else did something?

What could have made Sam forget?

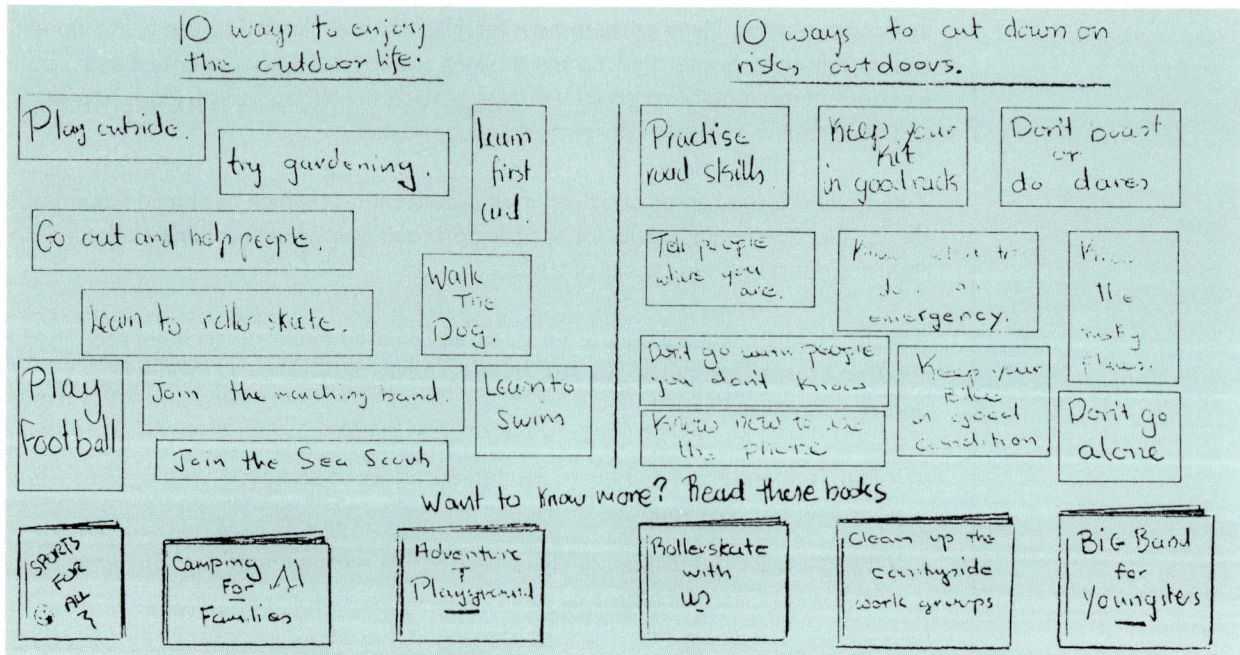

This activity could provide opportunities for children to think and talk about the skills they are learning and set realistic targets for themselves when mastering outdoor activities of all kinds. How can these skills help to minimise risks? What lifestyles, skills, and targets do local and national sports personalities aim for?

Content box 5 Focus on people

Who do I see when I am out and about? Who has the job of keeping me safe? What can we do to make their jobs easier? What does being responsible mean for me? Who can I trust? How can I tell what kind of a person someone is? How can I learn to keep safe from, and cope with, threatening people? **When am I most at risk?**

This section of the work can form one strand in a range of topics, focussing on the locality, the community and the people who work there. **Cross-curricular links** can be made with:

— children's literature.

— history.

— geography.

— environmental studies.

Activity I *Who has the job of keeping me safe?*

- Talking together. Describing. Interviewing. Reporting. Drawing and painting.

- Class or group and individual activities.

Remind the children of their work on Content box 4 when they explored the hazards, risks, refuges and safe people in their neighbourhood.

Ask the children to think about the journeys which they take. Who do they see regularly on these journeys? For example, shop keepers, stall holders, postal workers, delivery van staff, crossing patrol people, retired people, other children, people walking their dogs, police, shoppers, paper boys and girls, window cleaners etc.

Ask the children to describe, draw and/or paint some of these people. How do they recognise them? What do they do or say?

Next, focus on the people who, in some way, share the responsibility for keeping children safe. For example, crossing patrol people, ambulance officers, firefighters, and the police.

Talk about the places in the neighbourhood where the children go. Encourage them to think about who helps to keep them safe in these places, and the different ways in which this is done. For example, is it someone's job to keep them safe? Do voluntary groups take on the task of keeping them safe?

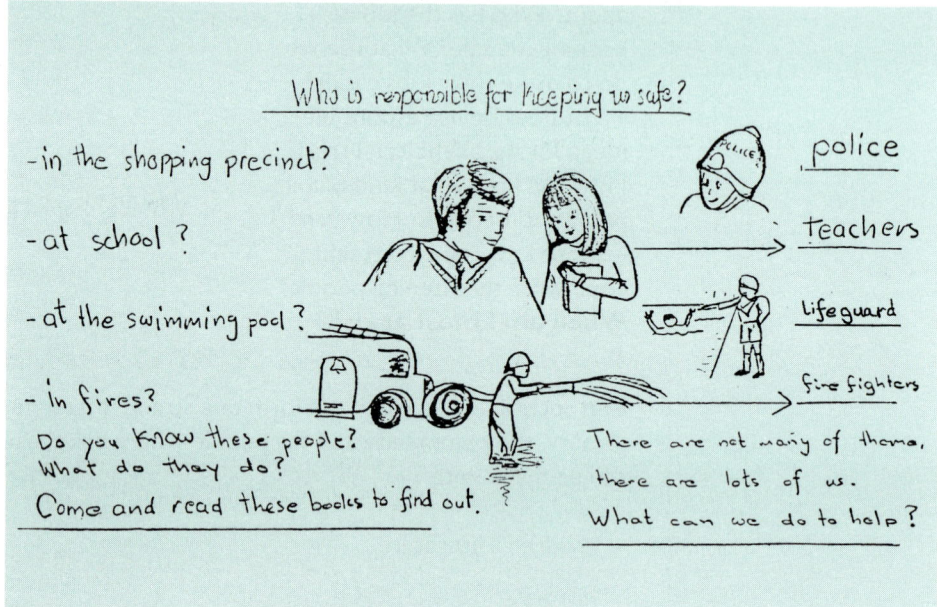

Ask the children to explore the jobs these people have. What risks and responsibilities are involved? Invite some of them to come into school to explain what they do. Organise visits so the children can see them at work. Encourage the children to use such occasions to develop their interviewing skills. Help them to prepare questions, take notes and use tape recorders. Ask them to focus on what responsibility means and how they can take on their share. They could collect and display books and other material relating to the work these people do.

Activity 2 ● *What does being responsible mean for me?*

- Talking together. Reviewing. Summarising.
- Class or group activity.

Revise Activity 1 with the children, and the work on outdoors and indoors. Talk again about the people who keep them safe and clarify what this involves and what responsibility means for them, for example:

- It's their job.

- They have to be there all the time.

- They have to think ahead.

- They get into trouble if they don't do it properly.

- They have to be prepared for people to do stupid or bad things.

- They must know the rules and risks.

– They must know where to get help.

– They must keep learning.

Explore with the children the ways in which *they* are responsible. What do they need to do? What skills do they need to be responsible? What can they do to make life easier for those with the job of keeping children safe?

Activity 3 ●   *Who can I trust?*

●   Talking together. Describing. Reviewing. Using literature. Media studies.

●   Class or group activity.

The children could gather their work on this theme into a personal folder or file. The aim of this activity is to help the children learn to evaluate how far they can trust people.

Ask the children, working in pairs or small groups, to look at some specific situations in which they might find themselves. For example:

– I'm feeling ill at school, at home, outside.

– I fall off my bicycle.

– I fall out with my best friend.

– I feel lonely, sad, worried.

– I have a bad dream.

– I feel scared, bullied, threatened.

– Someone says I've got to keep a bad sort of secret.

– I get lost.

– I lose something important.

– I get told off.

– Someone tells me to go off with them.

– I can't decide what to do.

Ask them to say to whom they would turn for help and guidance. Who can they trust? Who can't they trust?

Come together to review the list of people the children think they would turn to. Why would they trust them? Ask them to compare their different views and look for explanations. Ask them to group the people in some way, for example, family members, other grown-ups, friends.

Explore with the children the characteristics of trustworthy people. You could write a 'circle of feelings' to describe the things they do and don't do. How do the children recognise them?

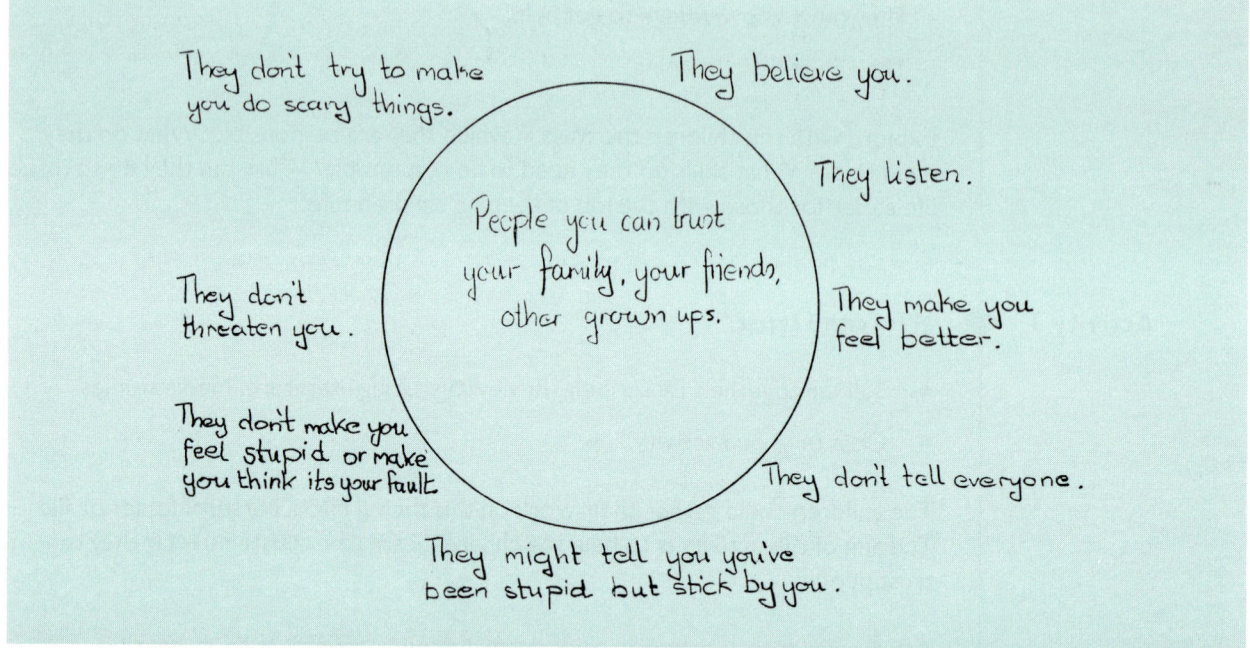

They don't try to make you do scary things.

They believe you.

They listen.

People you can trust your family, your friends, other grown ups.

They don't threaten you.

They make you feel better.

They don't make you feel stupid or make you think its your fault

They don't tell everyone.

They might tell you you've been stupid but stick by you.

Ask the children to differentiate between their special people and people who are there to help everyone.

Cross-curricular links: you could relate the children's views and experiences to stories, poems, television programmes, and current news items in which trust is connected with keeping safe.

Opportunities may occur for you to talk with the children about occasions when bullying, violence and child abuse mean that the child may have to think again about trusting the people involved.

Activity 4 ● *What kind of person is this?*

- Collecting and sorting pictures. Drawing. Writing. Talking together. Describing. Role-play.

- Class or group and individual activities.

Ask the children to help you make a collection of pictures of stereotyped characters as shown in comics or cartoons. For example:

– teachers with cap, gown and cane.

– doctors in long white coats, with stethoscopes.

– villains and other dangerous people with beards, eye patches, 'swag bags', evil facial expressions and guns.

– heroes and heroines who are young, superhuman and attractive.

Invite the children to check these stereotypes against the way these people look in reality. Ask them to draw a doctor, or a teacher, or a nurse, or a policeman whom they have met.

Invite them to add to the list by drawing and describing other characters, such as, a bully, a gang, a burglar, a vandal, a glue sniffer, a safe person, a stranger, a priest, rabbi, nun or paramedic.

Ask the children to group these characters into people they can and cannot recognise by appearance. For example:

People recognisable by appearance	*People not recognisable by apearance*
— traffic wardens	— friends
— crossing patrols	— strangers
— soldiers	— dangerous people
— Boy Scouts and Girl Guides	— bullies
— uniformed policemen	— vandals, hooligans
— some gangs	— burglars
	— safe people
	— glue sniffers
	— drug pushers

Ask the children to think of other things which help them recognise people who are not in uniform. What kinds of things do these people say, do or try to persuade others to do? Encourage them to use this type of exercise to create a method for evaluating people safely.

With the children, look at ways of dealing with hazardous situations in which they, and some of these not easily identifiable people, are involved. Help them to practise dealing with these situations using role-play and working in pairs or groups.

Action Planner
Keeping Myself Safe

10&11

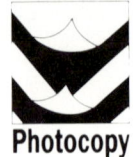

Photocopy

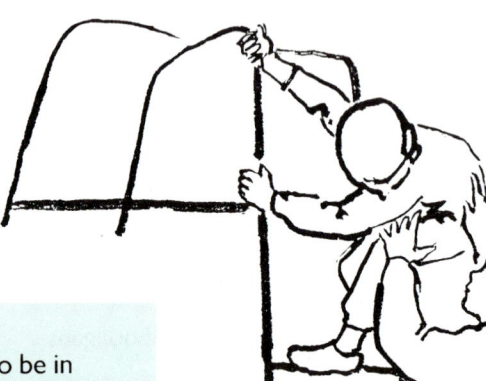

1 Focus on feelings

What does it mean to be in charge? Does it mean being grown-up? Is it always safe for me to be in charge? What do I do if I need someone to take over? Why do I always seem too young or too old? What do people mean when they tell me not to get hurt? Are there rules to stop my feelings from being hurt? How do I feel when I'm in danger? How does this affect my ability to keep safe? Can I learn to manage my feelings?
When am I most at risk?

2 Focus on me

How do I see myself, especially in risky situations? How do others see me? What do I think I have to keep safe from? Do I have imaginary fears or fears for the future? How do I keep myself safe? Which skills do I need to learn? What gives me confidence? Can I be over confident? Why does my family want to know where I am and who I'm with? What would I do in an emergency? What life-saving skills can I begin to master?
When am I most at risk?

3 Focus on responsibility and risk

Who is responsible for keeping me safe wherever I am? What do all these people think they are keeping me safe from? How do they try to keep me safe? How can I practise being responsible and using my judgement? What affects people's judgement? What do I believe when people tell me different things about keeping safe? How can I tell which are facts, opinions, half truths or fiction?
When am I most at risk?

4 Focus on places and situations

Which places do I like going to? Where do I go with my family? my friends? other people? alone? What are the rules and the risks? How can I get there and back safely? Do the risks change according to the time, day or company? Which accident is most likely to happen in the home? What can I learn from statistics? What causes accidents? How do alcohol related accidents happen to children? Can I practise avoiding accidents? Could I cope in an emergency?
When am I most at risk?

5 Focus on people and pressures

Who are the people I trust? What are the rules for getting on with them? What should I do if someone changes the rules, or makes me feel unsafe? Who else can I turn to? What can I do when no one will listen? Who are the people I admire? Should I set an example to younger children? How do people persuade others to do things? How can I cope when people persuade me to do something risky? When is it best to tell secrets? Is this the same as telling tales? What can I do to keep myself safer?
When am I most at risk?

Classroom Strategies and Activities for Ages 10 and 11

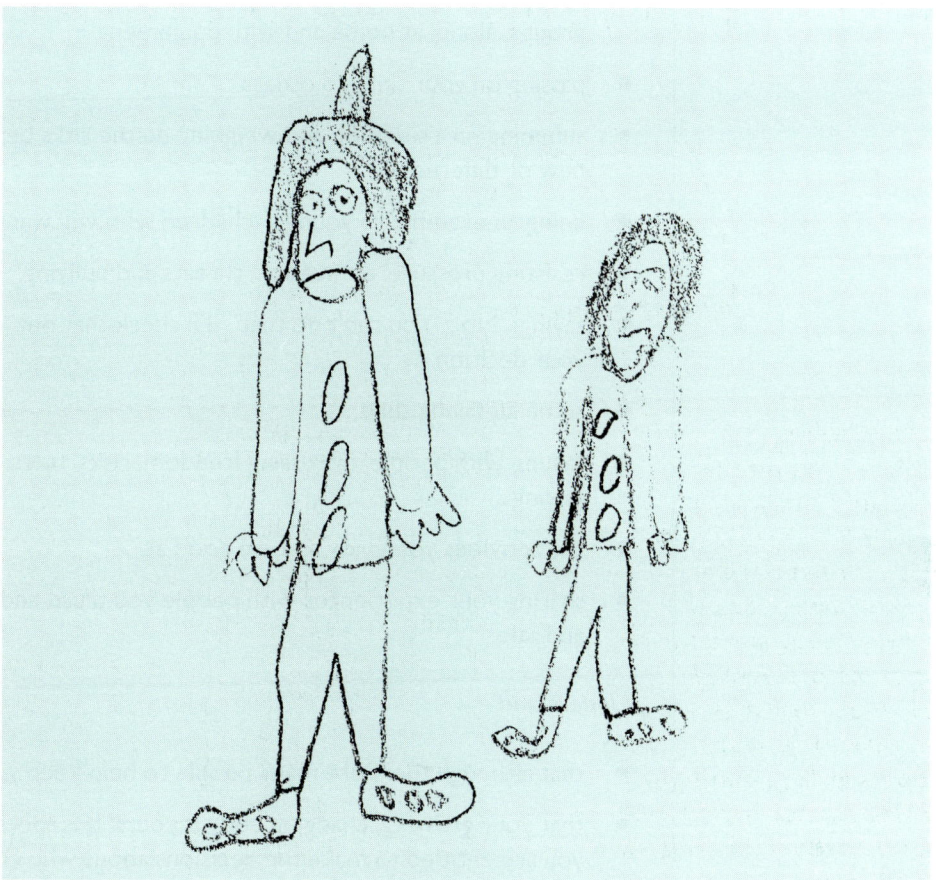

Key messages ● *Learn:*

- as much as you can about yourself, where you live and what kind of a person you are.

- who your friends are and where they come from.

- who is the leader, who is the authority and who are the followers.

- where you are, how you got there and how to get away safely.

- how to contact home, get to your home, get help, report an accident and not panic.

- who are the safe people to ask for help, the people you can trust.

- who or what can cause an accident, or a dangerous situation.

- about things which can affect your judgement, for example, excitement, unhappiness, tiredness, alcohol, and other drugs including medicines.

- the facts about accidents which happen to young people, especially alcohol related accidents.

- that different families, groups and places have different rules, and that the rules can be 'changed' by some people to suit their purposes.

Practise:

- safety skills which will enable you to cope in traffic, near water, in crowds, in groups, alone, at home and with equipment.

- passing on your skills to others.

- summing up a situation and weighing up the risks before you do something new or different.

- being an example to younger children who will want to copy you.

- resisting pressure, persuasion, threats and bullying.

- saying: 'No', 'You can't do that', 'I'll check that out', 'I'll ask', and sticking by your decision.

- some lifesaving skills.

- talking with people, discussing freedom, risks, rules, your feelings, their feelings,

- the activities you enjoy and are good at.

- sharing your experiences with people you trust, and who make you feel good, and safe.

Understand:

- that although there are many people to help keep you safe, it is also your job.

- that your growing, changing body is yours. It is special and valuable, and that you are entitled to make the decisions about who comes very close, and who touches it.

- that saying: 'No', 'I don't want to take that risk', 'I'll check that out' and 'I'll ask', are wise safety strategies, even though they may appear to upset or even anger people at the time.

- that threats, promises, information and secrets can be based on bias and opinion, and can be used to pressure you into doing something.

- that family concern and affection may look like over-protection or disapproval.

- that wanting independence and freedom is part of growing up, but involves taking on some personal responsibility too.

Content box 1 Focus on feelings

What does it mean to be in charge? Does it mean being grown-up? Is it always safe for me to be in charge? What do I do if I need someone to take over? Why do I always seem too young or too old? What do people mean when they tell me not to get hurt? Are there rules to stop my feelings from being hurt? How do I feel when I'm in danger? How does this affect my ability to keep safe? Can I learn to manage my feelings?
When am I most at risk?

Activity 1

What does it mean to be in charge?

- Talking together. Describing. Hypothesising. Summarising. Drawing. Writing. Role-play.

- Class or group, pair and individual activities.

Ask the children to explore the meaning of the phrase 'in charge'. As a starting point, ask them to think about what is involved in being in charge:

- of younger brothers or sisters?

- of a pet?

- of a class, a group, a team?

- of apparatus or materials?

- of a project?

- of a place?

- of their own belongings?

Help them to think of situations where they may have to keep things tidy and safe, care for people, keep order, prevent accidents, solve problems, make plans and decisions, supervise and organise others.

Invite the children to talk about what it is about being in charge that makes them feel good. What are the drawbacks?

Ask the children to explore the idea of 'being in charge of yourself', and see whether the same comments, advantages and disadvantages apply.

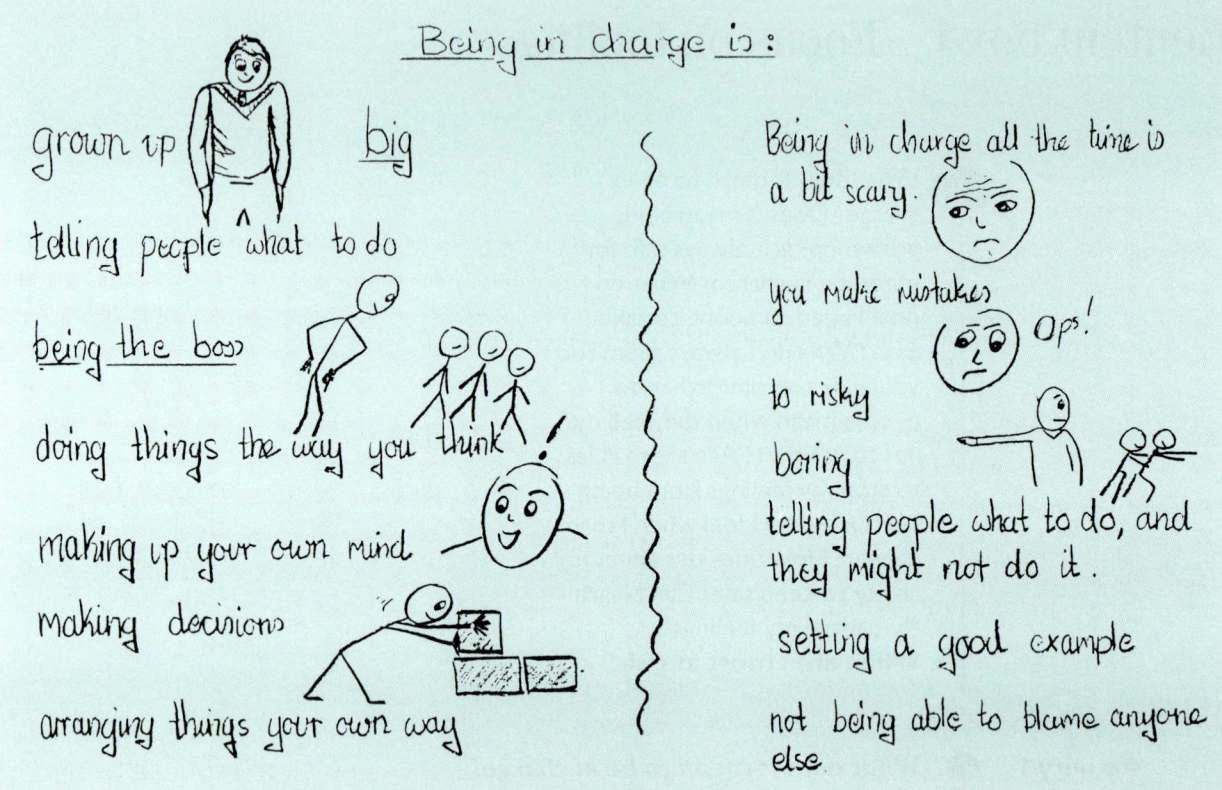

Ask the children to make a list of situations when other people tell them they are not old enough to be in charge. Why, particularly in the area of keeping safe, is this so? The situations they could consider might range from going out alone, choosing companions, clothing and leisure activities, to wider issues such as friendships, smoking, using alcohol and other substances and driving motorcycles and other vehicles.

Invite the children to work in pairs or groups, and to illustrate and write about being responsible for themselves in different circumstances. Ask them to concentrate on describing their good feelings, and their feelings of unease.

Invite them to include one or more illustrations with the caption: 'This is me wishing someone else would take charge here' and to share these with other groups.

Explore potentially dangerous situations using questions such as: How would you feel if someone asked you to take charge of:

— a young child you had not seen before?

— a bicycle you thought might have been borrowed or stolen?

— some cigarettes, alcohol, tablets, pills or powders?

— a meeting in which something dangerous or unkind is planned?

Ask them: What would you say or do? Would you take charge or ask for help? Whom would you ask? What would you say? Help the children to explore these situations using role-play and to think about the possible problems and different outcomes.

Activity 2 ● *How do I feel when I am in danger?*

- Drawing. Writing. Talking together. Describing feelings and situations.
- Class, group and pair activities.

Invite the children to draw themselves (working in pairs or small groups) looking and feeling as if they are in danger. Ask them to label their physical sensations, and to write about how they cope with them. It is important that the children realise that most people, including adults, share these feelings.

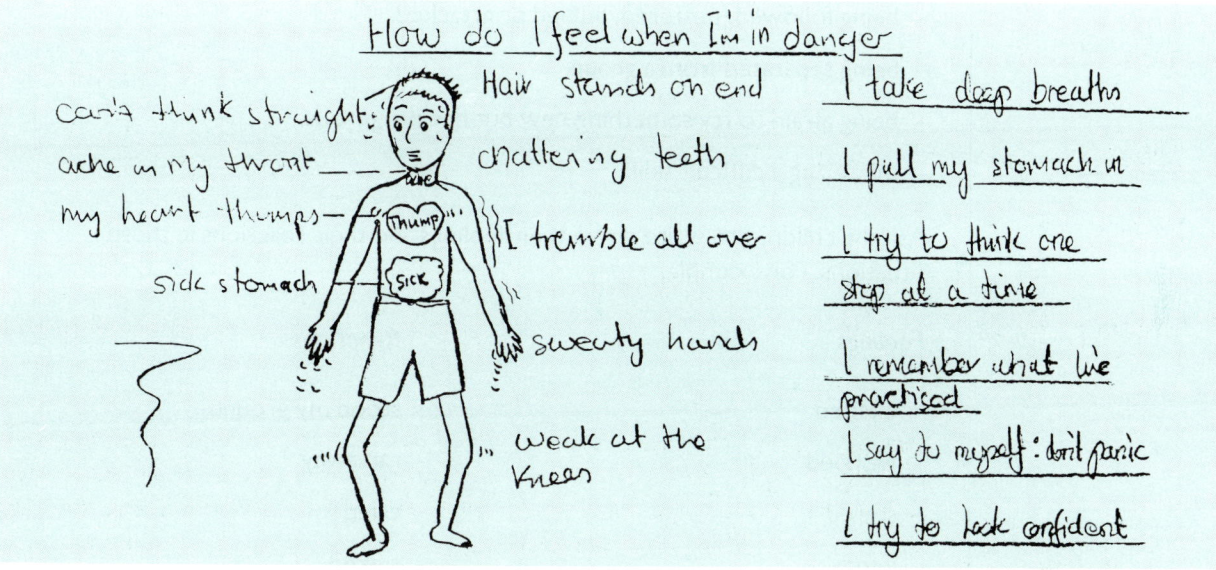

How do I feel when I'm in danger

can't think straight
ache in my throat
my heart thumps — THUMP
sick stomach — SICK

Hair stands on end
chattering teeth
I tremble all over
sweaty hands
weak at the knees

I take deep breaths
I pull my stomach in
I try to think one step at a time
I remember what we practised
I say to myself : don't panic
I try to look confident

Invite the children to share their experiences of dangerous situations, the feelings they experienced and the coping strategies they used. What feelings were experienced after successful, and unsuccessful situations?

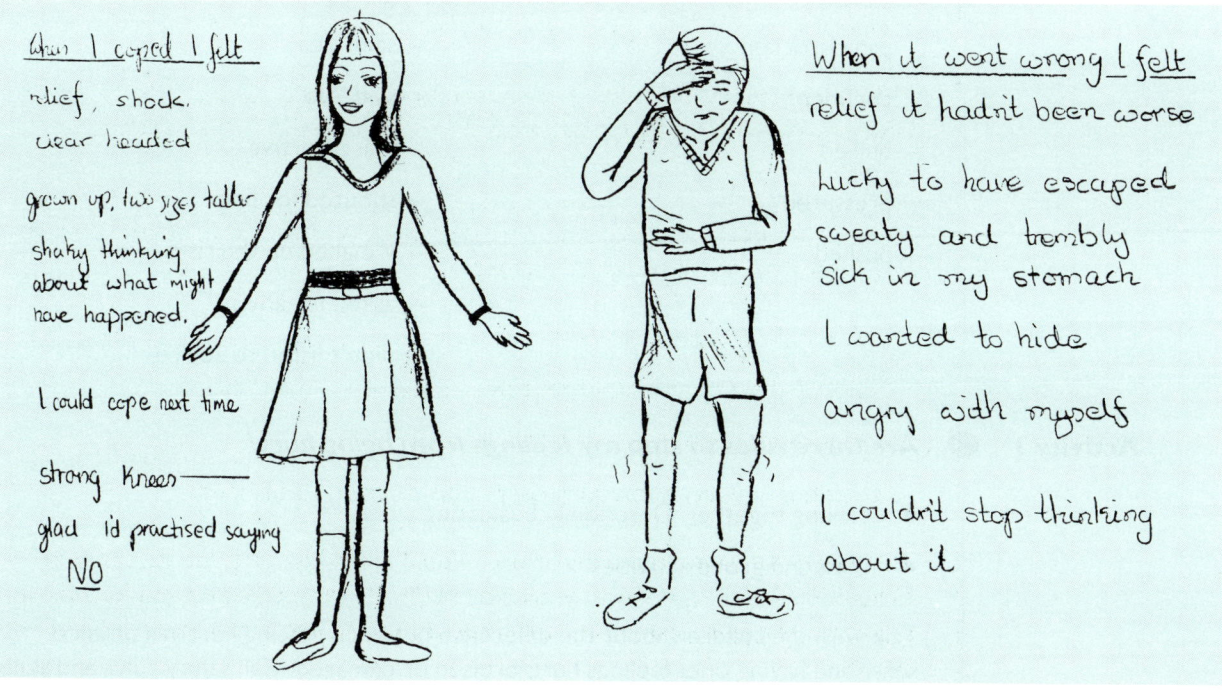

When I coped I felt
relief, shock.
clear headed
grown up, two sizes taller
shaky thinking about what might have happened.

I could cope next time

strong knees —
glad I'd practised saying
NO

When it went wrong I felt
relief it hadn't been worse

lucky to have escaped
sweaty and trembly
sick in my stomach

I wanted to hide

angry with myself

I couldn't stop thinking
about it

Emphasise that different people with different personalities, will chose different ways of coping and that it helps to know the kind of person you are, how you are likely to act and what skills you need to practise.

Invite the children to put themselves in a situation where they have lost something which is very important. What do they do? How do they react? Does what they feel affect the way they behave or their chances of finding the object? Repeat the activity with these situations:

- being pressured to experiment (by an older or peer group)

- being followed, pestered, bullied or attacked.

- being separated from a group.

- being afraid to try something new but not dangerous.

- mastering a difficult skill.

Ask the children to write down their feelings and their reactions in these situations. For example:

Feelings	*Reactions*
– excited	– stood my ground
– worried	– ran away
– scared	– cried
– jumpy	– sulked
– flustered	– froze
– careless	– moaned
– boastful	– gave in
– panic stricken	– said 'Yes'
– confident	– said 'No'
– bullied	– was assertive
– pressured	– shouted for help
– pushed	– weighed up the risks
	– asked for advice
	– didn't listen to advice

Activity 3   ● *Are there rules to stop my feelings from being hurt?*

● Talking together. Describing. Evaluating.

● Class and group activities.

Talk with the children about the difference between getting hurt in a physical sense and having ones feelings hurt, bruised or damaged. Can safety rules and skills be applied to feelings? How might the rules and skills be different? Emphasise how important it is to talk about one's feelings, to find someone to listen and help, and to have a wide range of words to use.

Activity 4 ● *Keeping a balance*

- Talking together. Evaluating. Drawing. Writing. Role-play.
- Class and group activities.

Invite the children to explore the life of a character who worried all the time about keeping safe. What would the person's lifestyle be like? Ask the children to get into groups to enact this lifestyle through role-play or to illustrate it using comic strip drawing and writing. Next ask them to think about the lifestyle of someone who never gave a thought to risks or to dangers at all. What would that lifestyle be like? Again, they could demonstrate this using cartoons and role-play. Emphasise that keeping a balance between these two extremes is part of growing up. We can avoid risks and still enjoy the thrills and spills.

Content box 2   Focus on me

How do I see myself, especially in risky situations? How do others see me? What do I have to keep safe from? Do I have imaginary fears or fears for the future? How do I keep myself safe? Which skills do I need to learn? What gives me confidence? Can I be over confident? Why does my family want to know where I am and who I'm with? What would I do in an emergency? What life-saving skills can I begin to master?
When am I most at risk?

Activity 1

How do I see myself? How do others see me?

- Talking together. Drawing and painting. Writing. Vocabulary work.

- Class or group and individual activities.

Invite the children to draw or paint their self-portraits. Ask them to add to the portraits words and phrases to describe the kind of person they think they are, and how they would respond in a dangerous or difficult situation. Build up a 'word box' of this vocabulary to share, re-use or extend. Ask the children to repeat the activity, this time drawing and writing from the point of view of an adult member of the family. How would this person see them reacting in such a situation? Talk about the different viewpoints.

Activity 2

What do I have to keep safe from?

- Talking together. Categorising.

- Class or group activity.

Ask the children to work in small groups, and to note down in a brainstorming session all the things they think they have to keep safe from, people, places, objects etc. Ask them to group their responses into categories such as:

– real and present dangers.

– imaginary or future dangers.

– physical dangers.

– dangers to feelings.

Explore responses such as: the dark, strangers, high places and getting told off, to discover more about their underlying fears. (Be prepared for questions about diseases, particularly AIDS.)

Invite the children to look back on early childhood fears. What at a young age did they think they had to keep safe from? Invite them to share these views, especially where there might be cultural differences to explore. This is a good opportunity to involve **families** and other relatives. The children could ask them to recall their childhood fears and perceptions of danger.

Ask the children to look for explanations as to how and why other people's views have changed as they have grown up. What have they discovered? learned? become better at? What experiences, good or bad, have brought about the changes?

Activity 3 ● *How do I keep myself safe?*

- Talking together. Summarising. Generalising.
- Class or group activity.

Remind the children of some of the strategies young children use, or think they should use, to keep safe. For example, stay with Mum, hold on, don't touch, don't go, hide your eyes, cry, run away, climb a tree. Are these the strategies 10–11 year olds would use? Why not? Remind the children that 5–7 year olds have a separate answer for every risk. For example, don't touch matches, don't touch fires, don't touch pans, don't play there, don't go there.

Emphasise that at 10–11 years old they have now learned to make rules which cover a whole range of risks and hazards. Ask them about the other things they have learned to do. For example, weigh up risks, see dangers before they happen, recognise the times when they are most likely to be at risk, become more confident.

Activity 4 ● *What gives me confidence?*

- Drawing. Collecting and sorting pictures. Talking together. Describing. Evaluating. Writing.
- Class or group activities.

Ask the children to draw or find pictures of people of all ages, who look as though they are confident. Help them to find pictures of confident people in a large range of activities and situations: coping with difficulties, and disabilities, involved in sporting activities, day-to-day jobs, emergencies, rescues etc. What makes them confident or makes them appear to be confident?

Explore with the children the specific, individual skills which can help them to feel and behave confidently. Ask them to work in groups and to write down these skills as a checklist, and to discuss their order of importance, for example:

– Swimming and lifesaving.

– Road user skills.

– Cycling skills.

– Skills for dealing with an emergency.

– Drug-wise skills.

– Skills for dealing with dangerous people.

– Safety-in-the-home skills.

– Skills which enable you to ask for help.

– Skills which enable you to tell people how you feel.

Explain to the children that they could use the checklist to decide which skills they need to practise, and how and where they could get help in doing this. The children could help you to display sources of information in the classroom, and organise relevant visits and visitors.

Talk with the children about the times when they and other people have to behave confidently, although they do not feel confident inside.

There is a **cross-curricular link** with the many stories from history and literature which you can use to illustrate this.

Activity 5 ● *What makes me feel less confident?*

- Talking together. Writing. Media study. Using literature. Vocabulary work.

- Class or group activity.

Invite the class to imagine themselves having just mastered a new skill – in the classroom, in the sports world or at home – which they are wanting to show others. Ask them to think of what might be said or done by the people who are watching which would make them feel confident and want to go on, for example, praise, advice (not too much), interest, attention, pleasure. What would make them lose confidence?

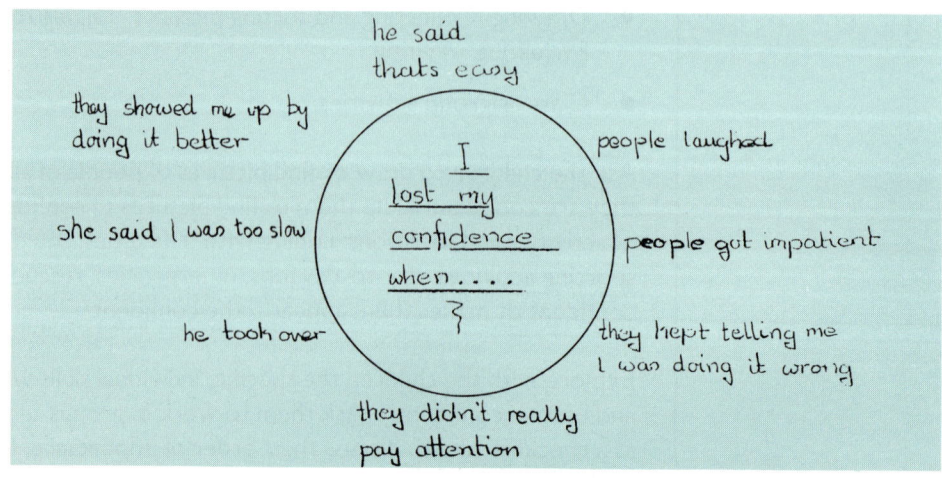

Invite the children to make a note of all those experiences when they lost confidence and to say why. Ask them to help you write a 'circle of feelings' to describe why they might lose confidence in this type of situation.

Ask the children to imagine that they are in a situation in which they are a newcomer to a class, a school, a club or a group of some kind, or they are trying out a new activity, going to a party, going on an outing or a camping holiday. How would they feel?

Talk with them about the different kinds of confidence which they need, for example, confidence to join in, confidence to retreat, etc. What helps them to find this confidence? Make a note of the children's suggestions. Encourage them to include strategies such as:

— learn as much as possible about the group, place and activities involved.

— be aware of the rules of the place or group.

— know someone in the group.

— be aware of the risks.

— make sure someone knows where I am and what I'm doing.

— remember that I can say 'No – it's not for me', and walk away.

Ask the children to help you write a 'circle of feelings' to describe why they might lose confidence in this type of situation.

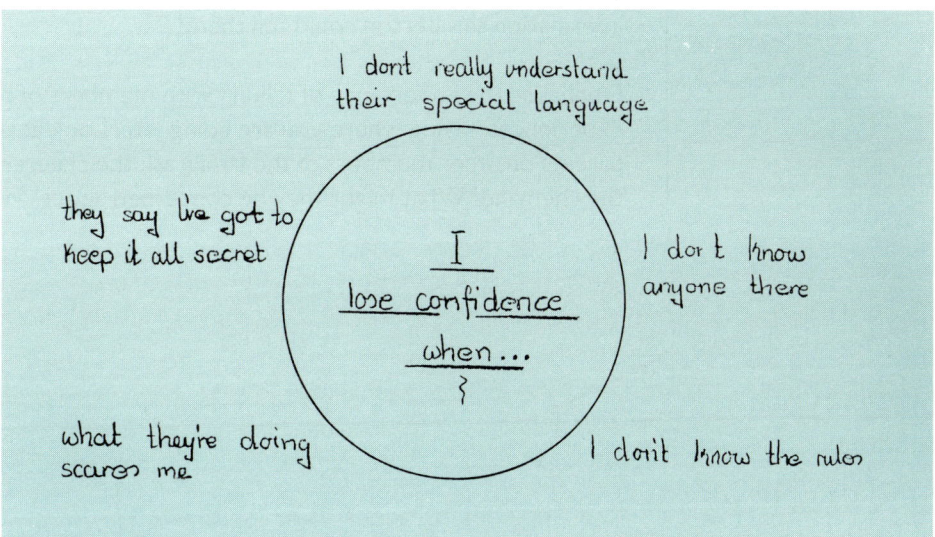

Look for examples of people being over confident in current news items, television programmes, and literature. What happened?

Ask the children if *they* have ever been over confident. What was the result? Tell them about your own experiences. What did you all learn from your experiences?

Emphasise to the children that there are areas in which most people at some time have experienced lack of confidence and over confidence, and that recognising this is part of growing up.

Activity 6 ● *Why does my family want to know where I am and who I'm with?*

- Talking together. Writing. Devising a questionnaire. Role-play. Drawing. Presenting information.

- Class or group and individual activities.

Remind the children that from childhood it is essential that people know, and are able to say or write:

– who they are.	– what time it is.
– where they have come from.	– where home is.
– who is with them.	– who is there.
– who is in charge.	– how they get in touch with them.
– where they are going.	– what time they have to get back.
– how they have got there.	– how they plan to get back.
– how long it has taken.	– with whom they will come back.

Ask the children to devise a questionnaire to test others on this knowledge. Provide opportunities for them to use it in the school and at home.

Ask the children to say why this knowledge is an important factor for keeping themselves safe. Invite them to put themselves into the role of someone helping a distressed person, especially a young person. Which would be the most important information this person could tell them?

Emphasise the importance of talking with members of the family, sharing experiences, saying where you are going, etc. Look at the kinds of questions which parents or other members of the family ask the children. What information do they demand? What might they be concerned about? What might they be afraid of?

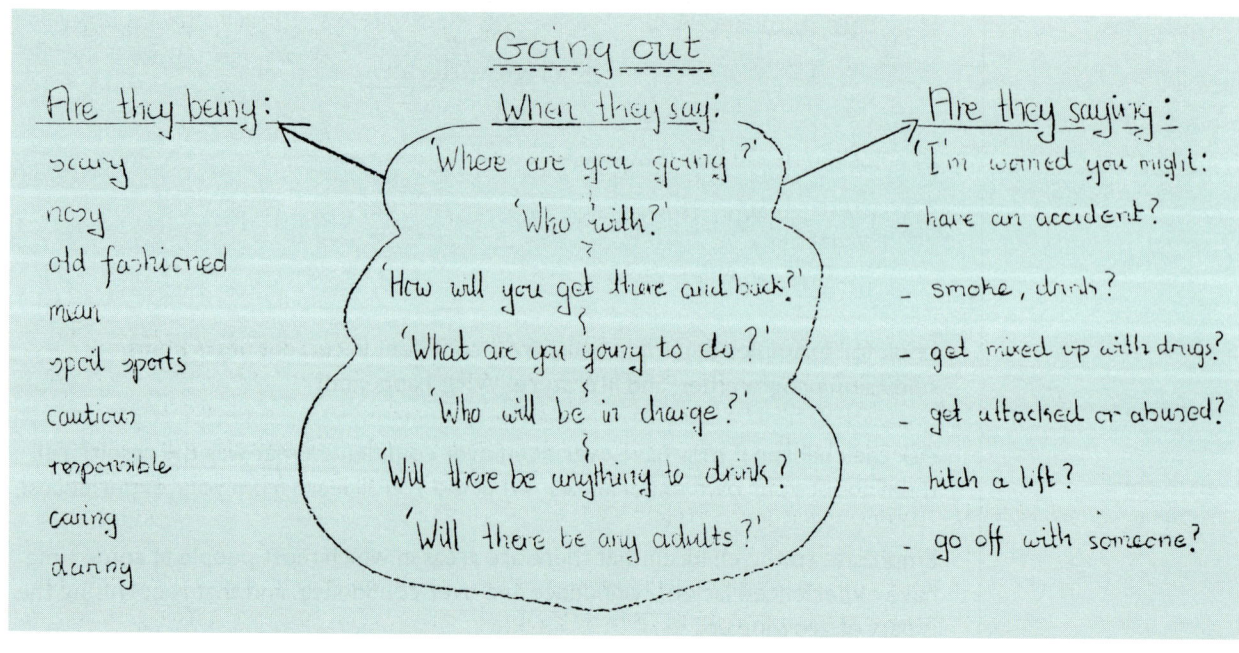

There is a lot of potential for role-play within this activity. Encourage the children to put themselves into, and explain, the parental role, and to reflect and role-play a range of alternative endings to role-play situations.

Emphasise the importance of having the confidence to sum up a situation, to decide whether or not to help or seek help, and whether or not to deal with an emergency.

Invite the children to imagine emergency situations, for example, an accident, a case of violence or abuse etc. Ask them to work in groups to explore the skills needed in these situations. Ask them to discuss the possible outcomes of using skills such as:

— deciding whether or not you can deal with the situation.

— finding adult help, persuading someone to listen.

— finding and using a telephone.

— describing a situation and location accurately.

— giving directions.

— staying calm.

— life saving.

Encourage the children to record their explorations of these situations in a variety of ways, for example:

— a sequence of pictures, speech bubbles or commentaries.

— a scenario for a play, radio or television programme.

— a 'What Would You Do?' game show.

— a newspaper report or television news bulletin.

Reinforce this work by asking the children to identify and categorise the skills which each one of them needs to practise.

Activity 7 ● ***How do my senses help me to keep safe?***

● Talking together. Role-play. Visits. Visitors.

● Class or group activities.

Explore with the children the highly developed senses that animals, birds and insects have, and the role these play in keeping them safe. Invite the children to consider how their own senses help them to keep safe (there are **cross-curricular links** here with science). How and when do they use sight, sound, touch, taste and smell to keep safe? When do they refuse to touch, taste or smell something in order to keep safe?

Explore with the children the role which our senses play in judging distance and speed, and in making decisions about retreating, taking over or seeking help.

Discuss the dangers of judging risks by what people say, or by their appearance. Invite the children to suggest and role-play situations in which this would be dangerous, for example, peer pressure, substance abuse, child abuse. Look at the importance of having more information, and going beyond what people say and how they look to what they are really saying or wanting.

Opportunities will occur for children to become more aware of how people whose senses are impaired learn to cope and compensate for their disability. There are **cross-curricular links** with community and environmental studies, visits and visitors.

Recall situations in stories or television plays in which people who have been blindfolded and taken to a strange place are rescued because they have been able to recall information imprinted on their senses, or the rescuers have been able to identify places through clues from the background noises in telephone or tape recorded conversations.

Ask the children to imagine themselves being blindfolded and led into a classroom in the school. How would they know which classroom it was? What would they hear? feel? smell? Invite them to choose other places in the school, at home or in the locality (including some potentially hazardous places), and describe what they think they would hear, feel or smell. Groups could exchange descriptions and try to identify the other group's location.

Content box 3   Focus on responsibility and risk

Who is responsible for keeping me safe wherever I am? What do all these people think they are keeping me safe from? How do they try to keep me safe? How can I practise being responsible and using my judgement? What affects people's judgement? What do I believe when people tell me different things about keeping safe? How can I tell which are facts, opinions, half truths or fiction?
When am I most at risk?

Activity 1   *Who is responsible for keeping me safe wherever I am?*

- Talking together. Categorising. Writing. Topic work.

- Class or group activity.

Invite the class to 'brainstorm' a list of people who may think they have some responsibility for keeping children safe. Ask the children to group together their responses using categories such as:

— People in our families.

— People at school.

— People outside school.

— People we know and see.

— People we don't know and don't ever see.

— People whose job it is to keep children safe.

— Friends.

— Ourselves.

(This activity could be extended to include a study of the jobs of a range of people in the local and wider community who provide people with a safer, happier and more healthy environment.)

Invite the children to express in a word or phrase what they think each of the people in the list is trying to keep children safe from. For example,

— pollution

— grown-up films

— drugs

— getting run over

— disease

— drink

— violence

— fires

— getting into trouble

— drowning

— war

— AIDS

— child abusers

— the wrong sort of friends

— gangs

— ruining our health

— accidents

This discussion is likely to provide an opportunity for you and the children to explore a wide range of sensitive issues.

Invite the children to look at ways in which people who are both known and unknown to them, attempt to influence their safety. Their responses might include:

— wanting to know where we are	— reminding us
— telling us	— teaching us how to do things
— nagging us	— treating us like babies
— advertising	— treating us like grown-ups
— television	— scaring us
— setting a good example	— making laws
— showing us proof	— making rules
— keeping us in	— catching criminals

Invite the children to review the list of people and what they do by considering these questions:

— Who, of all these people, knows me best?

— Who knows my feelings and fears?

— Who knows what I'm good at, or not so good at?

— Who knows who my friends are?

— Who can keep an eye on me and my safety wherever I am, all the time?

Introduce the idea that the children are the people who are best qualified to keep themselves safe.

Who is there all the time? Me!
Who knows I'm afraid of the dark and bullies? Me!
Who knows friends push me around? Me!
Who knows I'm learning to lifesave at swimming? Me!
Who knows my friend's brother bothers me? Me!
Who knows I get upset and forget the keeping safe rules? Me!
Who knows I'm afraid of things on T.V.? Me!
Who knows I'm getting better at saying No? Me!
Who knows I'm scared of turning right on my bicycle? Me!

Whose job is it to keep me safe? mine!
* It's my job to help to keep me safe *
— I am responsible _ _ _ _ Fred Biggins

Activity 2 ● *How can I be responsible?*

- Talking together. Role-play. Vocabulary work. Reviewing.

- Class or group activity.

Explore with the children the meaning of the word 'responsible'. Point out that it is a similar word to 'response'. Look at situations within the life of the school community, in local and national events or in literature and history, when people have attempted to respond to what is happening. What did they do? Did they 'respond' in a 'responsible' way? Invite the children to suggest situations in which they might have to decide whether to respond or not, and how to respond. Examples of these situations may include:

- bullying.

- vandalism.

- lack of tact.

- racism or sexism.

- an invitation to experiment with drugs.

- an invitation to go with someone to an unknown or dangerous place.

Ask the class to split into groups to role-play some of these situations. Invite the children who are watching to consider responsible and irresponsible outcomes in each case.

Look at areas of responsibililty in the classroom, around the school, in the home and in which children are already involved. Group these under headings such as:

- animals.   - resources.

- plants.   - people and their safety, well being or behaviour.

- places.   - personal safety.

- materials.

Ask the children: 'Who trained you for this responsibility?'

Ask the children to consider who else is responsible for the safety of the school, the playgrounds and the occupants. Ask them to find out who is the safety officer, what checks are made and when, what fire regulations and procedures are recommended, who deals with first aid and emergencies, and what training these people had. Have the children had any training in being responsible?

Invite the children to talk to each other about the responsibilities they have at home. How do the demands made on girls and boys differ? Talk this through. Which areas of responsibility do the children enjoy, feel confident to take on and wish to extend? Which responsibilities so far denied them would they like to take on? Which responsibilities cause them concern or unease, or place them in difficult or risky situations? Who can help in these situations?

Invite the children to brainstorm their answers to the question: 'How do I get better at doing things?' Focus on practical activities, for example, riding a bicycle, dancing, cooking, swimming, reading and baby sitting. Talk about responses such as:

– practise.

– get together with other people who are learning.

– put some time aside each week.

– read it up.

– watch the experts.

– ask someone how.

– keep at it.

Extend the discussion to include activities such as managing pocket money, keeping belongings in order, and organising homework in order to focus on skills such as planning ahead, foreseeing the problems, pitfalls and pressures and organising help.

Ask the children to review the skills, pitfalls and pressures involved in being responsible for their own personal safety. Help them to make an improvement plan.

Activity 3 ● *Using my judgement*

● Collecting pictures. Drawing. Talking together.

● Class or group and individual activities.

Ask the children to collect pictures of judges, particularly those involved in judging sporting or leisure activities.

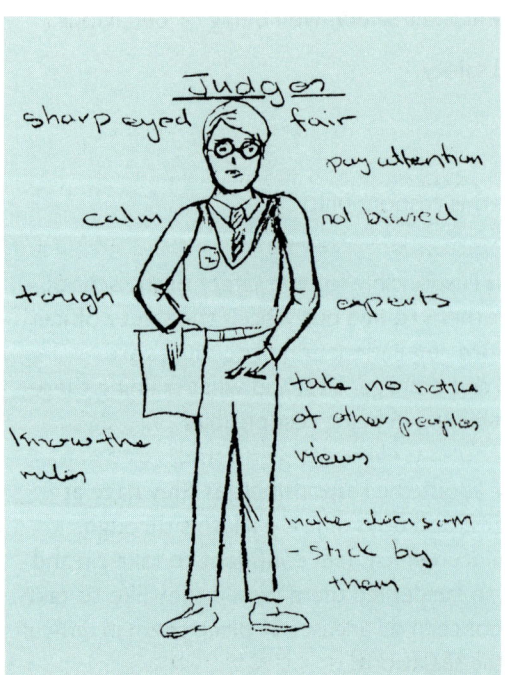

Invite the children to group judging activities into those which are rule based, and which could be verified later (for example, by camera, television, etc) and those which are based on personal views or assessments of performances.

Ask the children to illustrate someone judging an event, and to write down the vocabulary that describes the qualities needed by this kind of judge.

Explore with the children times when they have been asked to judge something. Were there rules to follow, or was an opinion asked for?

Encourage the chidren to recognise the extent to which their own practical judgement has developed. Ask them to think about how they use it in everyday activities, for example, judging distances, time, space and speed, although they are often unaware of what they are doing.

Invite them to think of times when they use their judgement, particularly when they have to assess the risks before making a decision, for example, before becoming involved in new activities, or more dangerous activities or activities with new people, or when they are being persuaded or pressured, to do something.

With the children, analyse a simple decision-making activity, such as jumping across a stream. Ask them to work out, and illustrate, the stages involved in making the decision.

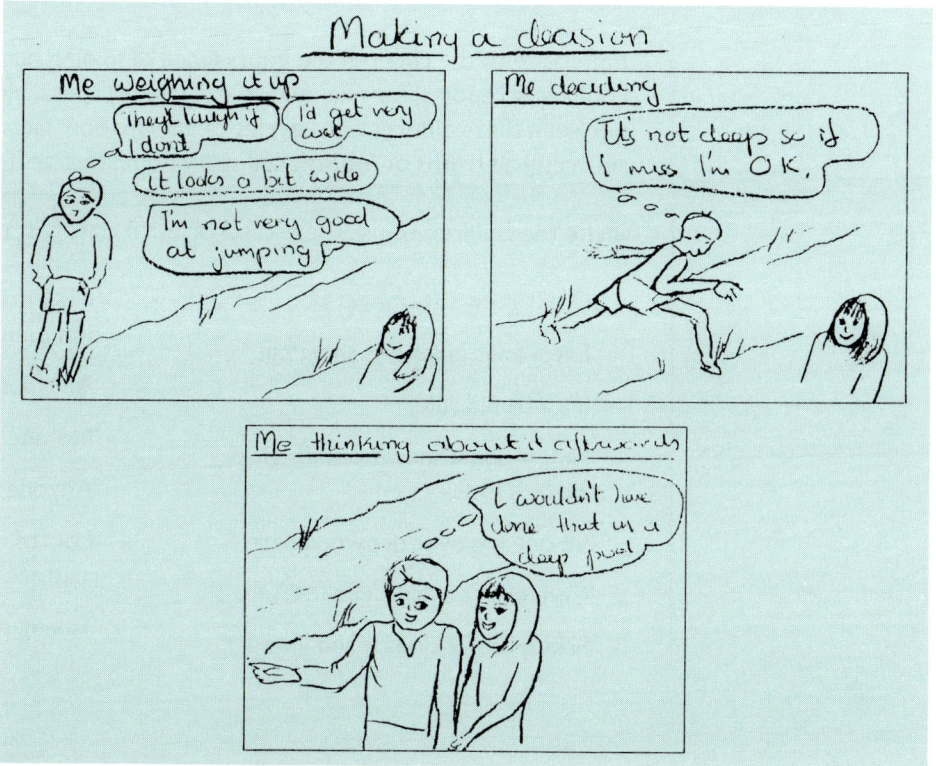

Invite the children to apply this type of analysis to other situations in which their safety could be at risk, for example:

— being pressured to experiment with smoking, alcohol, and other substances.

— being persuaded to go to a hazardous place, or into a hazardous situation.

Ask the children to put themselves in the place of a judge at a sporting event, who has to make a very important decision, and who is surrounded by people shouting advice, threats, and comments. How might the judge feel? How can he or she deal with this, remain impartial and keep the rules.

Invite the children to take this further and to imagine the impact on the judge of emotions such as anger, worry and excitement. How might tiredness, overeating, medicines and alcohol affect her or his judgement? Would someone's judgement still be sound after someone had tried to threaten or persuade them to do something?

What impact might these things have on *our* day-to-day decisions? This is an opportunity to focus on the relationship between alcohol and accidents.

Activity 4 ● *How can I tell the difference between facts, opinions and fiction?*

- Using literature. Talking together. Reading. Evaluating.
- Class or group activity.

A useful starting point would be to share with the class some myths, legends or traditional tales from various cultures which set out to explain difficult concepts through simple story lines. Invite the children to explore country lore and old wives' tales, and beliefs and traditions from different communities.

Emphasise to the children the importance of finding out the facts and weighing up conflicting reports, for example, in daily newspapers. Help them to distinguish between these different categories of information: facts, information from reliable sources, half truths or 'not the full story', opinions, attitudes and fiction.

Invite the children to use these categories to classify statements such as:

- 'Don't go with strangers.'
- 'Everyones takes this short cut.'
- 'It's a stupid rule.'
- 'I know someone who sniffs glue and he's OK.'
- No one has ever drowned here.
- 'Coffee isn't a drug.'
- 'Frizzo on TV does it and likes it.'

- 'Cigarettes are harmless if you don't inhale.'
- 'All rules are stupid.'
- 'No one will find out.'
- 'Anyone can do it.'
- 'Lots of children our age get hurt in road accidents.'
- 'Taking risks is fun.'

Content box 4   Focus on places and situations

Which places do I like going to?
Where do I go with my family?
my friends? other people? alone?
What are the rules and the risks?
How can I get there and back
safely? Do the risks change
according to the time, day or
company? Which accident is
most likely to happen in the
home? What can I learn from
statistics? What causes accidents?
How do alcohol related
accidents happen to children?
Can I practise avoiding accidents?
Could I cope in an emergency?
When am I most at risk?

Activity I ● *Which places do I like going to?*

- Drawing. Mapmaking. Talking together. Describing. Evaluation.

- Class or group or individual activities.

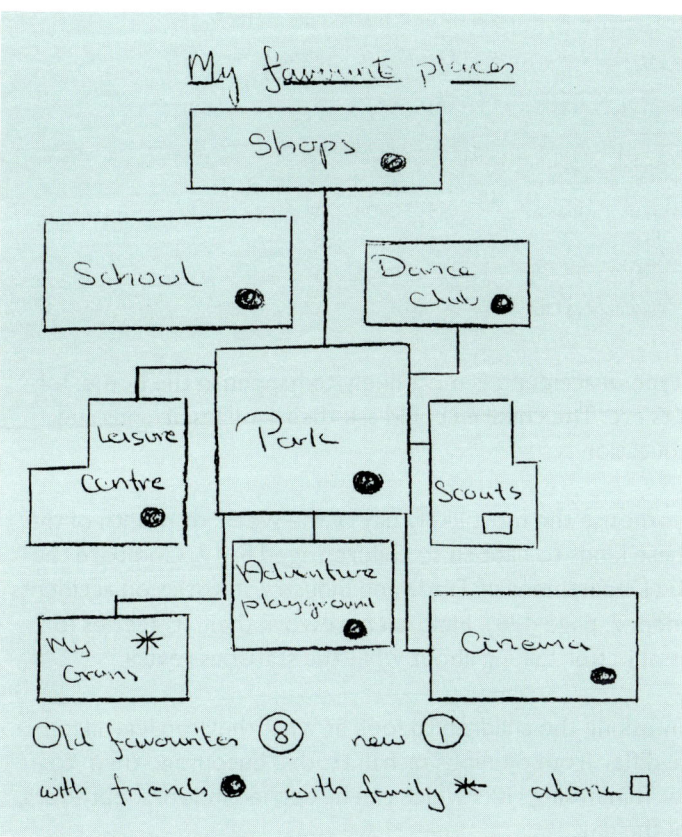

Ask the children to draw a picture or plan of their favourite places. Ask them to include places that they go to with family and friends, and places where they go alone. Where do they go to meet old friends, or make new ones? Where do they go to work, or to play?

Ask the children to identify their favourite places, and places which have only recently become popular. What do they enjoy doing most?

Ask the children to work in small groups and think of the risks connected with these places. What are the rules, written and unwritten, which help to make their activities safer and lessen the risks? Which are the skills they use most often to keep themselves safe?

Invite the children to look at the routes which they take from their homes to these places. Suppose someone needed instructions for the safest route to one of these places. Invite the children to describe the safest route to take by day, by night, alone or with a group, identifying the high risk places on route. What additional hazards would they point out if the person asking for directions was a child? On which days, or at which times of the day would the risks be highest for a child? You could ask the groups to present their work as a set of illustrated maps of the locality. There is a **cross-curricular link** here with environmental studies.

Activity 2   ● **Which accident is most likely to happen in the home?**

- Writing. Drawing. Survey work. Using statistics. Talking together.
- Class or group activities.

Ask the children to take part in a class survey in which they must respond in writing or drawing to this question: 'Where in the house are the most dangerous places for children of our age?'

Invite the children to analyse and present the results, and to suggest ways in which they could take on the responsibility of minimising the risks.

> We did a survey about the most dangerous places in the house
>
> We thought the dangerous places were:
> * the kitchen
> * the sitting room
> * the stairs
>
> This is what we thought We could do to bring down the risks.
> - learn to use things safely
> - mind little children
> - don't fool with electrics
> - don't leave things on the stairs
> - don't play around
> - know the risks

Ask the children what type of accident, is most likely to happen in the home, for example, falls, burns, cuts etc. The children could ask their families, friends and other classes the same question.

Ask the children to hypothesise the most likely day of the week, or month of the year, for accidents of these kinds to happen to children aged 8–12. Compare the children's views with the Department of Trade and Industry statistics on accidents in the home (see Appendix 2, page 426). Help them rework their strageties for minimising risks if necessary after talking about what the statistics reveal.

Conclude this activity by asking the children to look at what they can learn from statistics. How do these differ from opinions or half truths? Encourage them to develop a set of rules for minimising risks which can be applied indoors, outdoors, and at different times of the day.

Activity 3 ●   *What causes accidents?*

- Talking together. Writing. Evaluating. Generalising.

- Class or group activity.

Divide the class into groups and present each with a brief description of an accident (not giving any clues to the cause), for example:

  – A road accident in which a child was knocked from a bicycle.

  – A fall in a playground.

  – A fire in a home.

  – A road accident in which a car crashed into a bollard.

  – A swimming accident, indoors or outdoors.

  – An accident involving machinery, indoors or outdoors.

  – An accident involving electricity, indoors or outdoors.

  – The loss of a child.

Ask the children to note down as many possible causes of these accidents as they can. Help them to identify causes which are specific to a situation, and causes which are more general. Discuss general causes of accidents, such as

  – being unaware of the risk.

  – not knowing the safety rules.

  – ignoring the safety rules or advice.

  – taking too great a chance.

  – showing off or boasting.

  – being affected by one's feelings, or by something which happened earlier.

  – making mistakes.

  – being with someone who makes a mistake.

  – not having the skills to cope with the situation.

  – being under the influence of alcohol or drugs.

  – a chain of events.

Ask the children if they, or someone they know, has been involved in or witnessed an accident. What could have caused it? Could the accident have been avoided? How?

Activity 4 ●   *Can I practice avoiding accidents?*

- Talking together. Drawing and painting. Evaluating.

- Class or group activity.

Invite the children to spot the differences between practising skills in order to *do something better*, for example, swimming, cycling, first aid or using machinery, and practising *not doing things*, such as not getting hurt, not getting involved in accidents or dangerous situations and not being threatened or pressured to take part in activities. Can you go out and practise *not* getting run over?!

Invite the children to describe the differences between talking, about accidents and dangerous situations in the classroom (and listening to experts, or watching films and videos, or role-playing on this theme) and actually being involved in an accident or dangerous situation oneself.

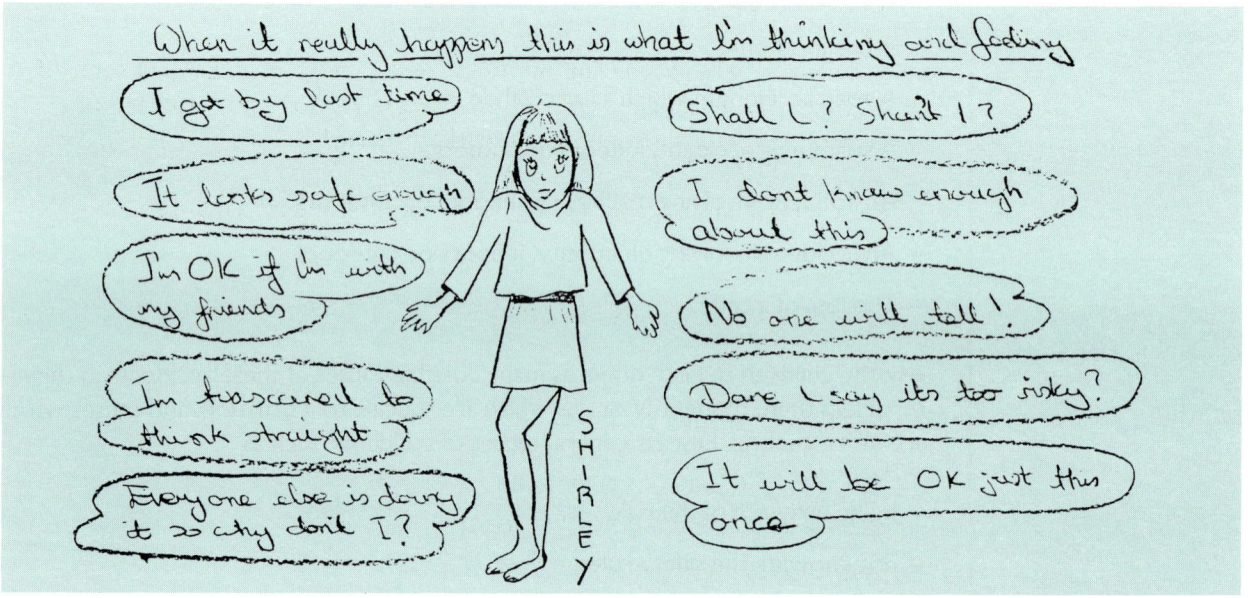

Talk about the ways in which accidents might be avoided. Invite the children to suggest coping strategies for avoiding the accidents described in Activity 3. Ask them to make an 'Anti-accident Poster' which promotes these strategies.

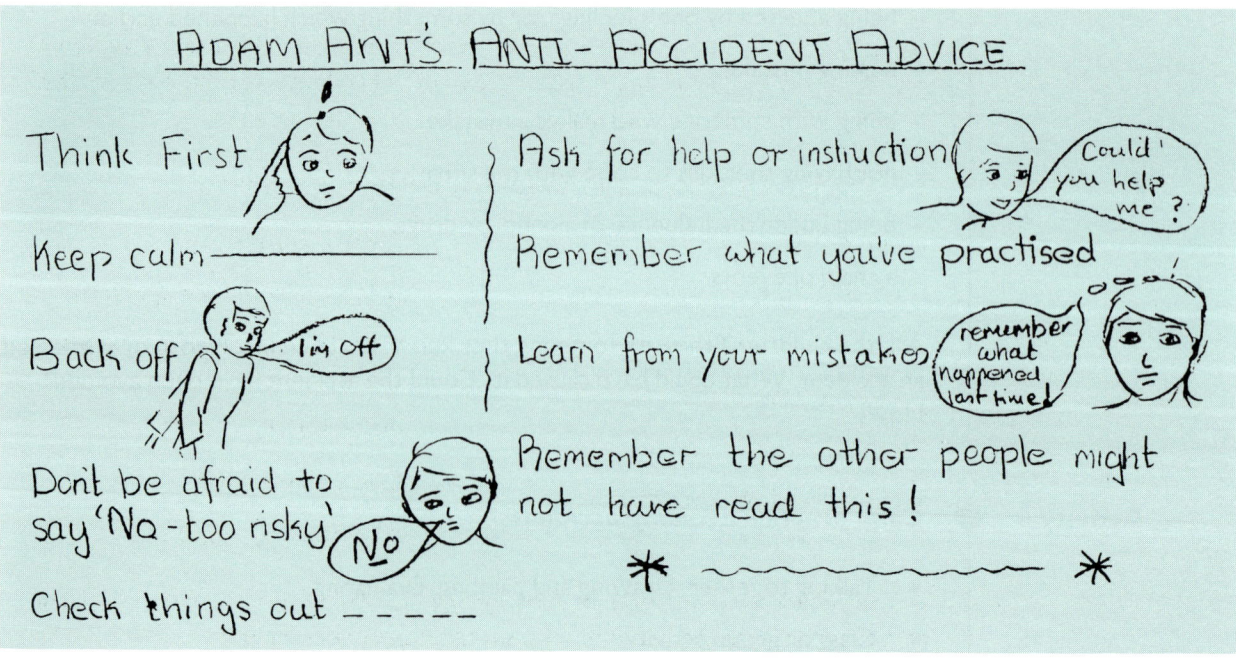

Opportunities may occur during this activity to explore coping strategies for a range of sensitive issues, including child abuse. It is also a good time to emphasise coping strategies for dangerous situations on the road, for example, in an illegally driven car, being offered a lift, hitch hiking etc.

Activity 5　●　*Could I cope in an emergency?*

- Talking together. Describing feelings and situations. Using literature. Television study. Role-play. Drawing.

- Class or group and individual activities.

Invite the children to try to identify what an emergency means. Look at some of the favourite places listed by the children in Activity 1. Can they imagine, or remember any emergencies happening in these places?

Ask the children to suggest emergency procedures for these situations:

– a fire.

– a child in danger in the water.

– a child being taken away.

– a child being threatened.

– someone being taken ill, fainting, or having a fit.

– someone inhaling a dangerous substance.

– a road accident in a country lane

– an accident in the school playground or in the park.

Talk through these situations with the children. What would they do? What would they *not* do? How would they get immediate help?

Look at stories, television programmes and news items in which the unexpected happens, or a seemingly safe situation gets out of hand. Look at the ways in which people deal with these situations.

You could invent two characters to help you explain coping skills:

Clem the Coper	*Sandy the Sad Sack*
– has practised emergency skills;	– is floored by the unexpected;
– knows how to get help;	– tends to panic: acts first, thinks later;
– doesn't panic;	
– can say 'No';	– sits and cries;
– has worked out the risks.	– follows the crowd;
	– takes the easy way out.

Ask the children to describe, or show using role-play, how each character might respond in an emergency, or when a situation got out of hand.

Invite the children to draw themselves just before the start of a concert or sporting event, in or out of school, and to add words and phrases to describe how they feel. What helps them to give their best performance? For example:

– practice.

– confidence.

– doing something I enjoy or feel good at.

– wanting to live up to people's expectations.

– wanting to succeed or reach the target.

– being alone.

– having my friends there.

Point out any conflicting views.

Look at 'performers' in the public eye. Are they always confident and interested? What keeps them going?

Ask the children to look at their responses again. How many of them also apply to coping in difficult or dangerous situations?

Ask the children to think about times when they feel they did not perform as well as they might. What could have caused this? For example:

– being out of practice;

– over confidence;

– over excitement;

– boredom;

– fright;

– lack of confidence;

– feeling pressured;

– feeling too afraid to say 'No'.

How many of these factors apply to coping in dangerous situations?

Content box 5   Focus on people and pressure

Who are the people I trust?
What are the rules for getting
on with them? What should I do
if someone changes the rules, or
makes me feel unsafe? Who else
can I turn to? What can I do
when no one will listen? Who
are the people I admire? Should I
set an example to younger
children? How do people
persuade others to do things?
How can I cope when people
persuade me to do something
risky? When is it best to tell
secrets? Is this the same as telling
tales? What can I do to keep
myself safer?
When am I most at risk?

Activity I   *Who are the people I trust?*

- Talking together. Describing people and situations. Writing. Visits. Visitors.

- Class or group and individual activities.

Remind the children of their work on favourite places (Content Box 4). Invite the children to make lists of their favourite things, and to include things which they do, remember, see and hear.

Now invite them to think about their favourite people. Who would go on this list? Invite them to share their responses and sort them into categories such as:

– People I know well.

– People I only know through television, magazines, etc.

– Imaginary people from stories, television dramas, fiction and history.

Invite the children to regroup their responses into categories such as:

– family.

– friends.

– others.

Explore with the children what it is about these people which makes them their favourites. Is it their appearance, performance and reputation? Is it the bond of trust and affection between them? Do the children like their favourite people because they have thought about good and bad points?

Ask the children to think about their relationships with their favourite real people. What makes the children feel safe with them and able to trust them?

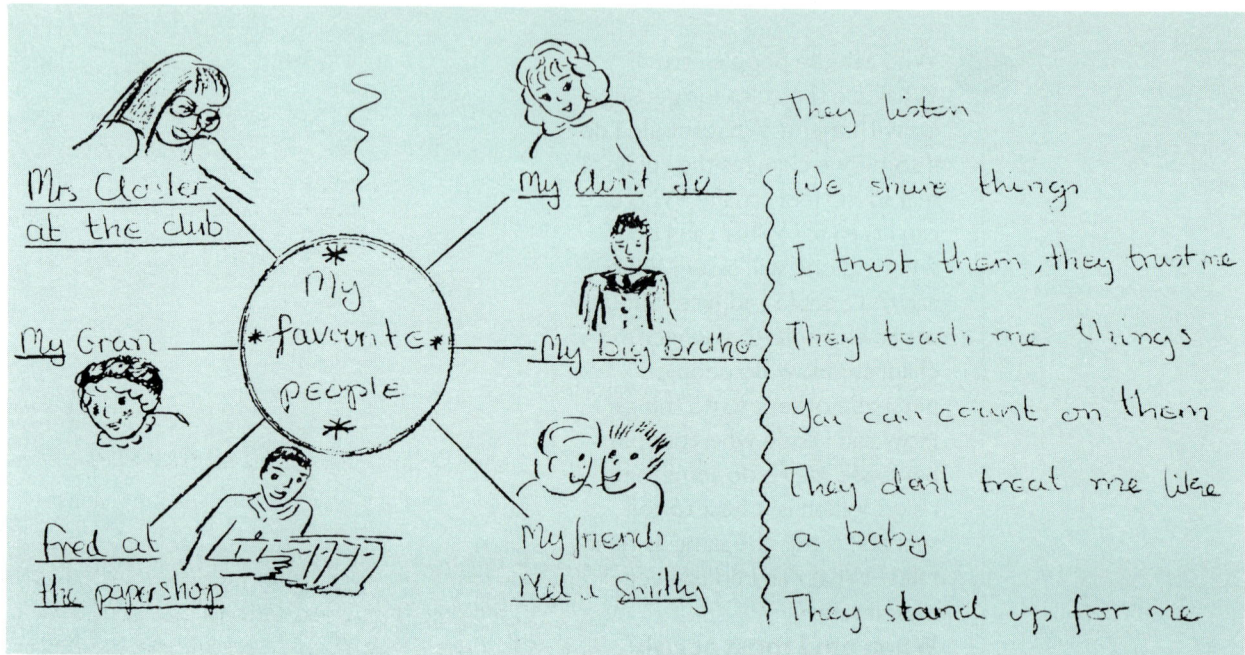

Ask the children to think about how they get on with their favourite people. What 'rules', both specific and general, must they keep in order to get along with them? For example:

- Rules for getting on with my Gran:
  visit her and talk to her.

- Rules for getting on with my big brother:
  don't borrow his best sweater, don't touch his records.

- Rules for getting on with Fred down the road:
  don't waste his time.

What happens if the rules are broken or changed, or if the relationship changes in ways which cause the child concern or unease, or which pressures them? This is an opportunity for the children to talk about concerns of many kinds, including abuse.

Recall the children's favourite places (Content Box 4) and the work on the recommended routes to and from these places. Invite the children to think of the people along the route to whom they could turn for help and advice if they were afraid, uneasy or in some kind of trouble. How would they find and recognise these people? What would they say to them? It would be a valuable experience for the children to go out and meet some of these people or invite them to school.

Suggest to the class that they make an illustrated book in which they could write about the people they could turn to. They could include in the book maps of safe routes. The book could be used as a resource for younger children in the school.

This could be a useful time to emphasise the importance of non-vandalised telephone booths.

Activity 2 ● ***What can I do when no one will listen?***

- Talking together.

- Class or group activity.

Explore with the children situations when they need adult help but the adults are too busy or preoccupied to respond, or they don't believe the child, or they say, 'Don't be silly', or they joke about it and tell other people or abuse the child's trust in other ways. Discuss what the children think might be done or said in order to convince the adults that they need help. What other safety strategies could they use?

Activity 3 ● ***Who are the people I admire?***

- Talking together. Describing. Evaluating. Using literature. Music. Drama. Visits. Visitors.

- Class or group and individual activities.

Explore with the children the lives of some of the people they are interested in and admire. Collect details of the lifestyles of these people: look at who is responsible for their safety, their risk taking and their decisions. Invite the children to summarise the lifestyles, and show what looks good and what may be the drawbacks.

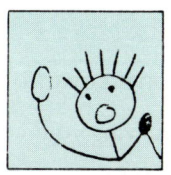 For example: Herby the Merby (lead singer of the Rock Planet).

His life looks good:

— He has the best food and drink.

— He travels the world.

— He has girlfriends.

— He has plenty of money.

— He has people to look after him.

— People think he's a great singer.

But:

— He has to practise for hours and hours.

— He has no time to relax.

— He smokes all the time.

— He has to sing whether he wants to or not.

— He is often offered drugs.

— He can't go where he wants to.

— Everyone knows him, so he has no privacy.

Help the children to analyse the lifestyles of the people they admire in more detail:

— What aspects of these lifestyles do they admire?

— Which skills would they like to have?

— What risks to safety and health are part of these lifestyles?

This could be an opportune time to look at people within the community who have special skills, interesting lifestyles and who may need to take risks, in order to widen the range of models the children can choose from. You could also use characters from the children's own historical roots, cultures and traditions, and from poetry, music, drama, stories, myths and legends generally.

Invite the children to describe or draw a grown-up. At what age do people become grown-up? When do people become middle-aged? When are people old? Explain to the children that they will appear to 5 year olds to be grown-up and will be their role models, just as they themselves look up to rock stars and sports personalities. Introduce the idea that they might have an obligation to act responsibly.

Activity 4 ● *How can I cope when people persuade me to do something risky?*

- Talking together. Role-play.

- Class or group and pair activities.

Ask the children, working in pairs, to suggest answers to these questions: How would you –

– make a dog come to you whenever you called?

– persuade the PE teacher to let you have an extra turn?

– persuade your friend not to start smoking?

– persuade your friend to stop going off on his own?

– persuade someone to stop teasing or bullying you?

– persuade your Mum to stop what she's doing and listen to you?

– persuade your little brother to learn to swim?

– persuade your friend to do something that scares him or her?

– persuade your Gran to show you how her lawnmower works?

Collect the children's answers and group them into categories such as:

– asking.

– telling.

– persuading.

– rewarding.

– being understanding.

– demonstrating.

– quoting facts.

– threatening.

– frightening.

Look with the children at the ways they think work best. (There is a link here with the work on 'persuaders' in *Health for Life 1*, page 94–96.)

Ask the children to put themselves in a situation in which someone is trying to persuade them to do something. What would they say? How would they feel?

What would they do if:

— someone tried to persuade them to go with them, without telling anyone first?

— the gang said they had to sniff or taste a secret powder before they could become a member?

— someone wanted them to keep something a secret?

— someone wanted them to help look for a lost child or pet?

Encourage the children to role-play one of these situations to the rest of the class. Ask the class to comment on how the 'persuaded' children are coping:

— How are they feeling?

— Are they disguising their fear or unease?

— Do they sound confident?

— How did they reply to the persuaders?

Activity 5 ● ***In what ways can people be dangerous?***

● Talking together. Drawing. Painting. Collecting and sorting pictures.

● Class or group activities.

Invite the children to draw and paint or collect pictures of people who appear to be dangerous. Look in particular at stereotypes in comics, cartoons and advertisements.

Display these pictures and invite the children to think of words to describe them. What kinds of people are included? Are they male, female, old, young or imaginary? How can one see that they are dangerous? Look at how stereotyping, gender and race are associated with danger.

Ask the children to be more specific about the different types of danger. Help them to group them into categories such as,

— physical harm.   — dares.

— threats.   — bribes.

— bullying.   — persuasion.

This could provide you with the opportunity to discuss the strategies for avoiding such dangers, or for coping with them, or for finding help. Discuss the question, 'When am I most at risk?'

Activity 6 ● *When is it best to tell secrets?*

- Talking together. Writing.
- Class or group activity.

Ask the children if they can complete the sentence: 'A secret is . . .'. Invite them to share their responses and discuss questions such as: What are the rules for secrets? When does a secret stop being a secret? Invite the children to make a list of the kinds of secrets they would not tell, and to say why. Is it because of trust? Friendship? Fear? What types of secret would the children want to tell, or would encourage other children to tell?

There are opportunities here to emphasise the importance of sharing one's fears, despite threats to the contrary, and that this is not 'telling tales'.

Explore with the children situations in which people might appear to be 'telling tales' and discuss what the hidden motive might be, for example:

– An adult sees you doing something risky and tells your family.

– A friend sees you doing something which is forbidden and tells the teacher.

– You and a friend are doing something which is against the rules and your friend tells his family.

Ask the children to think of other situations in which they might feel a need to tell someone something. Whom would they tell? Ask them to remember their list of favourite people. Help them to extend these personal lists to include people in the community who would be prepared to listen and to advise them, and who would when necessary, keep their intervention a secret.

Family Worksheet Masters

The worksheet masters in the following pages are photocopiable so you can give them to the children to take home and work through with their families. The worksheets can also be used by the children with the teacher in a one-to-one session, or in group work. However, home use brings to your health education programme the important benefit of family involvement.

The worksheets vary in difficulty, and begin with worksheets for the younger children. They have not been age-graded as you will probably prefer to select them according to the needs of your class.

A photocopiable letter has also been provided which you can send home with the worksheets. This explains to the parent, or family, the purpose of the worksheets and suggests ways in which they could be used. You may wish to adapt this letter to your own needs.

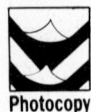
Photocopy

Dear

Family Worksheets

These worksheets are an important part of your child's health education. We would like you and your child to work on them together. They will show you some of the ways in which the children are learning to keep themselves safe. We are trying to make them aware of danger and to show them the best ways to avoid or cope with it.

The children are bringing these worksheets home so you can share in the work they have been doing at school. You can help them to get the most out of what they have learned. This is not the kind of homework which is taken back to school to be marked, it is family work, everyone can share in it. We think you will learn a great deal from the way your child thinks about health and explains it all to you.

When you sit down with your child to start a worksheet, one way to start is to ask your child to explain what has been happening in health education sessions at school. The next step is to work together through the activities on the worksheet. Remember that there are no right and wrong answers. The important thing is to talk together. Don't worry if your child's drawings are not very clear, you can always ask her, or him, to tell you about them. Read the worksheet *with* your child or read it *to* your child, but don't make the reading a struggle. Write for your child if that is what she or he would like you to do. Most importantly, feel free to contribute some questions of your own, and think of other things to talk, draw and write about.

This school is working to promote health and your child is sharing that with you at home. This is your chance to help bring important health messages home to your child.

We hope you enjoy sharing these worksheets with your child.

Keeping Myself Safe

Family Worksheet

My name is ....

1

Who am I?

Draw yourself.

This is me

I know my name.

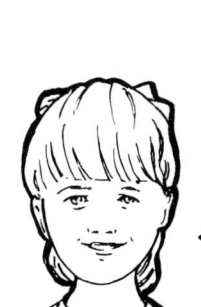

My name is

Draw your house.

This is my house.

I know where I live.

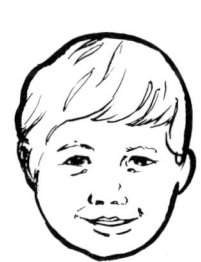

I live at

Draw your family.

This is my family.

I know my family.

I know their names:

_____

I know what to do if I get lost:

_____

Keeping Myself Safe

My name is ....

Keeping myself safe outdoors

Draw yourself keeping safe coming home from school.

Talk about some of the things you have to keep safe from.

Can you draw some of them?

Draw yourself keeping safe playing outside.

Talk about some of the things you have to keep safe from.
Can you draw some of them?
Talk about the best ways to keep safe outdoors.

Keeping Myself Safe

My name is ....

Keeping myself safe indoors

Draw yourself keeping safe in this kitchen.

Talk about some of the things you have to keep safe from in your kitchen.

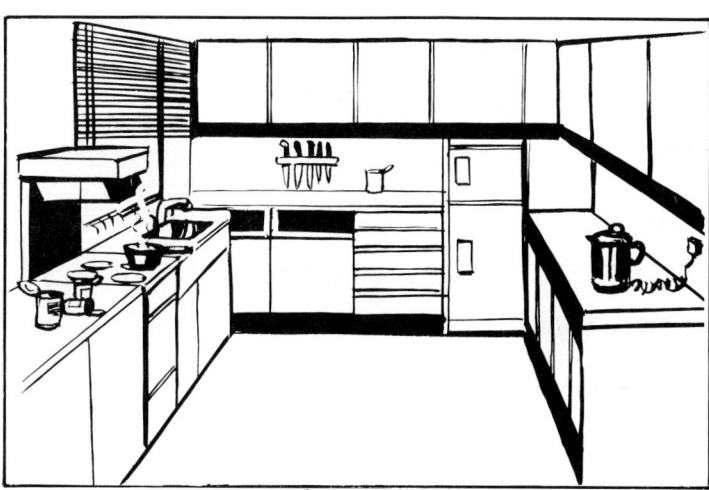

Draw yourself keeping safe on these stairs

How are you keeping safe?

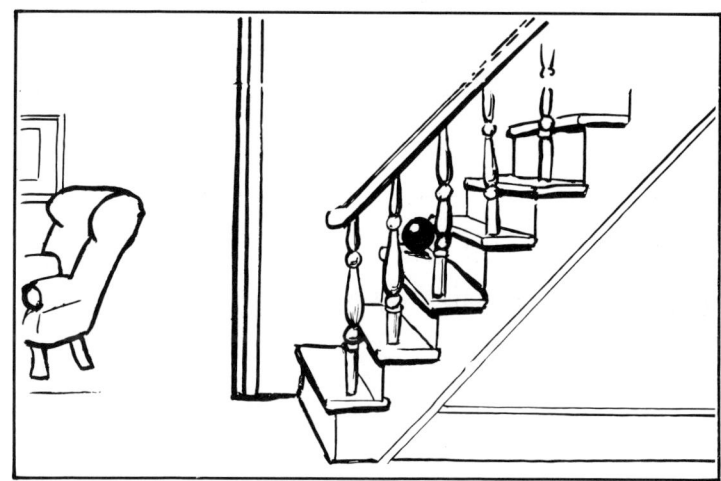

Draw yourself keeping safe in your house.

How are you keeping safe?

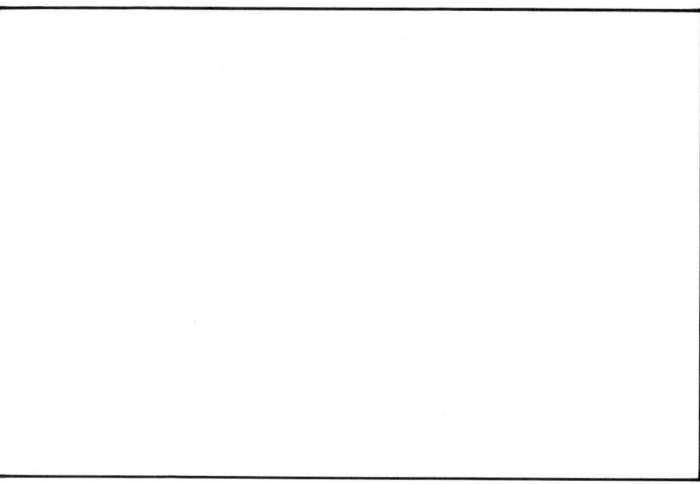

Talk about some other places in your house where you have to keep safe.

Keeping Myself Safe

My name is ....

How can these children keep safe?

Look at the pictures.
How would Tammy and Sammy keep safe here?

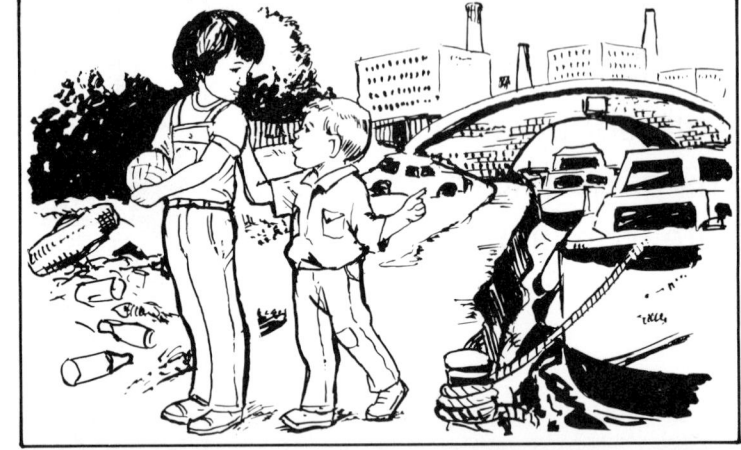

_____

What would you tell them to do?

_____

How would Lisa and Joey keep safe here?

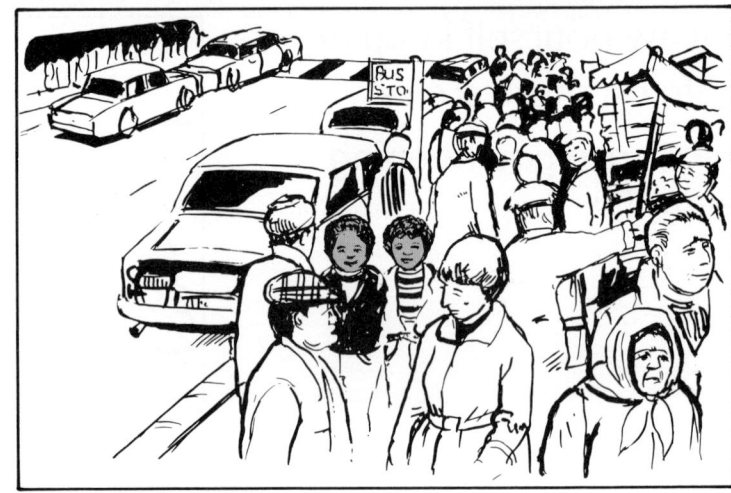

_____

What would you tell them to do?

_____

What is happening here?

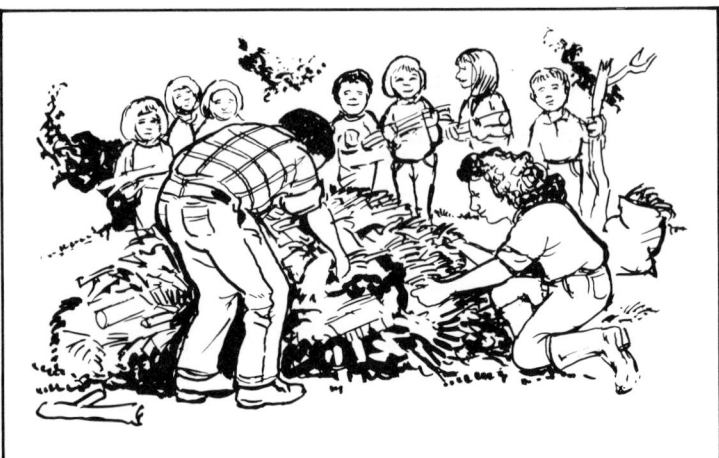

_____

What would you tell the children about keeping safe?

_____

Talk about some other places outdoors where you have to keep safe.

Keeping Myself Safe

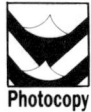
Photocopy

My name is ....

Keeping Benny safe

Benny is playing all alone here.
Is this a safe place for Benny
to play?

What would you say to Benny?

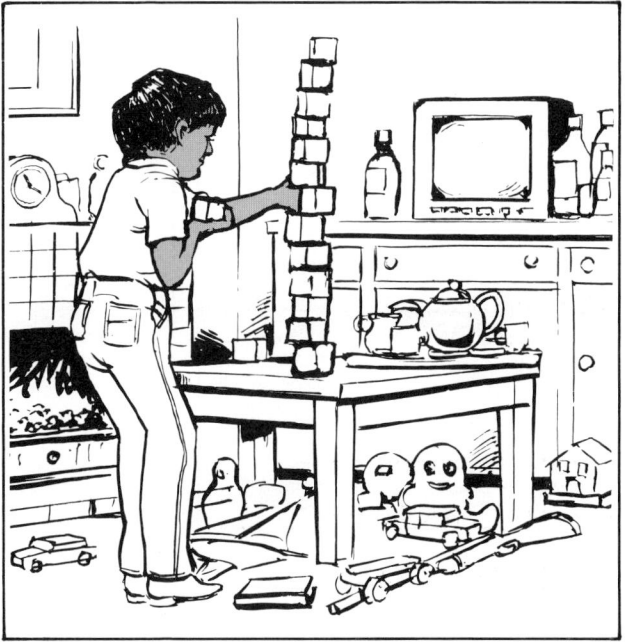

Benny is playing all alone here.
Is this a safe place for Benny
to play?

What would you say to Benny?

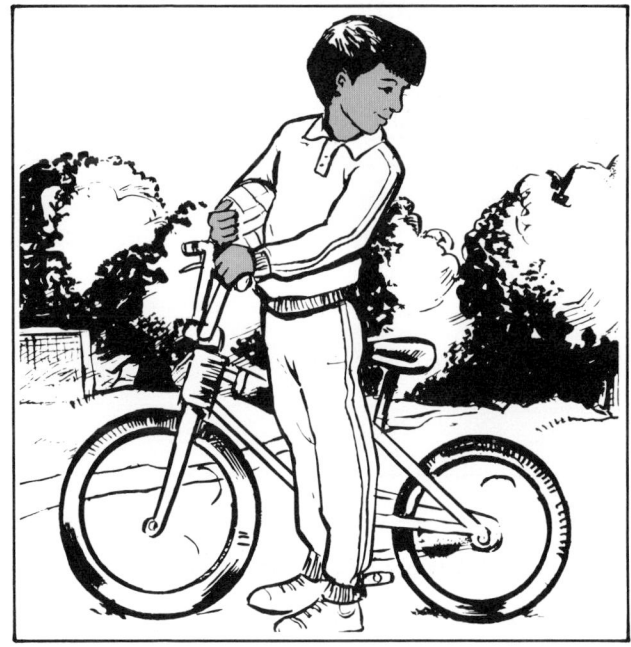

Talk about the places where you play alone.
How do you keep yourself safe?

Photocopy

Keeping Myself Safe

My name is ....

What frightens us?

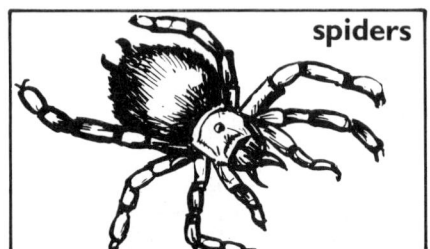
spiders

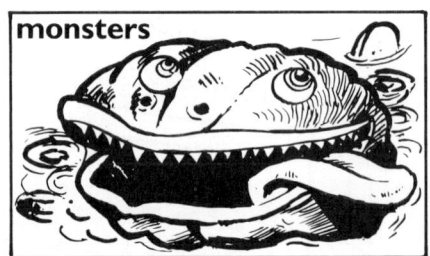
monsters

These are some of the things that frighten Sammy.

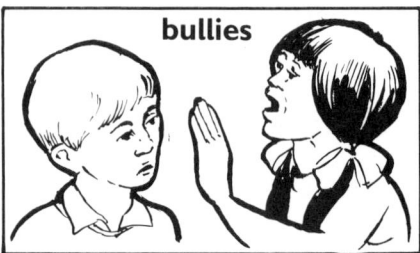
bullies

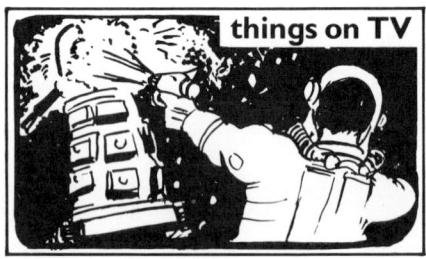
things on TV

What would you say to Sammy to help him feel better?

Talk about some of the things that frighten you. Can you draw some of them?

Talk about some of the people who frighten you. Can you draw some of them?

What can you do to make yourself feel better?

What can you do to keep safe from them?

Draw a safe person to tell.

© Health Education Authority 1989

Keeping Myself Safe

 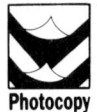

My name is ....

What can we do if we get lost?

Lisa is lost.
She is looking for a safe
person to tell.
What would you tell her to do?

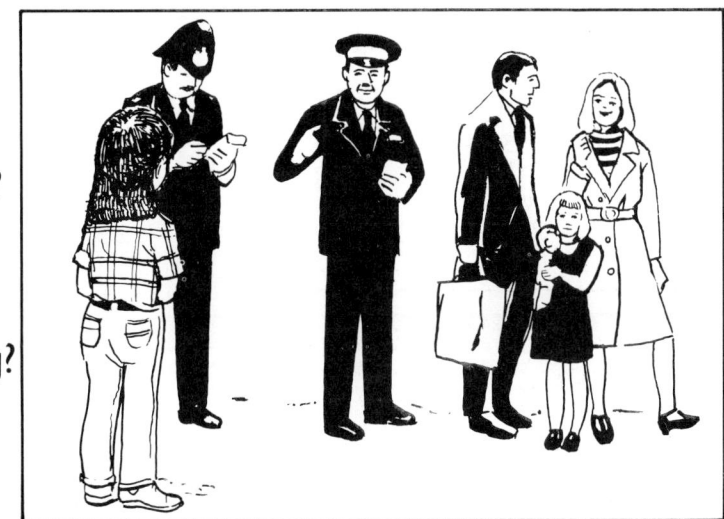

_____

What would you tell her to say?

_____

Draw yourself telling a safe
person that you are lost.
What are you saying?

_____

Someone has frightened Joey.
Talk about what you think
has happened.
What would you tell him to do?

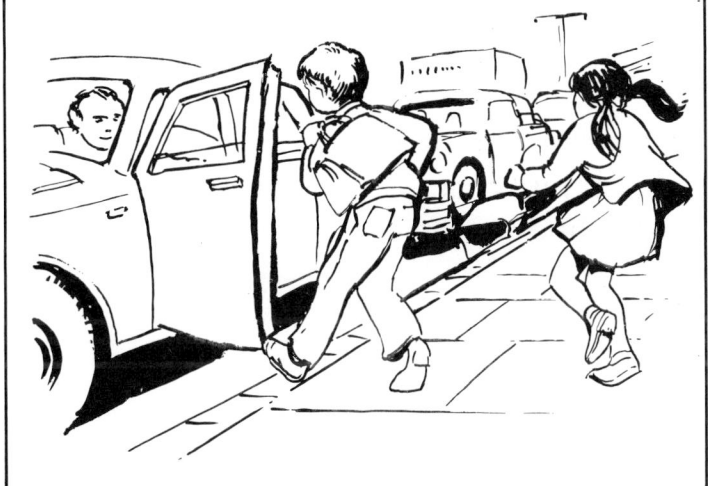

_____

What would you tell him to say?

_____

© Health Education Authority 1989

Photocopy

Keeping Myself Safe

My name is ....

Secrets

Sandy and Joey have got a good secret in their heads.

Can you guess what it is?

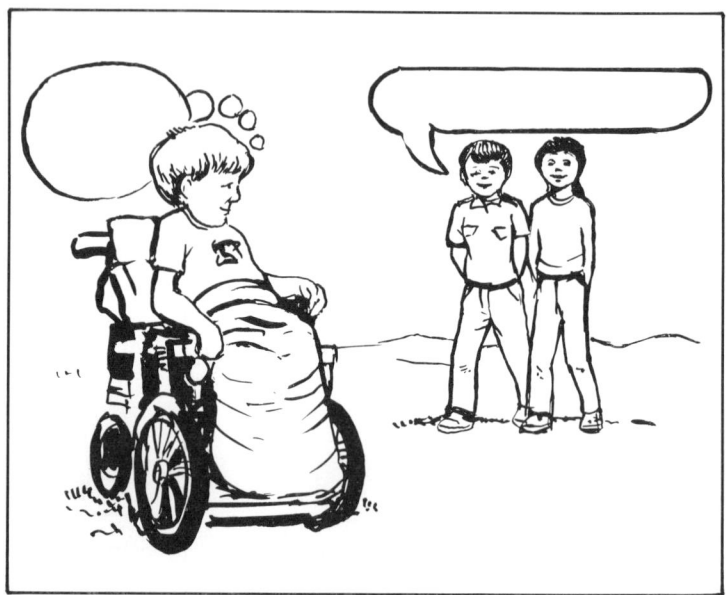

_____

How are they all feeling?

_____

Talk about some good secrets you have had.

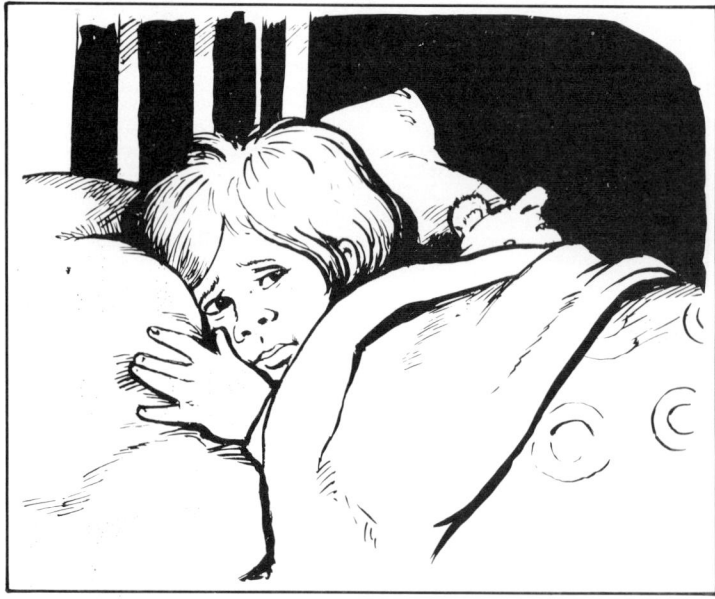

Mandy has a bad secret in her head.

Talk about what it could be. How is she feeling?

_____

What would you tell her to do?

_____

What would you tell her to say?

_____

Talk about what you would do if someone asked you to keep a bad secret.

_____

Who would you tell?

_____

Keeping Myself Safe

My name is ....

Who helps to keep me safe?

Talk about the people who help to keep you safe.
Can you draw some of them?

The people who help to keep me safe are . . .

How do they help you to keep safe?

_____

What do they say to you? What do you say to them?

_____

How do you help them?

_____

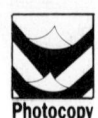
Photocopy

Keeping Myself Safe

Family Worksheet (10)

My name is ....

Who is in charge?

Who is in charge . . .

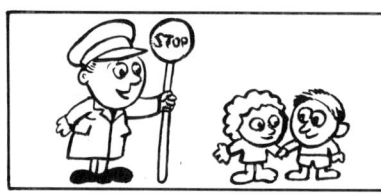 . . . at the crossing? ....

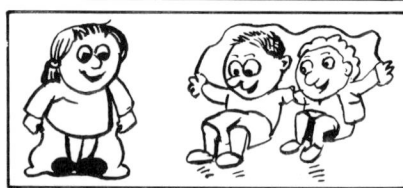 . . . in the school playground? ....

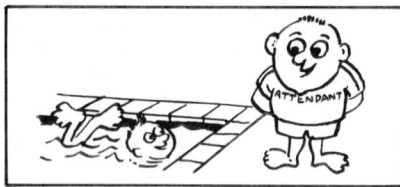 . . . at the swimming pool? ....

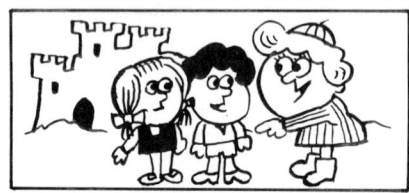 . . . on a school trip? ....

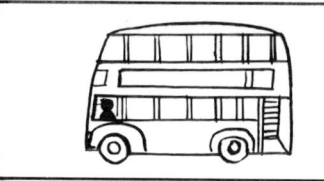 . . . on the bus? ....

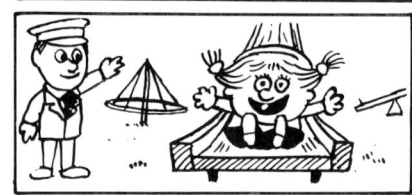 . . . in the park? ....

How do I help them?

_____

How do I ask them to help me? What do I say?

_____

Keeping Myself Safe

Family
Worksheet

 Photocopy

11

My name is ....

Going to school

My house

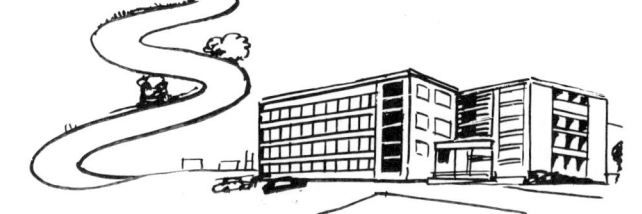

How do you get to school? (tick the box)

I walk	I go on a bus	I go in a car	I go on my bicycle

School

Who do you go with? (tick the box)

I go with a grown-up	I go with friends	I go alone

Draw the most dangerous places on your way to school.

What makes them dangerous?

_____

How do you keep yourself safe?

_____

Talk about who could help you if you needed help.

© Health Education Authority 1989

Photocopy

Keeping Myself Safe

My name is ....

How can I keep safe?

How would you keep safe from . . .

Draw and write.

. . . people who want you to try something dangerous.

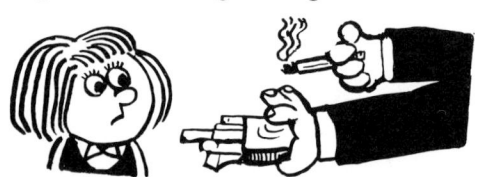

. . . people you don't know who ask you to go off with them.

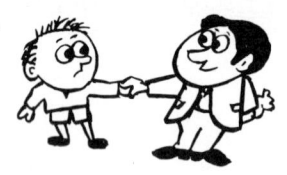

. . . people who want you to do stupid, dangerous things.

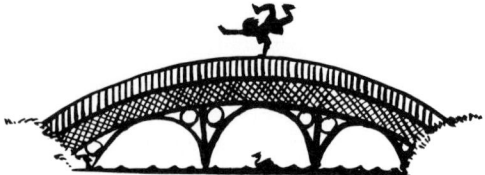

. . . frightening things you see on TV.

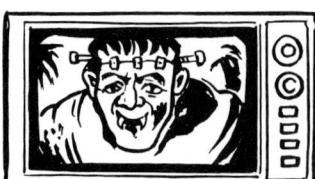

. . . ghosts, aliens, monsters, witches, gremlins.

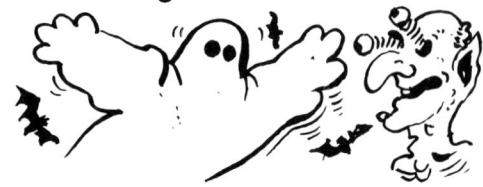

Keeping Myself Safe

My name is ....

How do accidents happen indoors?

Draw an accident in the kitchen.

Can you finish this poster?

Accidents happen in the kitchen when . . .

What made the accident happen?

Talk about other accidents which could happen there.

Write a keeping safe message for grown-ups who use the kitchen.

My keeping safe message to you is . . .

Write a keeping safe message for children who go into the kitchen.

My keeping safe message to you is . . .

Keeping Myself Safe

My name is ....

How do accidents happen on the road?

Draw a road accident in which someone on a bike has been hurt.

What made the accident happen?

Can you finish this poster?

Accidents happen to children on bicycles when . . .

Write a keeping safe message for children who ride bicycles.
My keeping safe message to you is . . .

_____

Can you think of some other places where an accident could happen?

_____

What do you think could make an accident happen there?

_____

What would your keeping safe message be?

_____   _____

Keeping Myself Safe

My name is ....

Keeping safe in different places

How would you keep yourself safe . . .

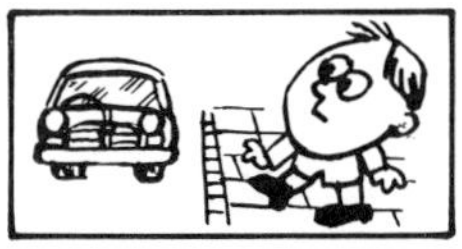

	. . . crossing the road?	....
	. . . on your bicycle?	....
	. . . by the river or canal?	....
	. . . in a crowd?	....
	. . . near the railway?	....
	. . . in the park?	....
	. . . out on your own?	....
	. . . out with your friends?	....
	. . . in the house on your own?	....

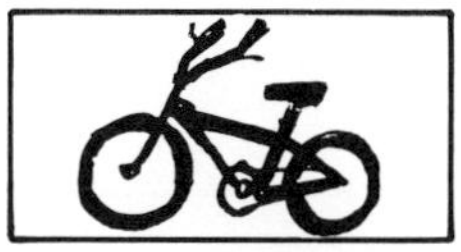

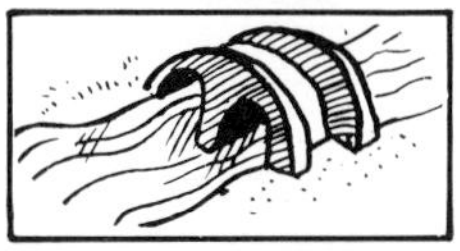

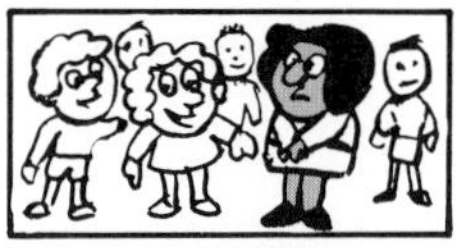

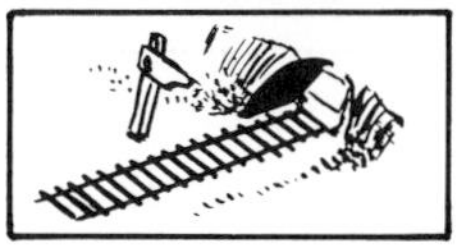

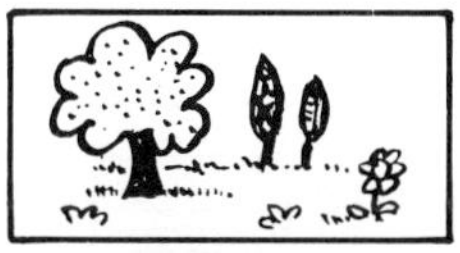

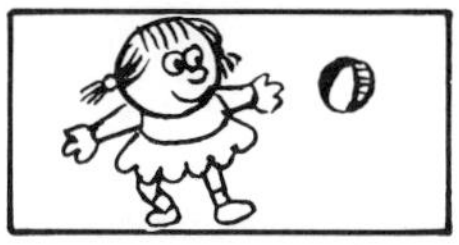

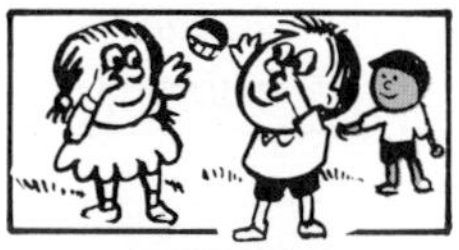

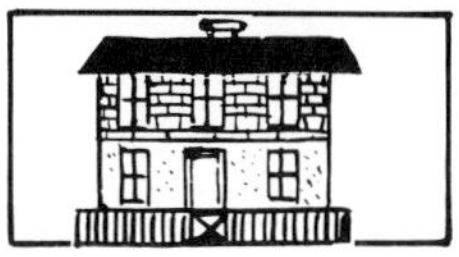

Here are some ideas to help you:

I can say 'No'

I think for myself

I keep the rules

I don't play about

I don't let people push me about

I say where I'm going

Keeping Myself Safe

My name is ....

Family Worksheet

16

Do's and don'ts

Accidents can happen on the stairs.
Can you make a list of do's and don'ts for keeping safe
on the stairs?

Do's	**Don'ts**
....	....
....	....
....	....
....	....
....	....
....	....

Choose another place and make a list of do's and don'ts.

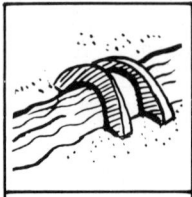
By the river or canal

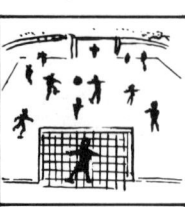
At the football match

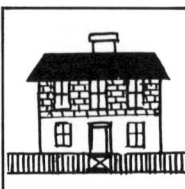
In the house alone

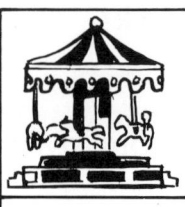
At the fair

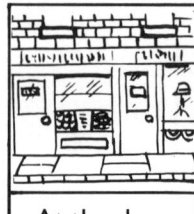
At the shops

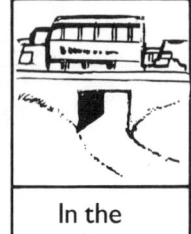
In the subway

Do's	**Don'ts**
....	....
....	....
....	....
....	....
....	....
....	....

Keeping Myself Safe

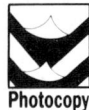
My name is ....

Keeping safe poster competition

The children in class 3 have been making posters about keeping safe.
You have been asked to be the judge. Look at all the posters carefully.
Which ones have the best keeping safe messages?

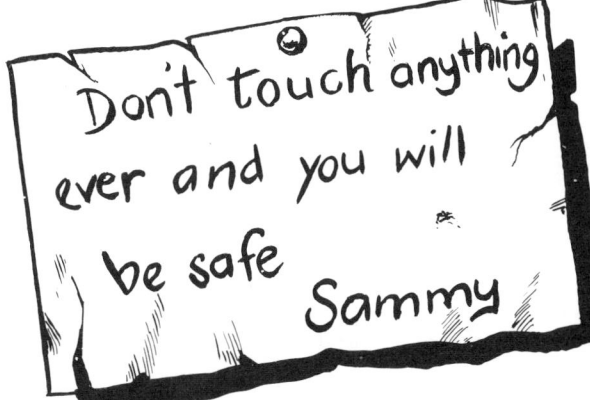

Don't touch anything ever and you will be safe   Sammy

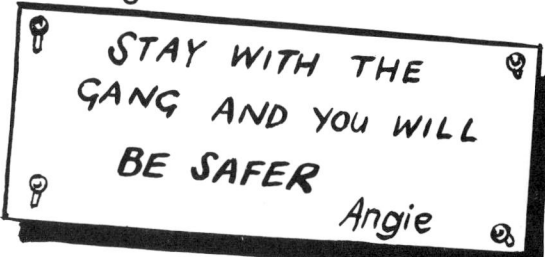

STAY WITH THE GANG AND YOU WILL BE SAFER   Angie

Always ask a grown up first   Rashid

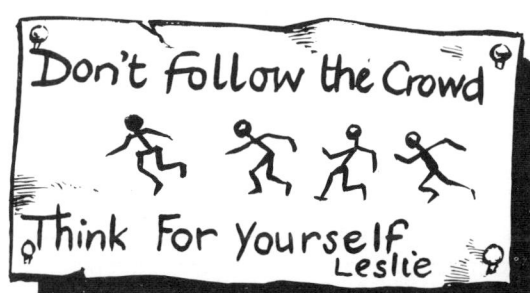

Don't Follow the Crowd   Think For Yourself   Leslie

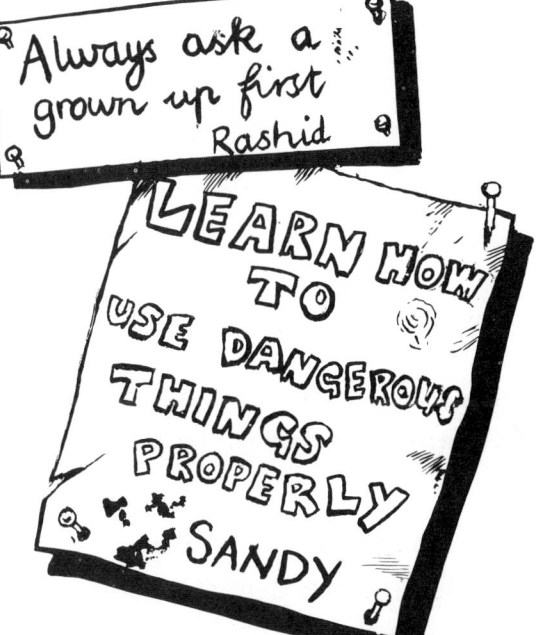

LEARN HOW TO USE DANGEROUS THINGS PROPERLY   SANDY

KNOW THE RULES OF THE PLACE AND KEEP THEM   Bobbie

First prize to:............................

because..

....

....

....

....

....

Second prize to:....................

because..

....

....

....

....

....

Keeping Myself Safe

My name is ....

What do people say to us about keeping safe?

Can you draw this picture?
Mum is mending the car. She
has left the children inside the
house. What would she say
to them about keeping safe?

Do	Don't
....	....
....	....
....	....
....	....
....	....

Can you draw this picture?

Dad is cooking the dinner.
The children are going to the
shop down the road. What
would he say to them about
keeping safe?

Do	Don't
....	....
....	....
....	....
....	....

Keeping Myself Safe

My name is ....

Photocopy

Whose job is it to keep you safe wherever you are?

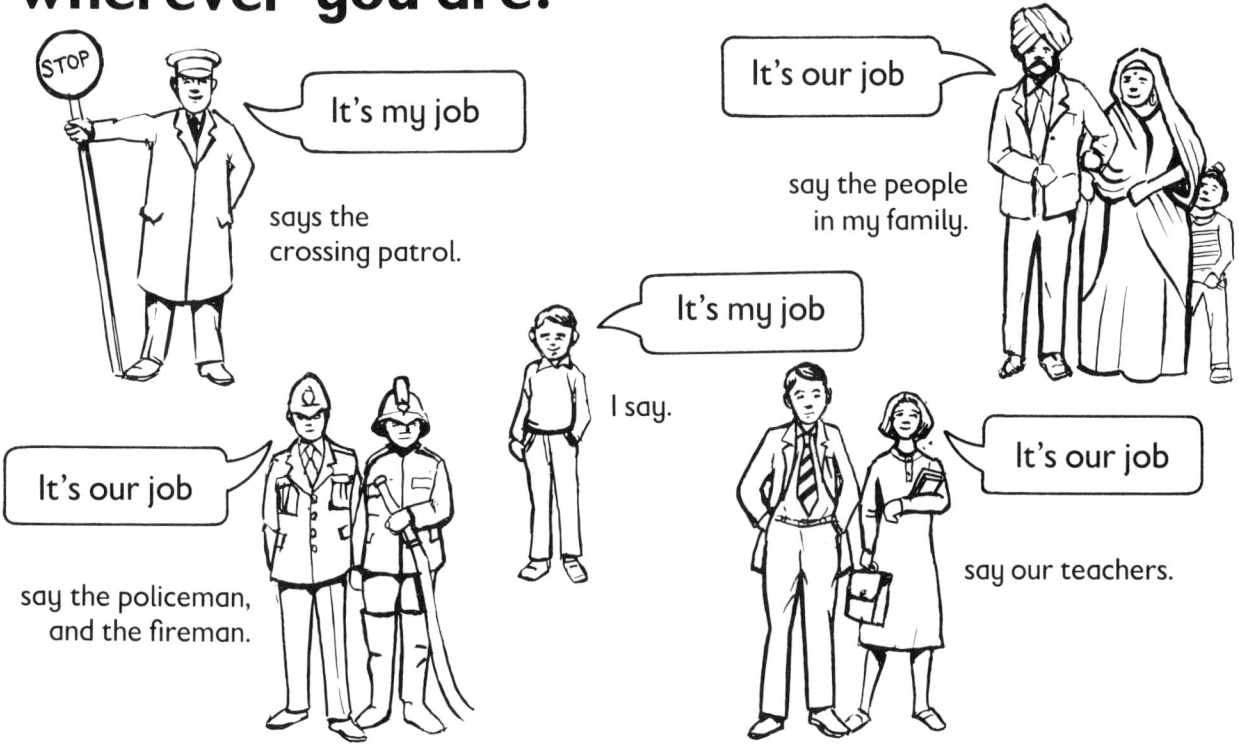

Can you think of any more? Draw them here. Say who they are.

I think the most important person is
because

I think the next most important person is
because

Photocopy

Keeping Myself Safe

My name is ....

Let's be safety experts

Try this safety experts test.
What would you say if you saw . . .

. . . a young child putting a cigarette in its mouth?

_____

. . . a bottle of pills with the lid off?

_____

. . . two children running across a busy road?

_____

. . . a friend going off in a car with a stranger?

_____

. . . your friends doing wheelies on their bikes down the main road?

_____

. . . some older people trying to make younger children smoke, sniff or taste something dangerous?

_____

Part Three
Me and My Relationships

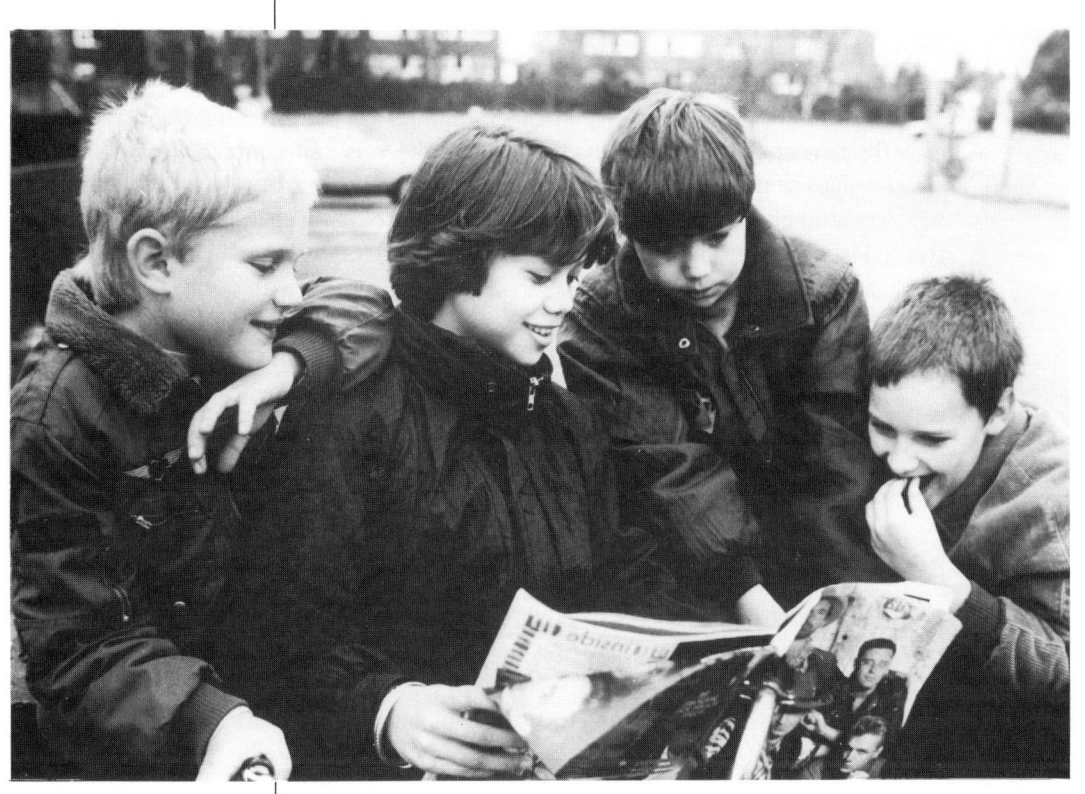

Introduction

Why we should teach children about relationships

When children come to school for the very first time they are embarking upon an important period of growth in their lives. Not only is this a period of intellectual growth, but equally important, it is a time when their rate of interaction with other children and adults will increase. Probably for the first time in their lives they are no longer the centre of attention – they have to share the teacher's attention with thirty or so classmates. They have begun to come to terms with the wider world of human and personal relationships.

The development of relationships with other people is a characteristic feature of what it means to be human. Our lives are continually influenced by the emotions stimulated by the networks of relationships we weave both consciously and unconsciously. Sometimes we are at the centre of these networks and at other times at the periphery, but we cannot easily avoid their effect upon us. Indeed, these 'memories' of past experiences help to shape our perception of ourselves and of the others to whom we relate. Relationships of various kinds, therefore, are central to our lives and it is unfortunate that the term 'having a relationship' has recently acquired sexual overtones. We have kept this in mind when framing the programme of work in this section and we have been guided very much by the children themselves.

The Health Education Authority's Primary School Project investigations showed how the perceptions of children change from the very self-centred view of relationships of the 4 and 5 year olds, to the 10 and 11 year olds' more sophisticated understanding of the need for reciprocity in relationships. We have the children's developing perceptions as a base line for teaching material in this book, and in this section we offer a range of classroom activities and family based work to encourage children to become more aware of their own networks and their places within them. The material also highlights how networks of relationships sometimes overlap, change and widen over time, often bringing tensions and difficulties which need to be resolved.

The following range of areas are explored in the material:

- making, breaking, ending and mending relationships.
- the role played by memory in the formation of self-image.
- loss, separation and grief.
- relationships with places and locations, including conservation, vandalism and pollution.
- attitudes to race, gender, special needs and age.
- aspects of child abuse.

While not offering a specific programme of sex education these materials do provide a supportive framework and context for its introduction. (For relevant materials see Appendix 2.) Under the Education (No 2) Act 1986, the governors of schools are responsible for deciding whether sex education should be given in their schools and in what form. Schools are advised to familiarise themselves with this Act and with the subsequent DES Circular 11/87 (Welsh Office 45/87) 'Sex Education at School'.

Clearly any work involving a closer look at relationships will need to be conducted with sensitivity and circumspection by the teacher, but with the help and involvement of their parents and families the children can develop deeper insights, skills and poise in their dealings with other people. In particular, teachers need to be sensitive to times when children are exposed to separation, temporary or permanent, for one or other member of their families due to divorce, death or some other cause.

The depth of understanding of the complexity of relationships demonstrated by children in the investigations was surprising. Children from the early years saw themselves as making people sad or happy by very specific acts, both through different kinds of behaviour and by the giving or withdrawal of material gifts. Specific activities continued to be important through to the age of 11. The growth of children's ability to generalise about the kinds of behaviour which affect relationships and to see the impact of their behaviour on other people was clearly indicated.

A surprising number of children associated happiness with a smiling face and indicated that the best way to make their special people happy was to entertain them. These indications persisted up to the age of 10 or 11. Although the largest percentage of children indicating this was in the 4 and 5 year old age group, it persisted throughout the age groups, gradually declining as the children grew older.

Children's awareness of love is particularly interesting. An important theme was the number of children for whom pleasing their special people, and being pleased by them, consists of the giving and receiving of love, expressed by hugs and kisses, etc.

Perhaps understandably the number of children who mentioned helping their special people as a way of making them happy grows throughout the age range with a significant leap between the ages of 6 and 9. When asked who was special to them, the children's responses varied from members of the nuclear family, to members of the wider family, or figures such as teachers, or Father Christmas or God. Some of the children's responses revealed complicated networks of relationships composed of stepfather, stepmother, half brother, half sister, 'uncle', 'two daddies', etc., but the children's ability to reflect on these and other differences in relationships was apparent. The responses showed something of the depth of the children's feelings about their 'special' people and although uninvited, some children expressed how they felt simply but starkly, for example, 'I love my Daddy', 'I hate my Mum'.

Relationships with friends, for instance, while important at every age, seem to have particular significance for the 4 and 5 year olds, approximately a quarter of whom listed them as people that are special to them. It seems likely that this may be due, in part, to the fact that they are choosing their own friends for the first time in their lives. Nearly half of the 6 and 7 year olds indicated in some form that their friends' willingness to play with them was what they liked most, and this kind of response continued through to the 10 and 11 year olds, although the number declined as the children grew older. Having someone to play with, and therefore avoiding the dreadful prospect of being alone or left out, is something that all children strive for.

As children grow older and become more independent friends are chosen without reference to parents. It may be that the giving and, especially, the receiving of gifts is tangible evidence of that friendship which is important at this stage. Around the age of 7 onwards children start to collect anything from conkers to toy cars, and will exchange and share these collections with friends. This is an important aspect of a maturing view of friendship.

Perhaps most interesting to note is the way in which children's perceptions of the qualities which constitute a true friend shift from those which serve to meet their egocentric needs to an understanding of the importance of character and personality in friendship. This is evident from the age of 8 onwards, but by 10 and 11 approximately half of the children indicate that these aspects are the most important. Mutual interests are also seen as significant, and the fun of friendship is also included.

Children develop and mature at different ages and stages but the study has revealed that they can understand from quite an early age that friendship involves both giving and taking, not just of material things, but of love, care, time and effort. In spite of their understanding about the qualities of friendship, the children still equated receiving gifts and being entertained with a happy relationship.

Taking on responsibility is an important theme. It develops slowly in the children's perception of making others happy yet it is there. A small sample of 4–7 year olds indicate 'independent' activities, such as 'going to the shops' or 'taking the dog for a walk' as those which make their parents cross, but from about the age of 7 and 8 onwards children are allowed more freedom and responsibility, and then they indicate that these activities please their parents.

The responses also revealed a universal respect for adult standards and requirements and an appreciation of the fact that to disobey will incur the wrath of parents and other adults. A rather sad note coming through the responses from children in every age group was that the best way to make their special people happy was 'to stay out of the way', or 'to go and watch TV' and 'be good'. Acts of disobedience, vandalism, stealing, telling lies, physical assault and accidental breakages were all things which made the children's special people cross.

Memories associated with family life grow in importance between the ages of 9 and 11. Some children demonstrated the ability to think in non-specific and abstract ways. They demonstrated clearly both their ability to remember what made them feel happy, and their wish to write or tell someone about these things.

There was a steady growth in the number of responses which showed the happiness of others making an occasion a happy one.

For the majority of the children in the sample, the saddest thing they could remember involved the death or loss of a close relative, or of someone they knew quite well, or of a much loved pet. 'When my Mum/Gran/Grandpa/Uncle/Aunt died' were typical responses, and many talked about 'when my Dad left home', 'when my Mum went away', and 'when my Mum and Dad separated'. The implications for teachers of the children's concern about death and loss are considerable because it became apparent that this is an area which generally remains unexplored by adults but which the children want and need to talk about.

Younger children appear to feel the effects of what other people do to them more keenly than any other group: 'when my mummy smacked me', 'when my friend broke with me', 'when my brother kicked me' were typical concerns of 4 and 5 year olds.

Indications that the children were saddened by the unhappiness of other people became more evident as the children grew older, and sometimes violent family rows were mentioned. Other people's illness or injury also made the children sad, although whether this is because they were genuinely saddened by the other's experience, or because they suffered in some way as a result, is unclear. What *is* clear is that children are acutely aware of their own sad feelings and increasingly understand some of the ways in which they can contribute to such feelings, both in themselves and others.

The study as a whole seemed to show that while there is considerable confusion amongst younger children between looking happy and being happy, between a momentary sensation and an established state, there is a growth in an understanding of what constitutes happiness, what contributes or detracts from it, and the importance of friendships and secure relationships as a major factor in achieving it.

Investigating children's perceptions of relationships in the classroom

Before beginning work on **the Me and My Relationships** activities, teachers might wish to use a Draw and Write Technique to discover the perceptions of the children in their class. This is the same investigation method adopted by the Project Team for their research. It is easy for the teacher to organise in the classroom, will reveal the children's knowledge of specific topics, and will provide a rich source of background knowledge from which starting points for the work will emerge. By using this technique before and after teaching the children it will be possible to chart their progress.

The analysis of the children's work can either be done quickly and simply to provide a quick overview of the children's perceptions, or extensively, to provide a detailed picture of their thoughts and ideas. Full details of this technique, suggestions for its administration and analysis are given in Appendix 1 on page 410.

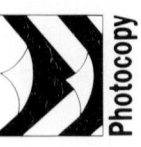

Me and My Relationships
Scope and Sequence Chart

Age	Children's changing perceptions of relationships	Suggested programme content	Suggested skills and strategies
4 & 5	We have both good and bad experiences with people. Our parents are our special people. We know we can make them happy, sad or angry by what we do. We don't really understand why they get worried when we try to be independent. When people ignore, tease or punish us we feel very sad or angry. We judge how adults feel by their facial expressions. We are aware of loss and separation. Our school friends are important to us because we choose them or are chosen by them.	Who loves me and helps me? Who are my special people? What makes them worried or cross? How can I show my special people I love them? How do they show me they love me? Why is my body special? What should I do if someone touches me and I don't like it? What should I say? Who can I ask for help? Who are my friends? What is good about having friends? Should I keep all secrets? How do I feel when a special person goes away? Where are my special places?	*Language skills:* Talking Listening Reading Writing Describing Recognising and naming Recording Categorising Illustration and presentation *General skills:* Observation Empathy Classroom play Decision making
6 & 7	We can use words like love, caring, and not caring to describe relationships	Who is special to me? How do we make each other sad or happy? What makes me	*Language skills:* Talking Listening

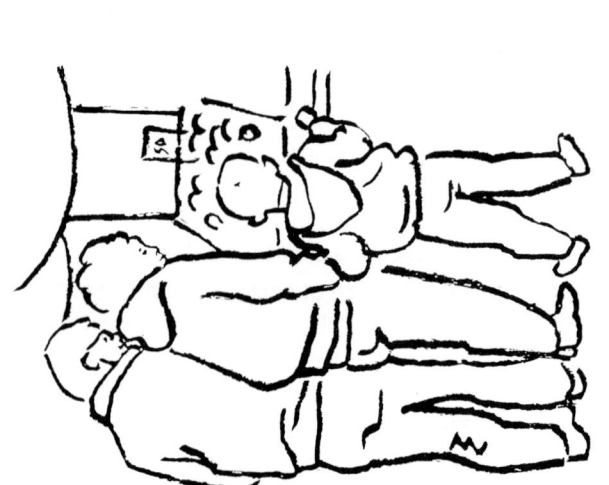

Classroom Strategies and Activities for Ages 4 – 11

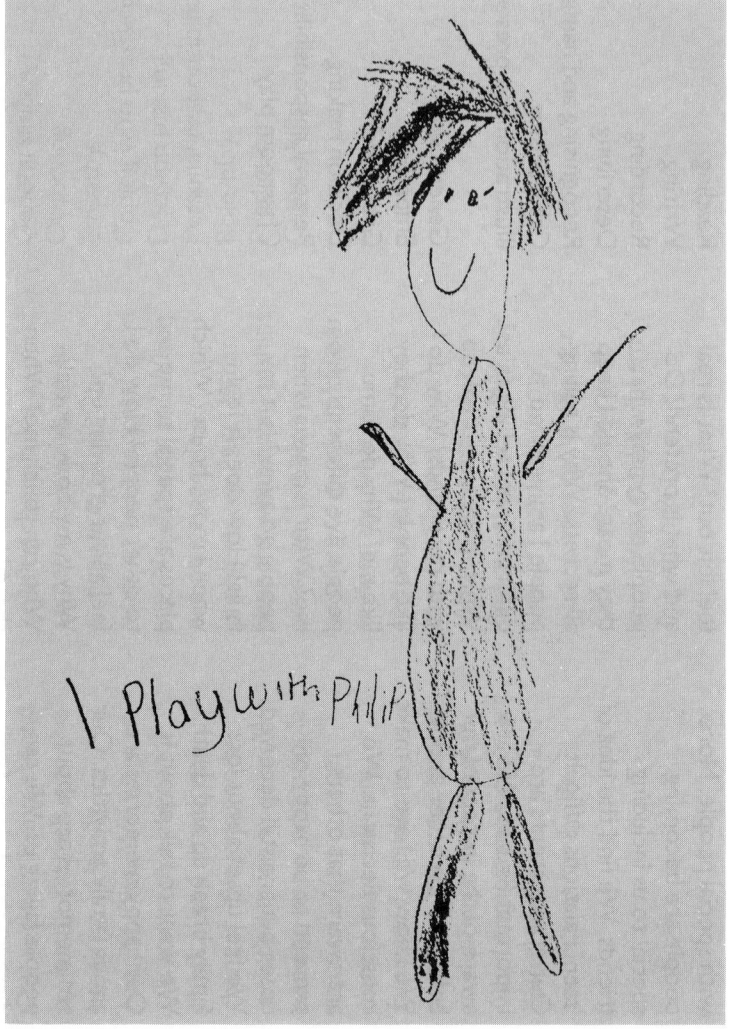

I Play with Philip

The activities in the following pages are based on the content boxes from the four Action planners for ages 4 and 5, 6 and 7, 8 and 9 and 10 and 11. There are five content boxes in each Action Planner, each of which has a distinctive theme, providing five themes which run through the activities:

Content box 1:   Focus on special people

Content box 2:   Focus on friends and friendship

Content box 3:   Focus on feelings

Content box 4:   Focus on memories and growing up

Content box 5:   Focus on special places

The content boxes suggest questions which are explored in detail in the activities. It is important that you select and modify these activities according to your needs. If you are devising your own programme on relationships you may be well aware of the health education priorities of your school and may already have selected the key themes you wish to explore with your pupils. If this is the case, you may find that the following activities are useful as examples, alternatively, you may wish to incorporate them as they stand in your programme.

4 & 5

Action Planner
Me and My Relationships

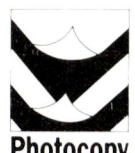

Photocopy

1 Focus on special people

What are the things I treasure most? When and how do I use them? How do I take care of them? How do I feel if I lose them or they get spoilt? How am I like other people? How am I different? How am I special? Who are my special people? What do my special people do to make me happy or angry? What do I do to make them happy or angry?

2 Focus on friends and friendship

Who are my friends? What do I like best about my friends? What do my friends like about me? Can grown-ups be my friends? Do I have to keep promises and secrets if my friends say so? How do I say 'No' to them? Are pretend friends OK – can a pet be a friend? How do I look after my friends?

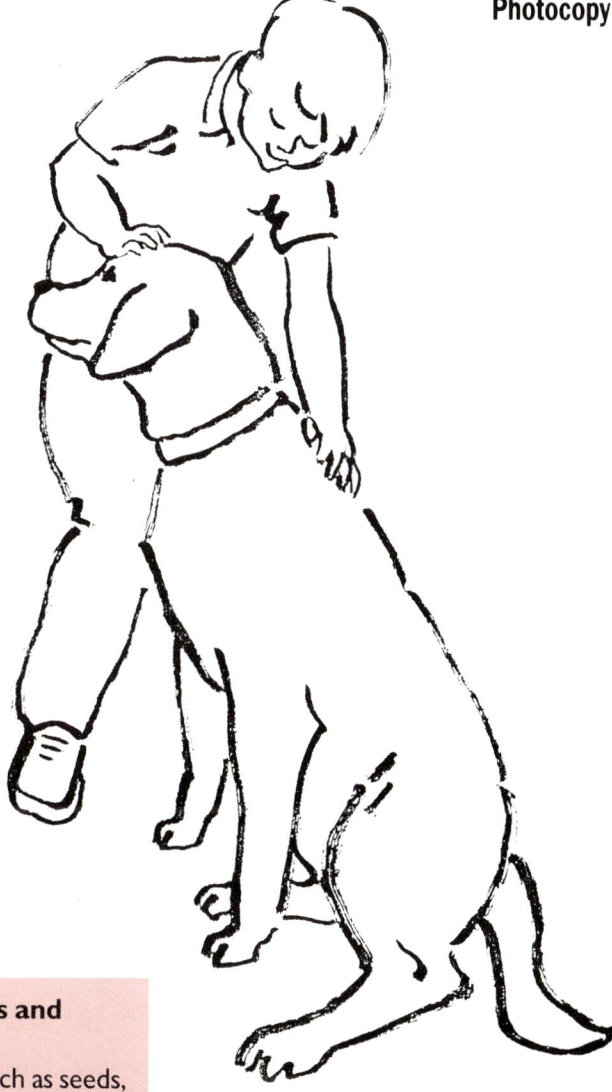

3 Focus on feelings

How can I tell how people are feeling? How can people tell how I am feeling? What kinds of things make me feel happy, sad or worried? Who and what makes us feel better? How do I feel when I lose something? How do I feel when my special people go away or die? Why don't people ask me how I feel? Who and what helps me when I feel like this?

4 Focus on memories and growing up

What makes things such as seeds, plants, animals and babies grow? What do they need to help them grow? What do I remember about being born and growing? What helped me to grow? What do other people remember about me? Do I remember the first time I did something? Who helped me? What is the happiest thing I remember? Who was there? Why was it so happy? Can my family and friends help me to remember things?

5 Focus on special places

Where are my special places in the classroom, at home and outside? What makes them special? What do I do there? Am I on my own, or with people? Is it safe to be there? Who knows I'm there? Is it a happy place? What keeps places special and happy? How can I help to keep my special places happy, healthy, clean and safe?

Classroom Strategies and Activities for Ages 4 and 5

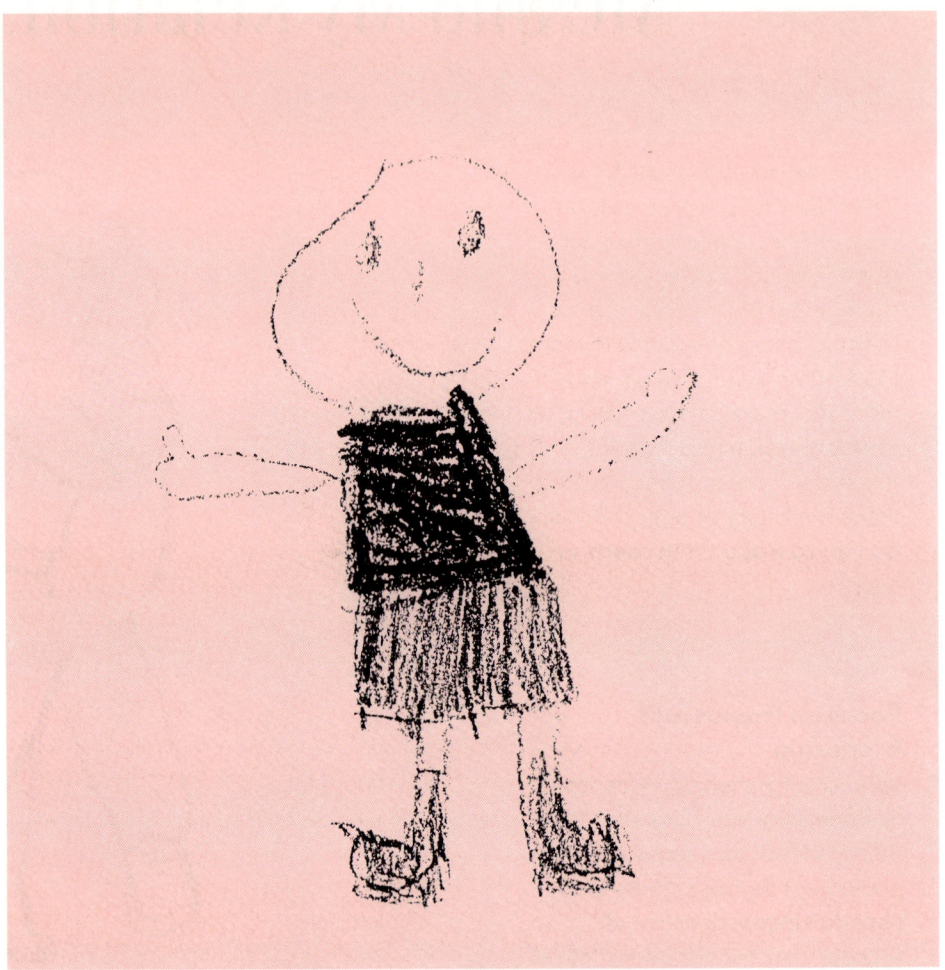

Key messages ● *Learn:*

- how to find and tell a safe person if people hurt and bully you.

- how to say 'No' if people touch you and you don't like it.

- to respect other people's special places.

- to talk to your special people about how you feel.

Understand:

- that just as your special people make you happy, sad or worried, you do the same to them.

- that most special people love and care for you all the time and will always help you.

- that when special people go away or die it may be very sad but it is not your fault.

- that people are born, grow up and grow old.

- that there is only one of you and that makes you very special.

Content box 1   Focus on special people

 What are the things I treasure most? When and how do I use them? How do I take care of them? How do I feel if I lose them or they get spoilt? How am I like other people? How am I different? How am I special? Who are my special people? What do my special people do to make me happy or angry? What do I do to make them happy or angry?

Activity 1 ● ***What are the things I treasure most?***

- Talking together. Display. Drawing. Writing.

- Class or group and individual activities.

Ask the children to help to make and display a collection of special things, both personal and classroom treasures, for example, a new toy, an old and much loved toy, a photograph, some shells, a stick, a tin, a special piece of clothing, a book, a 'jewel'.

Invite the children to name and talk about these treasures as they are collected. Ask them to try to put into words what it is that makes seemingly ordinary things special to someone: point out the ones which are shiny and new and easily recognised as 'treasures', and the ones which are old, worn out and broken, but are still valued.

The items could be labelled, for example: 'This is special to Alice', and grouped, for example: 'These are old', 'These are new' etc. Talk with the children about their treasures: Where do they come from? When do the children need or want them? Do they share them, hide them, or keep them for their own use?

Ask the children to talk, draw and write (using you as their 'scribe' as necessary) about the way they take care of their treasures. How do they keep them safe? How do they feel if they lose them or they are thrown away? How can they explain to other people that these things are so special?

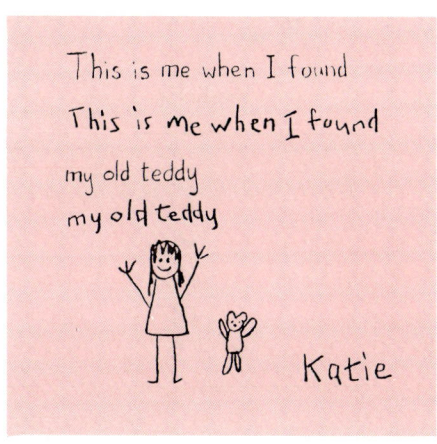

Activity 2 ● *How am I special?*

- Talking together. Drawing and painting. Family work.

- Class or group and individual activities.

Talk with the children about their classroom. How is it different in appearance from other classrooms? How is it different because of the people in it? What happens there? Look with the children at the people in the class who make us smile, laugh, bring things to show us, tell good stories, and jokes, sing, help, paint exciting pictures and look after the plants and animals.

Invite the children to contribute paintings, drawings and photographs of themselves and to help you make a collage on the theme of 'our class'.

Ask the children to try to think what is special about each person in the class, for example, their names, what they are good at, what they like doing, etc.

Talk with the children about the things they can do for themselves, and about the things they are getting better at. These can either be practical or emotional achievements, for example, not getting upset. This activity could be extended through **family work**, to include the things children are learning to do, or need help with, out of school.

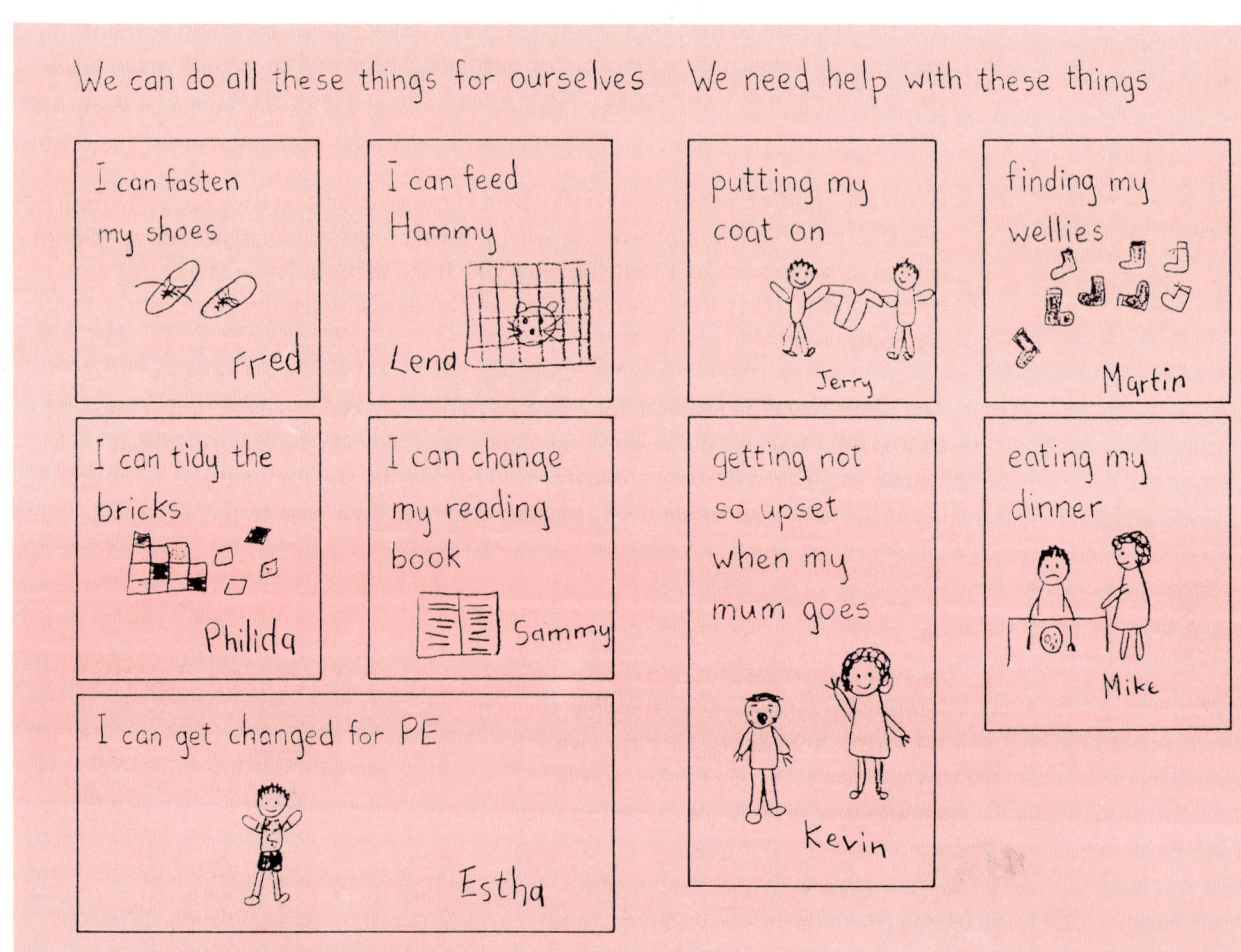

Activity 3 ● *Who are my special people?*

- Talking together. Drawing. Writing. Language work. Family work.

- Class or group and individual activities.

This is a way of introducing the children to the idea of themselves at the centre of a network of special people (who also have their own networks).

Talk with the children about all the people who are special to them. Ask them to draw and label them. Invite them to tell their group or class about their special people: at home, at school or elsewhere. What do they do together? What do they share? What do they say to them? How often do they see them? What do they look like? How do they speak, etc.

Help children to make their own books or charts about themselves and their network. These could be displayed or shared so that the children can see that, while they are often similar to each other, each of them is unique.

There are **cross-curricular links** with language work here.

Extend the children's vocabulary of relations and relationships by providing them with opportunities to talk about their extended families, including the people they have left behind and the people who are new.

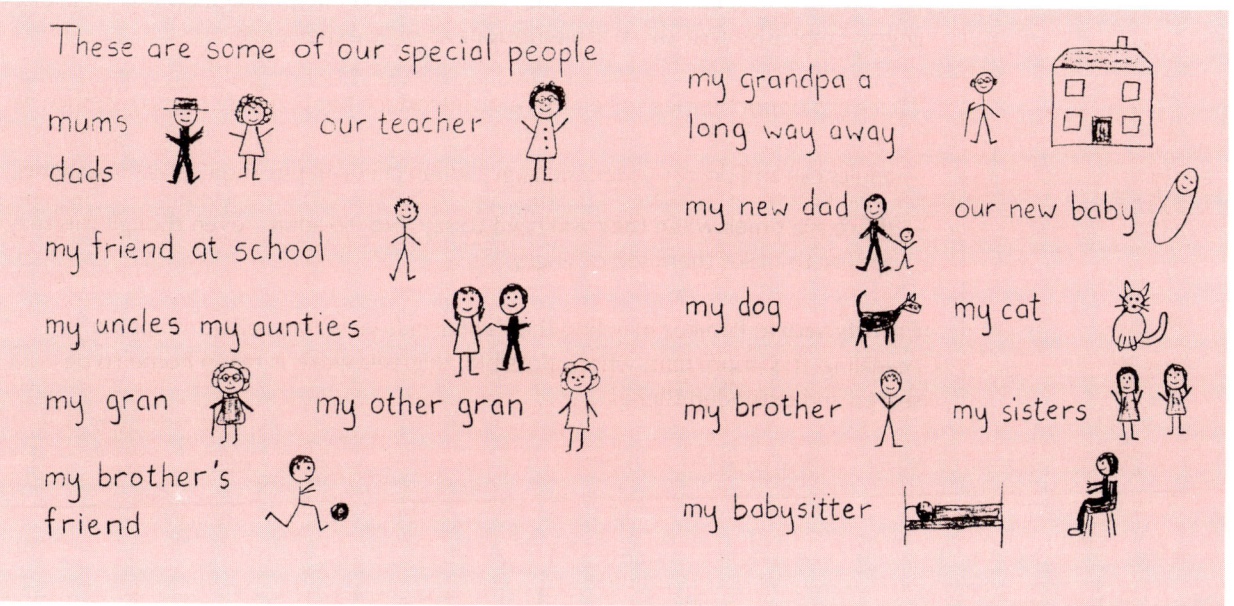

Ask the children this question: 'What do your special people do to make you happy?'. Their answers may focus on material things, such as, giving presents and sweets, or be more concerned with playing together, loving, caring, not teasing or not getting cross. Next, you could explore what the children think their special people do to make them upset, sad or angry. This is an opportunity to widen the vocabulary the children use to describe their feelings, and to deepen their understanding of the impact of other people's behaviour on themselves. Opportunities may arise for children to reveal experiences which frightened or threatened them or made them uneasy.

Invite the children to talk about their special people, or person, and what they do to make their special people happy. Record the children's ideas in a way that enables their views to be easily shared among the children and their families.

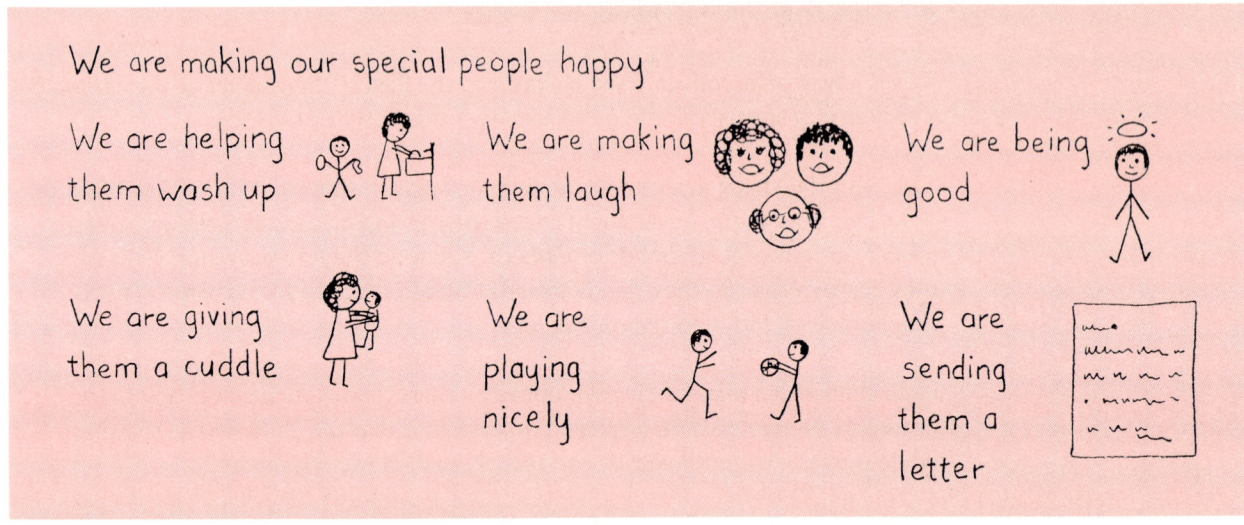

This could be an opportunity to explain that pressure from people, special or otherwise, to make them happy in ways which cause the children distress must be resisted and reported.

Explore what the children think they do to make their special people sad, upset or angry. Emphasise that these are emotions all of us experience.

There are opportunities to reinforce or introduce keeping safe messages, such as:

— adults can and do get upset and angry when children put themselves in danger.

— there are times when they will have to say 'No' to adults, even though this may appear to make them sad or angry.

Family work: families may find their children's views on relationships very revealing. It is important, where possible, that this work is taken home to be shared and extended there.

Content box 2 Focus on friends and friendship

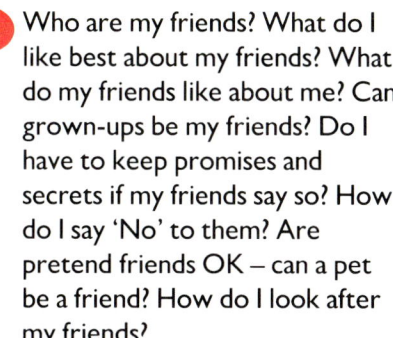 Who are my friends? What do I like best about my friends? What do my friends like about me? Can grown-ups be my friends? Do I have to keep promises and secrets if my friends say so? How do I say 'No' to them? Are pretend friends OK – can a pet be a friend? How do I look after my friends?

Activity 1 ● *Who are my friends?*

- Talking together. Drawing. Family work. Links with literature.
- Class or group and individual activities.

The opportunity to choose one's own friends is an important step in the first years of school. Some children may previously have been told or expected to make friends without being given any choice. Others may have been told that the arrival of a new baby or new brothers and sisters will mean having new friends and this may not have been so. It can be helpful to children to begin to explore their own views of what a friend is and does, and what friendship means.

Imaginary or fictional friends may have been, or may still be, part of the children's fantasy life, and this can be a starting point for exploring aspects of friendship. **Cross-curricular links** with literature: many picture story books, stories and poems for young children have friendship as a theme, featuring both real and imaginary friends. Children will enjoy thinking about the stories to discover why a character needed or wanted a friend, whether or not that friend was found, whether or not it was a real or imaginary friend, the difference which the friendship made, etc.

Invite the children to ask their families if they had imaginary friends when they were young.

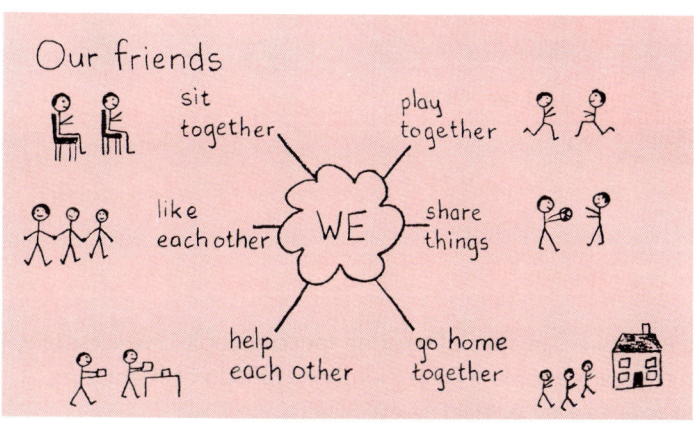

Invite the children to draw the friends they have at school, and to talk about them. Who are they? What do they do together? What do they share with them? Help them to make a 'friendship chart'. The children could contribute their own illustrations, or pictures from magazines, to the chart.

Ask the children what they like best about their friends. (Answers are likely to include aspects of appearance and personality.) A more difficult, but important question to ask them is: 'What do your friends like about you?' In answering this question, the children will have opportunities to reinforce positive images of themselves as people who are valued. For example: 'I always play with her', 'I wait for him', 'I'm good at helping him', 'I lend him my things', 'I make him laugh', 'She likes me'.

Activity 2 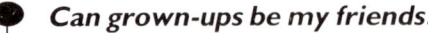 *Can grown-ups be my friends?*

- Talking together. Literature.
- Class or group activity.

Explore with the children the idea of having grown-ups as friends. Include people inside and outside their network of special people, and people met on a more informal basis. Talk about what makes these people so special. What do they do with the children? (For example, do they take them out on special occasions?) Where do they go? What makes them special friends? Could they go to them if they were lost or upset?

Our grown up friends

The crossing lady
She knows our names
She talks to us when
she sees us in Tesco
She keeps her things
at school

My big brother
Alexander He
takes me to see
football and he
buys me a hot dog

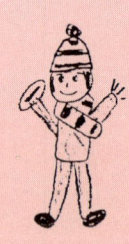

My aunty Rose next door
She babysits me and
we stay up late. I keep
it a secret

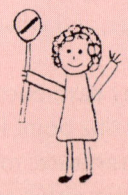

Mrs Kalinsky
She takes us to
church in the
minibus every
week and sings
all the time

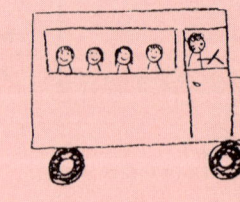

My uncle Phil
He takes me fishing
He lets me do it .
I'm good at it

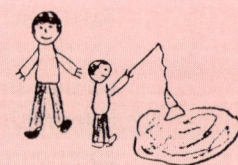

This could be a time to introduce the idea of trusting special people. For example, special people they can trust are people who are kind, are fun, don't frighten or threaten them and who stop teasing or tickling etc. when asked.

The children could go on to explore what these special grown-up friends help them to do, for example, learn and see new things. What do the grown-ups ask them to do? For example, keep secrets. How does this make the children feel grown up? This would be a good time to look at keeping secrets, and promises. (See Keeping Myself Safe, page 134–5.)

Explore with the children the times when apparent friends turn out to be not such good friends after all. **Cross-curricular link**: children's literature can provide a good starting point here.

Some children may want to talk about times when people turned out to be not such good friends, they may have broken their promises, threatened, bullied or abused them in some way.

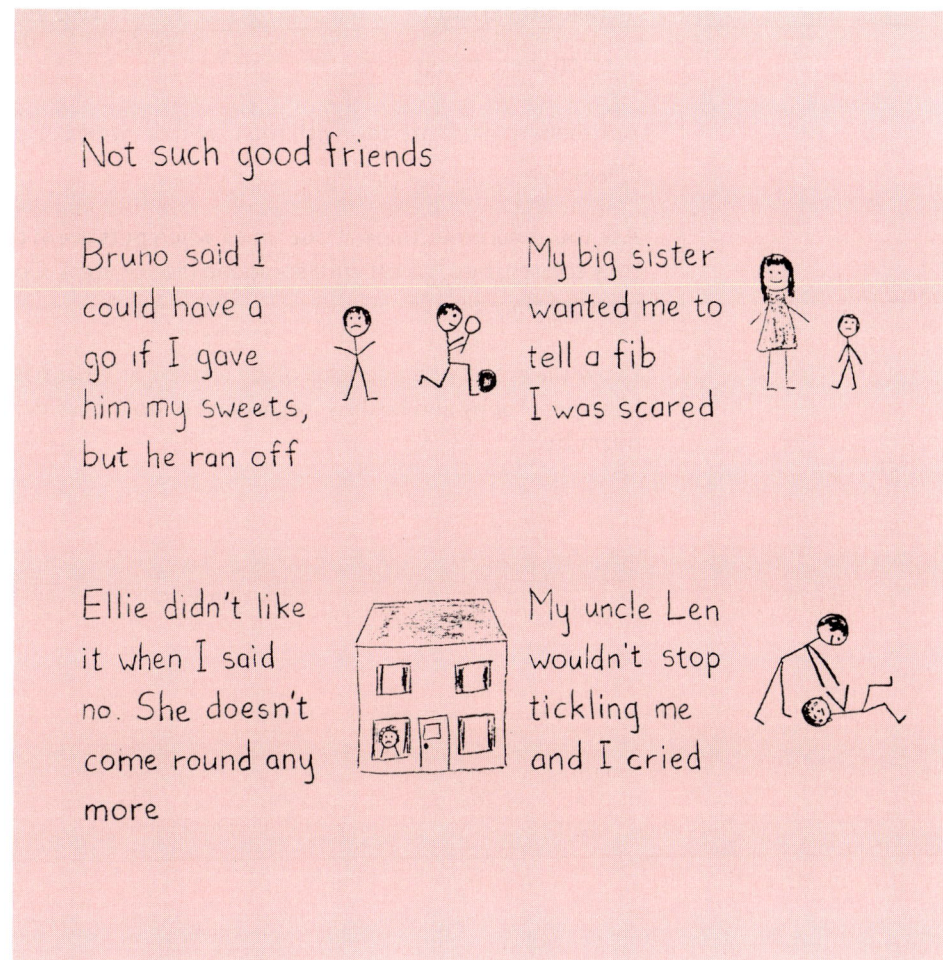

Not such good friends

Bruno said I could have a go if I gave him my sweets, but he ran off

My big sister wanted me to tell a fib I was scared

Ellie didn't like it when I said no. She doesn't come round any more

My uncle Len wouldn't stop tickling me and I cried

Activity 3 ● *Can a pet be a friend?*

- Talking together. Drawing or painting. Collecting and sorting pictures.
- Class or group and individual activities.

Invite the children to talk about domestic and classroom pets. Who looks after them? When? How? Ask them if they know of people in the neighbourhood who have pets, particularly people who live alone and have a pet as a companion.

Remind the children of all the things they said that they could do and enjoy with their friends. Can pets do the same things, or more? For example:

You can:	Pets can:
— play with them.	— make you laugh.
— talk to them.	— listen to you.
— cuddle them.	— love you.
— share sweets.	— look after you.
— go out with them.	— keep you company.
— stay in with them.	— play with you.
— look after them.	— make you cross.
— teach them things.	

Ask them to illustrate this with their own drawings or paintings or pictures from magazines.

Ask the children to think about times when pets seem to be bad friends: when they scratch, bite, go off with someone else or steal. Contrast this with the fun and pleasure they give us.

Draw the activity to a conclusion by looking at what has to be done every day to keep pets happy and healthy, regardless of how busy or tired the pet's owners might be.

Content box 3   Focus on feelings

How can I tell how people are feeling? How can people tell how I am feeling? What kinds of things make me feel happy, sad or worried? Who and what makes us feel better? How do I feel when I lose something? How do I feel when my special people go away or die? Why don't people ask me how I feel? Who and what helps me when I feel like this?

Activity 1

How can I tell how people are feeling?

- Talking together. Drawing and painting. Collecting pictures. Display.
- Class or group and individual activities.

A useful resource for exploring and deepening children's understanding of feelings and emotions is a collection of pictures of people laughing, crying, looking sad, worried, angry, lonely, frightened etc. This collection can be a starting point for small group activities, in which children are encouraged to talk about some of the pictures, thus increasing their vocabulary for describing emotions.

Invite them to sort the pictures into groups, using their own criteria to do this. Provide labels for each group for example 'These are laughing faces'. The children could add to this collection with pictures they have painted, photographs and pages from magazines etc.

Explore in mime and movement the facial expressions and body language of laughter, sadness, unhappiness, anger, fright etc.

Invite the children to paint pictures of themselves or other people showing some of these feelings and to display these as a wall story or collage.

Talk with the children about times when they have felt like this. Discuss when and why they feel like that. When they felt unhappy, what made them feel better?

Activity 2

How do I feel when I lose something?

- Talking together. Classroom play.
- Class or group activities.

Suggest themes for the playhouse or play area on losing something, for example, a pet, a toy, a parcel or something special and important. Encourage the children to reflect on some of their feelings when they discovered a loss. What do they say? How is the problem solved?

Write for the children a circle of feelings, using speech bubbles, based on this activity. Invite the children to illustrate it, using pictures from the collection they made in Activity 1, or their own drawings and paintings.

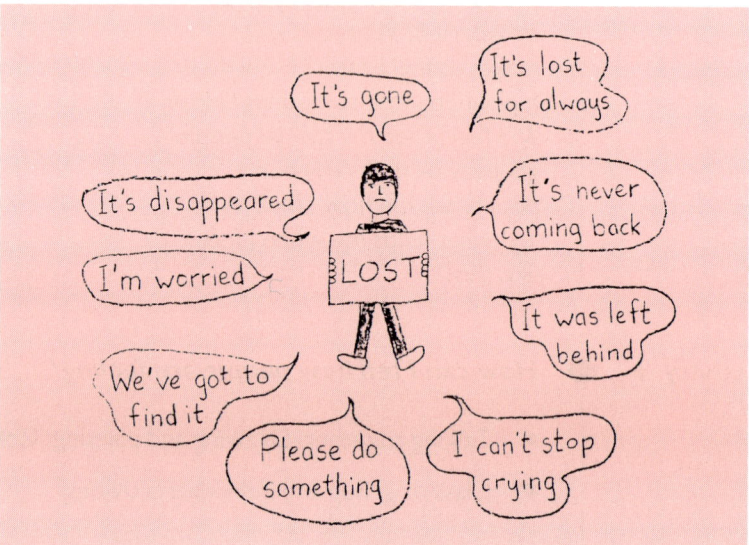

Encourage the children to talk about how they feel when their special people leave them or go away for some reason (permanently or temporarily or die). This is particularly important since many young children in situations such as these may be excluded or protected from expressions of grief, or given compensatory presents to distract them. This can result in feeling they have been left out of something important, and leave them with many unanswered questions, such as: 'Was it my fault?'

Talk with them about what makes them feel better. Responses might include:

'My dad told me what had happened. We had a cry together.'
'My granny gave me a big hug.'
'My best friend said I could stay over at her house'.
'I told my teacher about it and she was sad too.'
'My Uncle Fred said I would feel better soon'.
'My Mum said it wasn't my fault.'

Content box 4   Focus on memories and growing up

● What makes things such as seeds, plants, animals and babies grow? What do they need to help them grow? What do I remember about being born and growing? What helped me to grow? What do other people remember about me? Do I remember the first time I did something? Who helped me? What is the happiest thing I remember? Who was there? Why was it so happy? Can my family and friends help me to remember things?

Activity I ● ***What makes things grow? What makes me grow?***

- ● Talking together. Drawing. Collecting pictures.

- ● Class or group and individual activities.

Cross-curricular link: this part of the work links with early science activities in which children can be encouraged to observe and categorise living things as they change and grow.

Look at growing things in and around the school and classroom: seeds, plants, animals, the children themselves. Are any of the children expecting the birth of a baby brother or sister? This might be a good time to talk about how new babies are born and cared for. Make a note of the children's ideas of what makes these things grow. Sort them into groups and help the children to illustrate them.

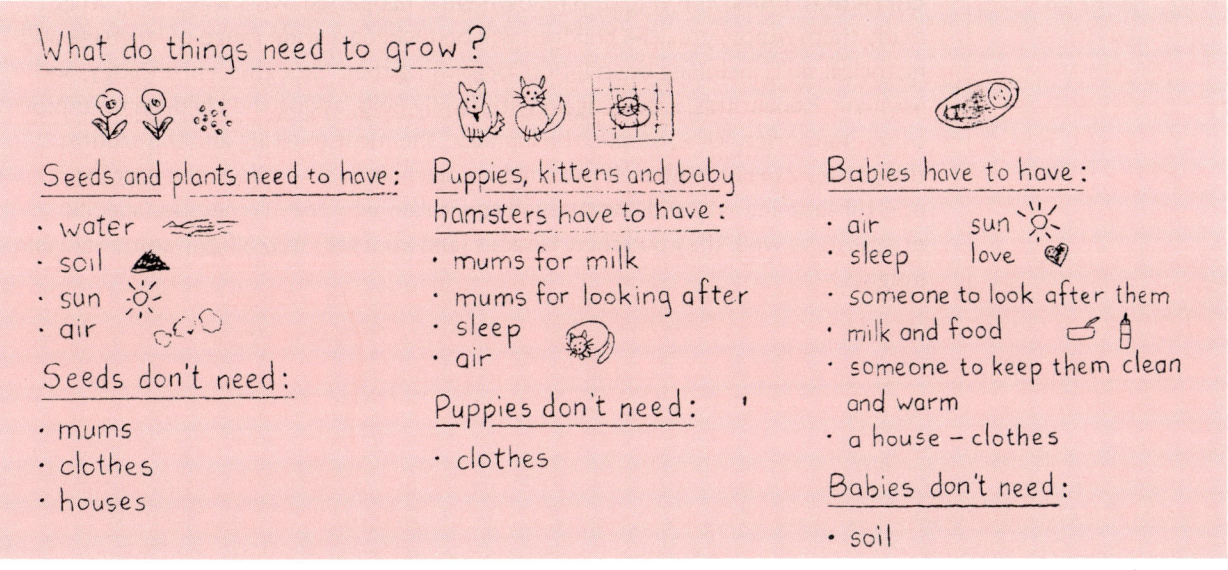

What do things need to grow?

Seeds and plants need to have:
- water
- soil
- sun
- air

Seeds don't need:
- mums
- clothes
- houses

Puppies, kittens and baby hamsters have to have:
- mums for milk
- mums for looking after
- sleep
- air

Puppies don't need:
- clothes

Babies have to have:
- air   sun
- sleep   love
- someone to look after them
- milk and food
- someone to keep them clean and warm
- a house – clothes

Babies don't need:
- soil

Invite the children to make a collection of pictures of babies and young children. They could include photographs of themselves, or their own drawings of themselves, when they were small. Display these as a starting point for talking about their memories of the people involved in helping them to grow up. What did people do to help them? For example, loving, caring, protecting, teaching and providing.

Activity 2 ● *What do I remember about being born and growing?*

- Talking together. Family work. Writing. Drawing. Language work.

- Class or group and individual activities.

Ask the children if they can remember being born or *before* they were born. (Some children will be certain they can, and these memories, if shared, can be very illuminating.)

Ask them if they can remember being in cots, prams or pushchairs. Do they remember learning to walk, talk, feed themselves, dress and undress, going on trains and buses, going to playgroup or the child minder, the nursery or hospital? Who was with them?

Family work: where appropriate, invite members of the children's families to contribute their memories of the child growing up. Memory and other people's memories form an important part of a person's sense of identity.

Exploring this aspect of growing up, can help each child to begin to be aware of the network of relationships he or she is involved in, and the place he or she holds in that network.

The children could make a class book, or set of books, of these memories.

Family work: ask the children and their families to remember some of their happiest moments. Encourage the children to share these memories. **Cross-curricular links**: in trying to pin down what happened, who was there, what made them happy, etc., the children will be tackling a wide range of language and historical skills including description, organising their thoughts, chronology, and listening. Repeat this activity again with family help, asking the children to explore other memories, for example, the funniest, the most exciting and the saddest things they can remember. If the children are helped to explore the past in a non-threatening way and encouraged to explain why they remember specific occasions so well, they and their families (and yourself) may all gain some valuable insights.

Content box 5   Focus on special places

Where are my special places in the classroom, at home and outside? What makes them special? What do I do there? Am I on my own, or with people? Is it safe to be there? Who knows I'm there? Is it a happy place? What keeps places special and happy? How can I help to keep my special places happy, healthy, clean and safe?

Activity 1   *Where are my special places?*

- Talking together. Drawing. Writing. Links with literature.

- Class or group and individual activities.

This part of the work has **cross-curricular links** with environmental studies and children's literature. A useful starting point would be a story or poem about animals who have their own special places to live in, hide in, or retreat to. Ask the children about the special places where their pets sleep. Ask them where their own special or favourite places are and why. Start with areas in the classroom, for example, by the radiator, in the playhouse, in the book corner etc.

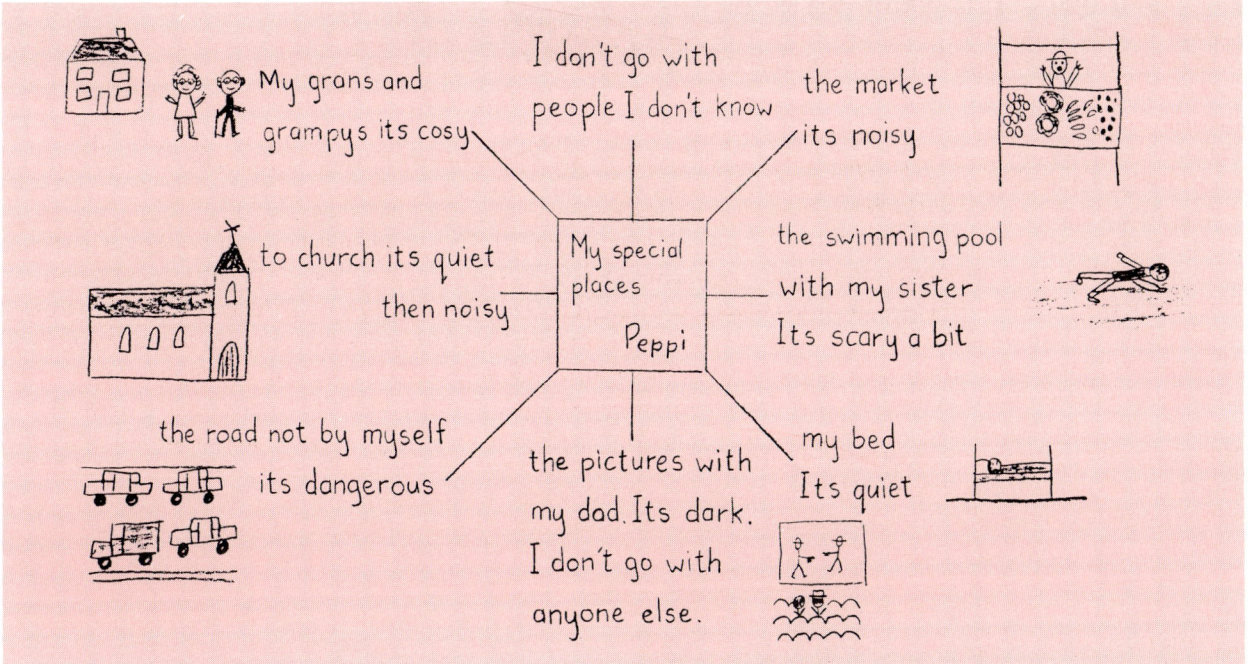

Ask the children where their other special places are, for example, at home, in the playground, in the neighbourhood. Talk with the children about what makes these places special and safe. Who takes them there and what do they do? Which people would they not go with? Ask the children to put this information on to individual charts. Write for them as necessary. Encourage them to take these home, and ask their families to add to them with drawing or writing.

Explore with the children what they do in their special places. What do they enjoy most? What makes the place a happy one? In what ways can they, or other people, make their special places happy, clean, tidy and safe?

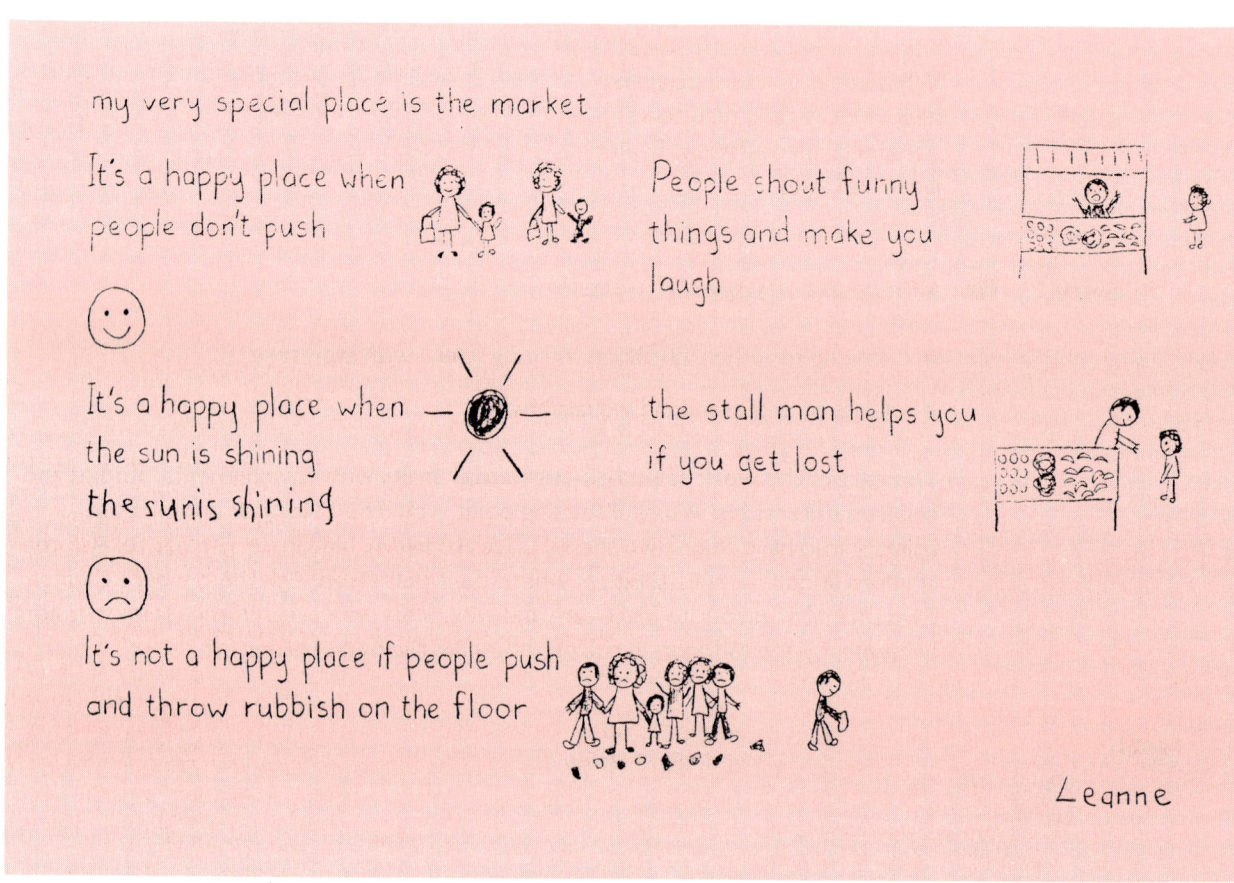

my very special place is the market

It's a happy place when people don't push

People shout funny things and make you laugh

It's a happy place when the sun is shining
the sun is shining

the stall man helps you if you get lost

It's not a happy place if people push and throw rubbish on the floor

Leanne

6 & 7 Action Planner
Me and My Relationships

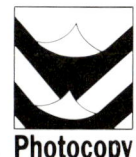

Photocopy

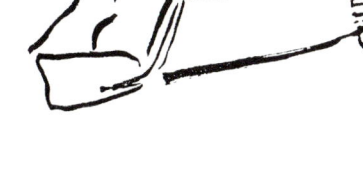

1 Focus on special people

Who are my special people? What do we do together? How do I know when people are special to me? How do we tell each other we are special? How do my special people and I make each other happy? How do they make me feel clever, excited, safe, or hurt? When is it OK to say 'No'? Who can I tell if saying 'No' is difficult? When is it OK to pretend and when is it dangerous? Do grown-ups pretend sometimes?

2 Focus on friends and friendship

What is a friend? Who are my best friends or my oldest friends? When have friends helped me? What good bargains have we made with our friends? What are bad bargains? How do I make friends? How can I get to know what people are really like? How do I feel when things get broken? How do I feel when friendships are broken? How can people stay friends? Are pretend people, or people from television programmes or stories, friends? What can I do about real people who might pretend?

3 Focus on feelings

When have I felt too excited to sleep or eat? Why did I feel this way? When did I feel this way? When have I felt bullied, upset, angry or scared? How did I cope? How do people look when they are angry? What happens when people around me quarrel? Do they mean what they say? How do I feel after I quarrel with someone? How do I feel when I am left out? How do I feel when my special people go away or die? How can I tell people how I feel?

4 Focus on memories and growing up

What are my special belongings? Who is allowed to touch them? Is my body one of these special belongings? Who is allowed to touch it? What is the difference between hurting my knee and hurting my feelings? What makes these hurts better? How can I help people feel better? What can I remember about growing up? What were the funniest, saddest or noisiest times? Who shares my memories?

5 Focus on special places

What makes some places special to me? What makes our classroom special? How do we keep it looking and feeling good? What spoils it? How do we feel if places are dirty or broken up? Where do I feel happy and safe? Which are the places I wouldn't go to? Which places are special to other people, or our pets? What can we do to keep their places happy for them?

Classroom Strategies and Activities for Ages 6 and 7

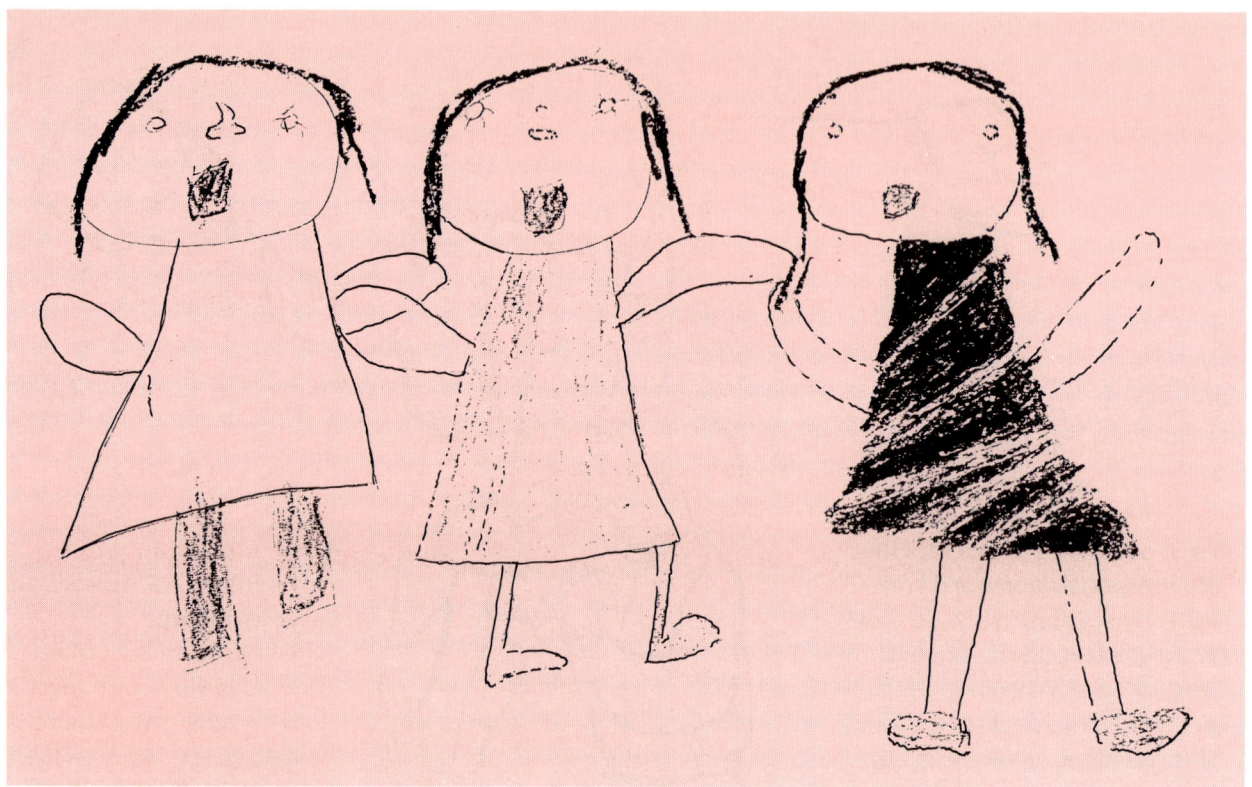

Key messages ● *Learn:*

- the names of your special people, both the names you know them by and the names they use for each other.

- how to make people feel better.

- how to tell a safe person you are frightened or worried.

- how to say 'No' if someone hurts or frightens you.

- about making friends and sharing things with your friends.

- to help people who don't have friends.

- that other people may live lives which are different from yours.

- that when we move house we have to build up another network of friends which can be hard.

- to respect other people's things and places.

Understand:

- that as you make more friends it is as if a network of people grows around you.

- that the people in your network are special to one another in different ways and sometimes you may feel left out.

- that you and the people in your network can make each other happy, sad or angry, but you can also make each other feel better.

- that people pretend or cover up their feelings sometimes in order not to worry you.

- that if pretending or keeping secrets is frightening you must tell someone you trust – it is not the same as 'telling tales'.

- that friendships can be broken but that they can also be mended again.

- that just as you like people for their qualities so they will like you for your qualities.

- that sometimes your family will not like your friends, and although this is worrying, it is best to talk about it.

- that when people in your network go away or die it is not your fault, it may be for reasons you don't understand.

- that babies are born, grow into children and become women and men, and we have to help the younger ones.

- that your body is your very own. Take care of it and keep it healthy and safe.

Content box 1   Focus on special people

Who are my special people? What do we do together? How do I know when people are special to me? How do we tell each other we are special? How do my special people and I make each other happy? How do they make me feel clever, excited, safe, or hurt? When is it OK to say 'No'? Who can I tell if saying 'No' is difficult? When is it OK to pretend and when is it dangerous? Do grown-ups pretend sometimes?

Activity I   ●   *Who are my special people?*

● Talking together. Drawing and painting. Collage. Links with literature.

● Class or group and individual activities.

The children could take as their starting point the central character from a story which you have read to them. With the children's help draw the character's network of special people.

Talk with the children about how the characters in the story related to one another? Which people knew each other? Who knew about each other but never met? Who didn't know about the others? Explore how the central character might have felt if people in the network had not liked each other.

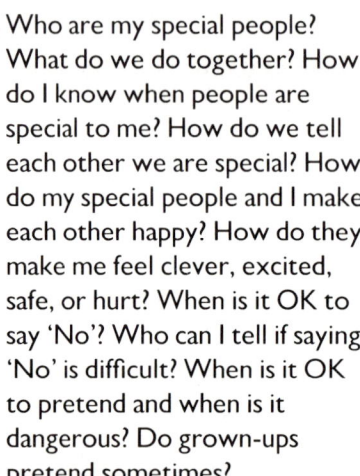

Grondpa's adventure
· Grandpa knew them all
· Grandma didn't know Barny or Tenko
· Grandma knew Jo, Jenny and the paper boy
· Tenko didn't know anyone but Grandpa
· Grandma wouldn't like Barny and Tenko
· Jo and Jenny would like Barny if they met him
· Grandpa didn't tell Grandma about Tenko or Barny
  She'd have gone mad!

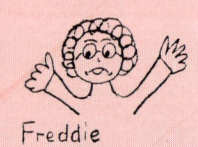

Freddie

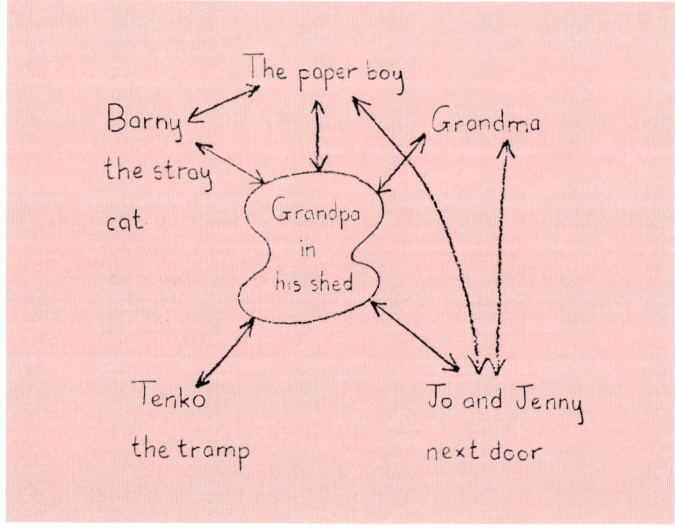

Help the children to understand that everyone lives within a network of people and that tensions between these people are common. Some children may be able to use the network of the characters in the story as a model for constructing and exploring their own networks.

Invite the children to draw pictures of their special people and the other people in their network, or to bring to school photographs of them, and make them into a collage or network chart. They could include in this network their immediate and extended families, people they see infrequently, friends at school and out of school. It is important to behave sensitively to children who have few special people, or no family, or families which are going through separation.

Explore with the children why these people are special. For example: 'We like each other'. 'We belong together.' 'We play together.' 'We look after each other.' 'We have special names for each other.' 'We have special ways of saying hello and goodbye.' The idea of unique relationships existing between and among people is not easy to grasp but the children's responses will indicate their level of awareness. Encourage them to illustrate their responses in drawing, painting and classroom play.

Talk with the children about how they are special: the unique way each of them looks and sounds, their unique role in their own special network. Help them to write down how they are special. Ask each of the children to draw a picture of herself or himself, with a speech bubble saying, 'This is me. I'm special.'

Talk about the ways in which people tell the children they are special without using the word special or without using words.

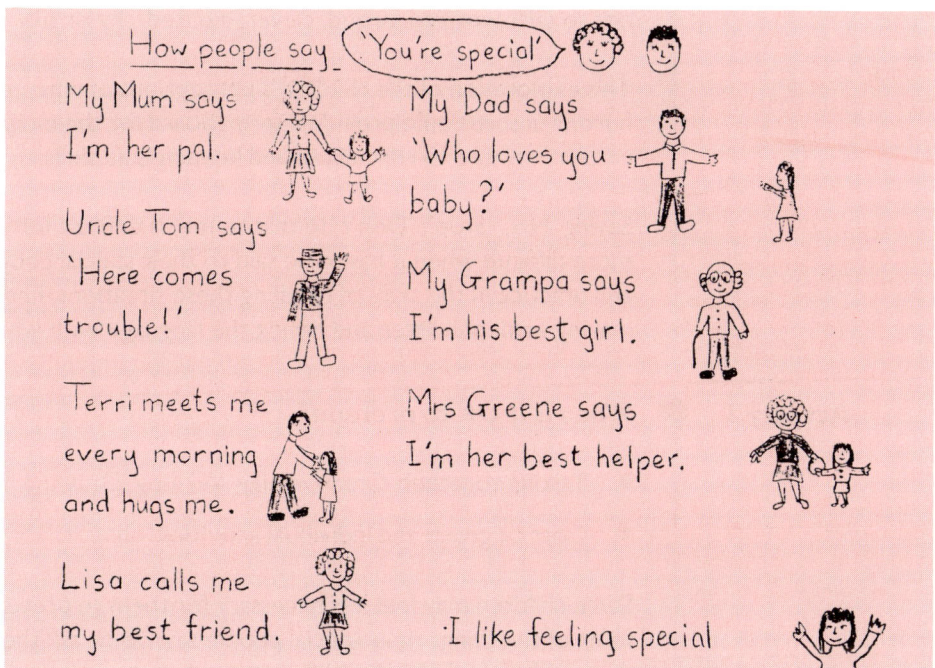

Ask the children to think of ways in which they tell their special people how special they are, in words or actions. For example: 'I say, "I love you"'. 'I say, "You make the best chips in the world,"'. 'I say, "I missed you"'.'I say, "I like it best when you are here"'.'I play with the baby to help.'

Activity 2 ● *How do my special people and I make each other happy?*

- Drawing. Writing. Making books. Analysing. Categorising. Talking together.
- Class or group and individual activities.

Ask the children (without any prior discussion) to draw themselves making their special people happy. Ask them to write at the side of each of their pictures what it is they are doing, or if they cannot write to whisper to you so you can write for them.

The children's perceptions of their roles in these relationships can be very revealing. (A simple method of analysis is provided on page 410.) The children could help you to analyse and present the results pictorially. Together look at the similarities and differences in their views.

This activity could be repeated by asking them to draw themselves making their special people worried, angry, sad or proud of them. The children could make individual illustrated books showing how their behaviour has an impact on their special people, and share them with other children to look for similarities and differences.

Invite the children to repeat the previous activity, this time looking at what their special people do to make them happy. Encourage them to share in analysing their responses. How many children are made happy by gifts? How many are aware that love, care and family life make them happy?

Repeat the activity asking them to draw their special people making them feel safe, not so safe, worried, proud, clever, excited, shy or silly.

This exploration of the children's perceptions of what makes them feel unsafe, hurt or unsure could provide a springboard for the introduction of more specific material related to child abuse and keeping safe skills.

Saying 'No', 'Stop', 'Don't do that to me' is difficult for young children, and is even more difficult when it has to be said to their special people. They will need help and practice in the skills of handling these situations, finding someone to tell, making someone listen and having the language with which to explain.

Activity 3 ● *When is it OK to pretend?*

- Talking together. Creative play. Writing. Drawing. Family work.
- Class or group and individual activities.

Some children may feel it is necessary for them to pretend not to be upset by some of the things their special people say, do or ask them to do. It is important that children be helped to differentiate between the pretending which is good, or fun, and pretending which is dangerous or potentially dangerous.

Invite the children to make small scale people using paper, card, scrap materials, wooden spoons etc. They could also bring their own puppets or Action Man style toys to school. Encourage them to use these to role-play imaginary and real stories of all kinds, with or without audience participation.

Talk with them about this kind of pretending, and about the fun of being the hero or the 'baddy', and being brave, clever and different. Ask them to remember times when they dress up as someone else, for example, when they take part in a class or school play.

Encourage the children to think about other kinds of pretending, for example:

– pretending something doesn't hurt, such as, a cut knee or an injection.

– pretending someone hasn't hurt your feelings, frightened you or made you worried.

– pretending you like being hugged, tickled, touched, picked up or teased.

– pretending you don't mind being called pet names or unkind names.

There are opportunities here to work on aspects of gender, exploring ideas such as: 'only girls cry', 'boys have to be brave', 'these are boys' clothes . . . games,' etc.

Invite the children to talk, illustrate and write about different kinds of pretending and to decide whether the pretence was good, or whether it could be dangerous.

<u>We are pretending</u>

I am pretending
I am the caretaker.
That's fun. :)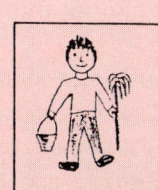

Our baby pulls my hair.
He loves it – I am pretending
I do. It's OK for him
– not for me.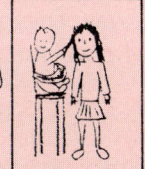

I am pretending I like
Sullah's cake. I don't
like to upset her
That's OK.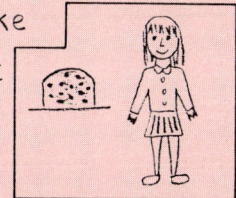

We are dressing up.
That's good. :)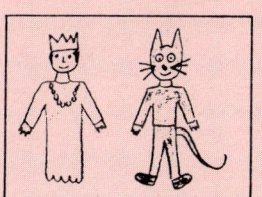

I am pretending my knee
doesn't hurt. I am being
brave. That's good.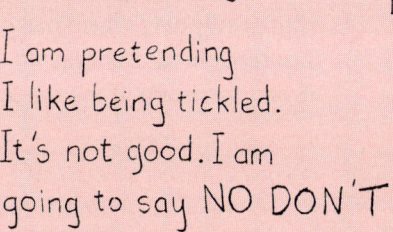

I am pretending
I like being tickled.
It's not good. I am
going to say NO DON'T
and tell my mum :(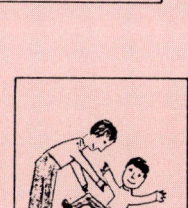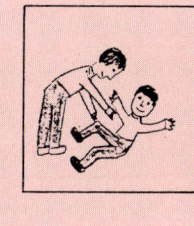

I am pretending I
like being called
Baby, but I don't.
That's stupid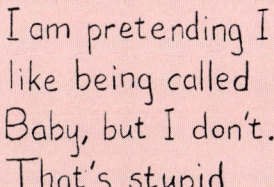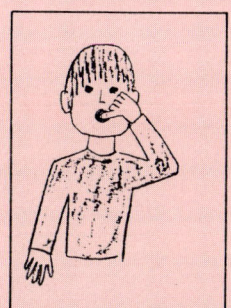

Grown ups pretend sometimes

Mrs Green pretends she's gone deaf because we shout That's funny.

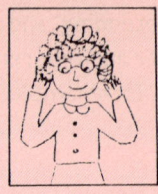

My mum pretends she's forgotten to buy our tea. I know she hasn't.

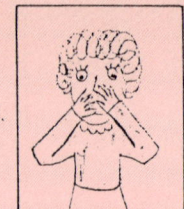

Auntie Lou pretends she doesn't know me because I've grown big. She does really.

My dad pretends he's a hungry bear and he's going to eat us up. I like it when he pretends.

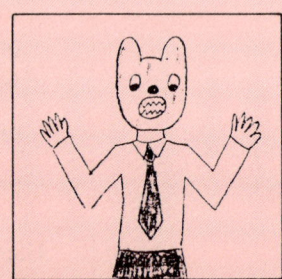

That's OK pretending

This could be an opportunity to reinforce keeping safe skills looking in particular at situations where strangers (and others) may pretend they need the children's help, or have messages for them, while having ulterior motives.

Family work: the success of the work on pretending requires that, wherever possible, it is shared with and reinforced by the children's family network and the wider community. The children will need constant reassurance, in and out of school, that saying 'No', 'Stop', 'That's not true' and 'I'll ask', is the way to deal with pretending which makes them feel uneasy or unsafe, and that they will not get into trouble for behaving in this way. They will need reassurance too that there is always someone in the school who will listen to their concerns.

Content box 2   Focus on friends and friendship

What is a friend? Who are my best friends or my oldest friends? When have friends helped me? What good bargains have we made with our friends? What are bad bargains? How do I make friends? How can I get to know what people are really like? How do I feel when things get broken? How do I feel when friendships are broken? How can people stay friends? Are pretend people, or people from television programmes or stories, friends? What can I do about real people who might pretend?

Activity I ● ***What is a friend?***

- Talking together. Drawing and painting. Collage. Movement and drama. Writing.

- Class or group and individual activities.

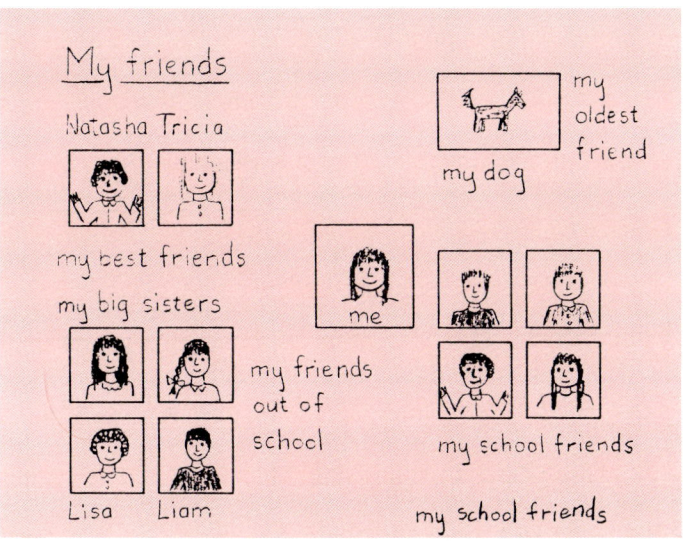

Talk with the children about the friends they have made in school, out of school or in other places. Ask them to make a picture or collage of their network of friends. They can start by putting their self-portrait in the centre and grouping around it photographs or drawings of their school friends, old friends, best friends, new friends etc.

Invite the children to share their work with others. Some children may have included imaginary friends, pets, older brothers and sisters and adults, and this can be the starting point for discussion of what friends are or can be.

It is important to be sensitive to the feelings of children who are new to the class, who do not make friends easily, or are shunned for some reason.

Invite the children to think about all the things friends do together with and for each other. Make a note of their suggestions and explore them using classroom play, painting, movement and drama.

The children could make a display of books, stories, poems and pictures about friends and friendship and add to it their own pictures and writing.

Talk with the children about the things good friends do for them. Invite them to recall times when a good friend, or someone in the family network, helped them. How did it feel to have a good friend? Ask the children to recall times when *they* acted as a good friend to someone else. How did it feel to be the good friend? Look for words to help children express the feelings and friendship.

Activity 2   ●   *Good bargains and bad bargains*

- Classroom play. Talking together. Literature.
- Class and group activities.

With the children use play to enact 'If you do this . . . then I'll do that . . .' situations, for example:

– 'If you are quick to tidy up, then we can have a story.' (Teacher and class.)

– 'If you help with the baby, I'll get your tea ready.' (Adult and child.)

– 'If you help me with this writing, I'll help you to glue your model.' (Children.)

Ask the children to invent more examples. Talk with them about keeping bargains such as these. Who feels good when they work? What are the results?

We made some good bargains this week.

Mrs Green said if we cleaned the hamsters out, we could play with them.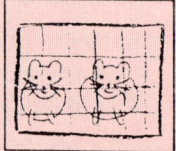

My dad made a bargain with me. I helped clean the car and he took me fishing.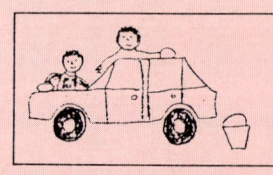

I helped Sammy with some work and she helped me make my puppet.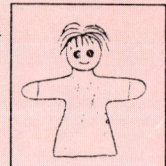

I made a bargain with Jo and Les. I wouldn't get in their way and they would stop teasing me.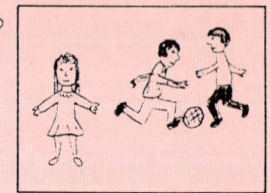

These are good bargains – We got lots done

Talk with the children about 'bad bargains', which are one-sided or threatening, and which people could use to lead children into danger or persuade them not to tell anyone. There are many examples of these in children's literature which you could use as starting points for a discussion with the children. They could make a collection of examples of 'bad bargains' in stories and from their own experience.

Activity 3 ● *Making friends and breaking friends*

- Classroom play. Talking together. Categorising. Writing. Drawing.
- Class or group and individual activities.

Set the scene with a story outline, for example, a new child has joined the class and is shy and knows no one. Using body language and role-play explore with the children how the child might look, speak, move and feel when he or she is without friends but wants to make friends.

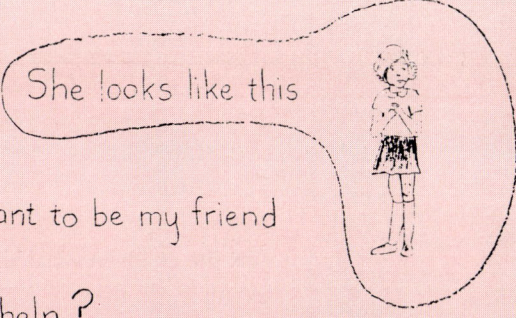

Tommy is new to the class.
She feels shy. She wants to
make friends.
She is thinking   Nobody is going to want to be my friend

She looks like this

What could we do to help?

We could say hello! Can I be your friend? Do you want to play?
We could share things – show her the way.
The dinner ladies could look after her.
We could say You'll like our class – it's the greatest.
Mrs Greene could tell her we're friendly.

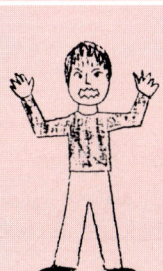

Jimmy looks
very big
and rough
I was scared of
him at first

inside hes
a bit shy
and very kind.
Hes my friend.

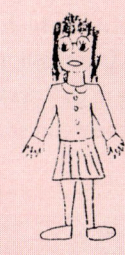

Leslie can't
talk very well
I couldnt tell
what she said
at first

inside shes so
funny and
makes me laugh
She plays good
games, shes my
friend

Sharon

Ask the children to explain how they decide to be friends with someone. What helps them to decide? Is the way the person looks important? How would they get to know what the person is like inside?

Invite the children to make a collection of broken things which they have found in the classroom, the neighbourhood and at home. Ask the children to group the items, using categories such as: 'Someone broke these', 'You can mend these', 'You can't mend these'.

Ask the children how they feel when they break things or when they see broken things. Make a note of the vocabulary they use and write it on the board in the form of a 'circle of feelings'. Invite them to draw and write about their own experience of breaking things or finding broken things.

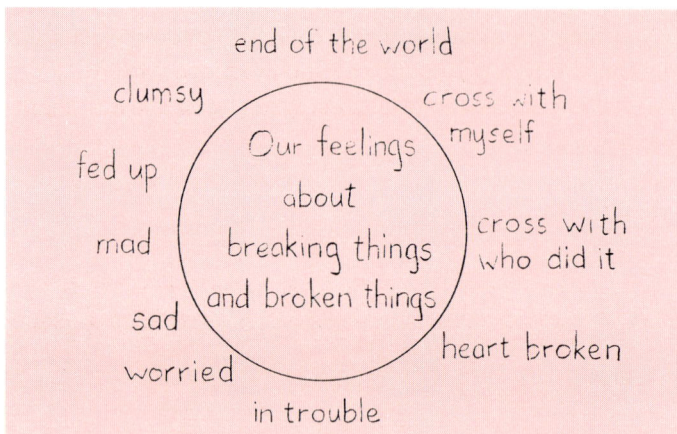

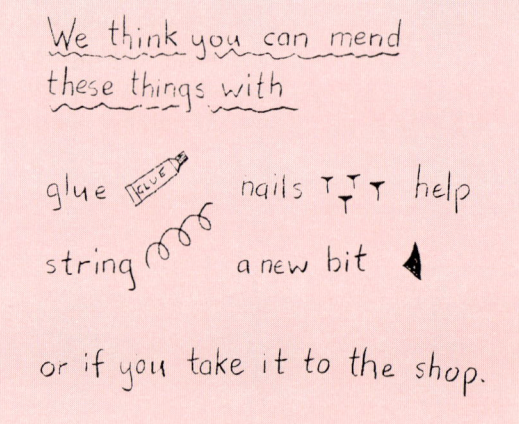

Ask the children what they do with the things which cannot be mended, for example, do they:

— keep the bits.

— throw them away.

— forget about it.

— keep remembering it.

— get a new one.

— cry.

— tell someone.

How do they feel?

Talk with the children (or begin by using a story or classroom play) about how it feels when a special friend goes away, moves house or changes schools. How does it feel to be the one left behind? How can they keep in touch and remember the friend and the friendship?

Look back with the children at their work on broken things. What else, besides moving house can break friendships? Help them to think about quarrels, misunderstandings, and the attraction of new friendships. How does it feel when friendships get broken? Can these be forgotten, or repaired with glue and nails? Explore with the children the ways in which they can stay friends with people, for example: We can stay friends by:

— not being bossy.   — not being unkind.

— saying 'Sorry'.   — helping each other.

— sharing and taking turns.

Activity 4 ● *Imaginary friends*

- Talking together, using literature and television programmes. Writing. Drawing.

- Class or group and individual activities.

Stories, poems, televison programmes, comics and cartoons often feature imaginary friends who are sometimes visible, and sometimes invisible. These friends may play important roles, providing company, good advice, a conscience and specific skills. Invite the children to make a list or collection of stories which feature this kind of 'pretend friend'.

Explore some of the stories to discover why the character needed a pretend friend and what their pretend friend did. Ask the children if they have had, or still have, pretend friends.

We have been playing pretend friends

Harry had a pretend dog in the story. He couldn't have a real one in the flats.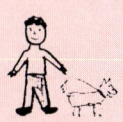

Micky had a pretend friend. He was scared of the dark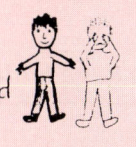

Naim had a pretend friend, so she always got two sweets

Louella in the film had a pretend sister. She really had 6 brothers.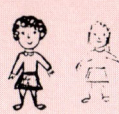

Grizelda had a pretend friend. It made all the mess.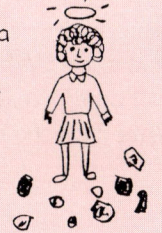

Someone wanted Smithy to be his secret friend, but Smithy said NO. It was on the video we saw. We all said NO.

Traditional stories and fables can provide a useful starting point for looking at the more threatening aspects of pretence, for example, 'bad' characters use a disguise. For example, Little Red Riding Hood. Invite the children to look beneath these characters' disguises and their seemingly innocuous actions, and think about their real motives.

Encourage the children to illustrate some of these situations. Use speech bubbles to help them describe what is being said and thought bubbles to capture the real intentions of the bad characters.

There are opportunities here to talk with the children about ways of avoiding potentially dangerous situations and places, and to practise keeping safe skills.

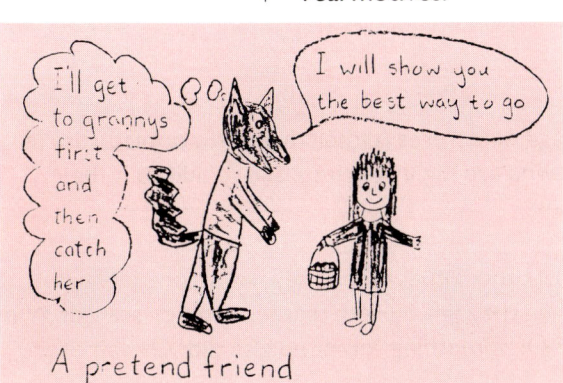

A pretend friend

Content box 3   Focus on feelings

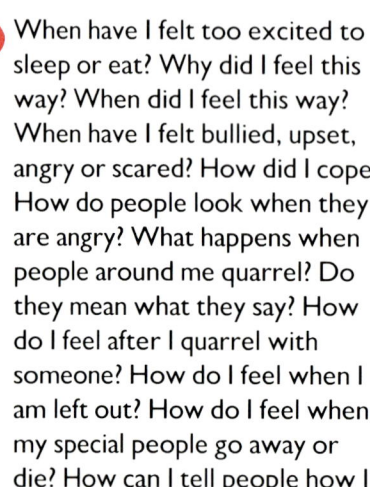

When have I felt too excited to sleep or eat? Why did I feel this way? When did I feel this way? When have I felt bullied, upset, angry or scared? How did I cope? How do people look when they are angry? What happens when people around me quarrel? Do they mean what they say? How do I feel after I quarrel with someone? How do I feel when I am left out? How do I feel when my special people go away or die? How can I tell people how I feel?

Activity I   ● *When have I felt too excited to eat or sleep?*

- Talking together. Language work. Painting and drawing. Collage. Writing.

- Class or group activities.

Talk with the children about the times when they have felt too excited to sleep or eat. How did it feel? When and why did they feel this way? Was it before or after some special time? What happened in the end? Make a note of the vocabulary they use, and write it on the board as a 'circle of feelings'.

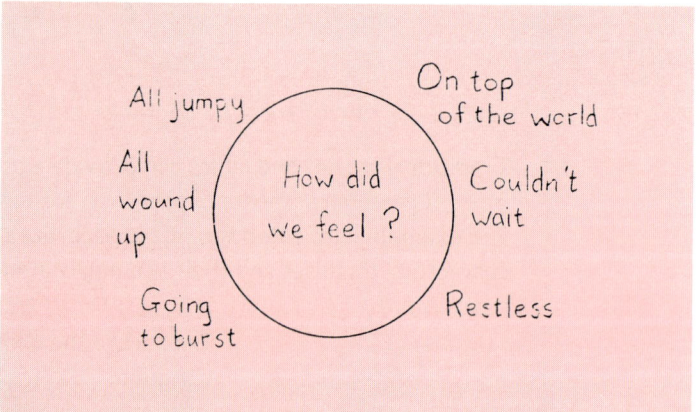

Invite the children to make a collage of pictures (either their own or pictures cut from magazines) showing people who are highly excited, and to add to it their own descriptive words and phrases.

Explore the children's memories of other times when they had strong feelings. Can they remember the times when they felt bullied, teased, upset or scared? Was it something they themselves did? Or something someone else did? Or something they were afraid might happen?

Activity 2 ● *What happens when people quarrel?*

- Talking together. Language work. Links with literature.

- Class or group activities.

Describe a situation in which two children are fighting, it could be in the playground, or in a classroom or at home. They look as though they are hurting each other, but when they are stopped by adults they say, 'We were only playing'. Invite the children to think about the adult. What made the adult think it was a quarrel? Was it the noise? Or the physical violence? Ask the children to talk about times when they have seen people who look as though they are quarrelling. Have they ever been mistaken?

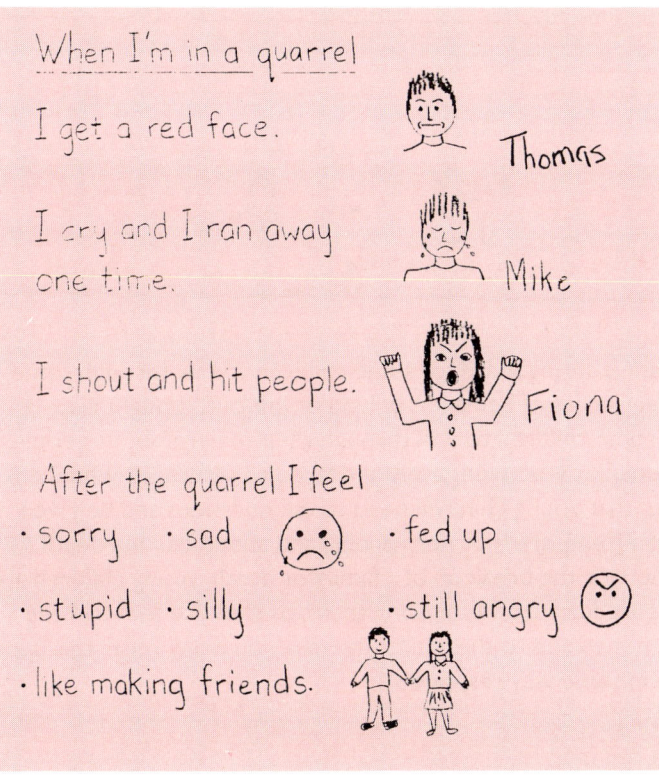

Talk with the children about how it feels to be in a quarrel with friends or grown-ups. What do they do? What do they want to do? How they feel afterwards? Make a note of the children's vocabulary and encourage them to broaden it. Some children may use the words 'silly' or 'stupid' frequently at this age to express a range of meanings.

This is an opportunity for children to talk about how they feel when quarrels happen around them, particularly in their networks of family and friends. It is important for the children to understand that quarrels do and will happen around them, and that they are rarely the cause.

There are many picture books and stories which you can use so the children can share the feelings other children have about quarrels and quarrelling. Ask them to look at how the characters in stories react and how they deal with the situation. What might they themselves have done?

Activity 3 ● *How do I feel when I am left behind or left out?*

- Reading. Talking together. Links with literature.

- Class or group activity.

Ask the children to look for poems, stories or news items which are about things or people being left behind. Encourage the children to contribute their own recollections, their paintings or drawings on this subject or pictures cut from magazines etc. Invite the children to put themselves in the place of some story character who has been left behind, and explore the situation through classroom play. How did they feel? Did they think they were left behind for ever? Encourage the children to think about why people and things get left behind. Help them to ask questions such as 'Was it because the person ran off?' 'Was it because the person was a girl?' etc.

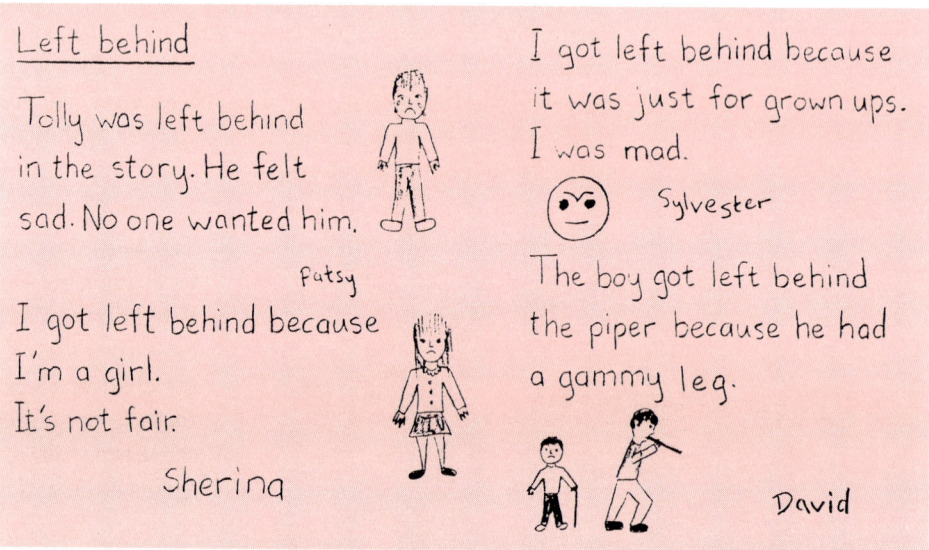

Left behind

Tolly was left behind in the story. He felt sad. No one wanted him.

Patsy

I got left behind because I'm a girl.
It's not fair.

Sherina

I got left behind because it was just for grown ups. I was mad.

Sylvester

The boy got left behind the piper because he had a gammy leg.

David

This activity could provide a springboard for some children to talk through some of their own hurtful experiences of being left behind or left out. It might also provide an opening for some children to talk through their feelings about people who were special to them, but who went away and failed to return, or who died. There is strong evidence that young children need to ask questions and be given answers about separation (temporary or permanent) and about loss and death. Where there is separation, or the break up of a family or death, young children are often excluded as adults are fearful of distressing them, or they are told to keep out of the way in order not to add to the adults' distress, and many recall this later as a sign that they were in some way responsible.

Content box 4   Focus on memories and growing up

What are my special belongings? Who is allowed to touch them? Is my body one of these special belongings? Who is allowed to touch it? What is the difference between hurting my knee and hurting my feelings? What makes these hurts better? How can I help people feel better? What can I remember about growing up? What were the funniest, saddest or noisiest times? Who shares my memories?

Activity 1 ● *My special belongings*

- Categorising. Talking together. Writing and drawing. Family work.
- Class or group and individual activities.

Ask the children to look in the box or drawer where they keep the things they use in school and to sort out what is there, grouping them into categories such as:

— These belong to the class.

— These belong to someone else.

— These are the things I share.

— These are the things which belong to me and are special to me.

Talk with the children about the special belongings which they keep at home and at school.

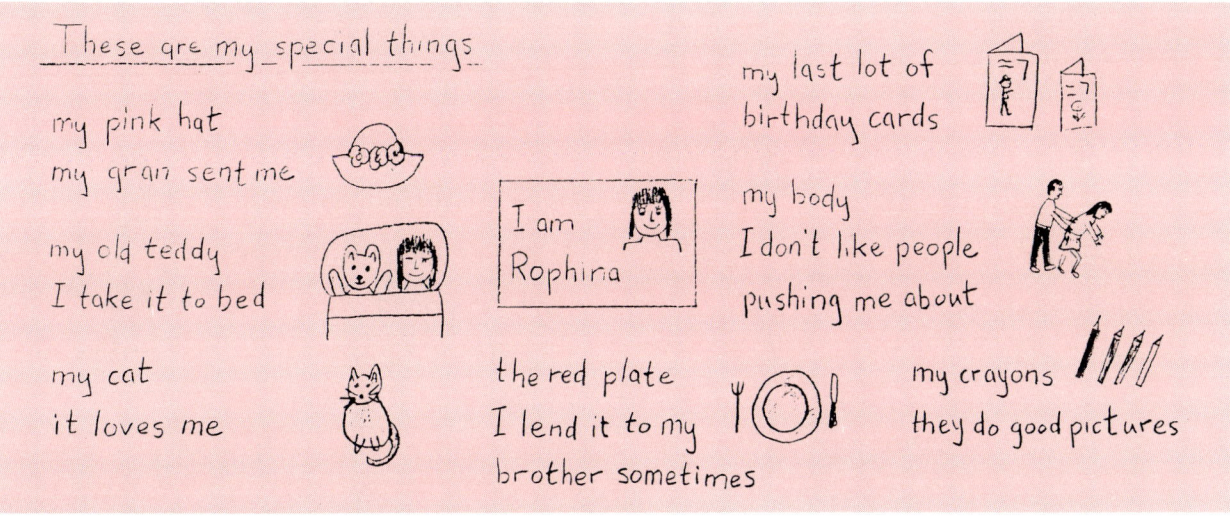

These are my special things

my pink hat
my gran sent me

my old teddy
I take it to bed

my cat
it loves me

I am
Rophina

the red plate
I lend it to my
brother sometimes

my last lot of
birthday cards

my body
I don't like people
pushing me about

my crayons
they do good pictures

Talk with the children about where they keep these special things, when they use them, whether they like to share them and let other people touch them, use or take them. Children do not find it easy to pin down what makes their things special but are very aware of their feelings of personal possession. Invite the children to make and illustrate their own charts like the one below, and to share them with others so that they can become more sensitive to other people's feelings.

Family work: the children could take home their charts, explain them to their families and ask them to add their comments and illustrations.

Take this activity one step further by asking the children to make charts showing the special belongings of members of their family network or their network of friends.

Encourage the children to explore ways in which they can show other people that they respect their belongings, for example, by not touching them, by asking the owner first and by taking care of them.

This activity could provide an opportunity to introduce or reinforce the children's understanding that their bodies (and the space immediately around them) are very special and belong to them alone, and that they can (and must) seek help if they are uneasy or frightened about the way others touch them.

● **What is the difference between hurting my knee and hurting my feelings?**

● Talking together. Classroom play.

● Class or group activities.

Recall with the children the work they did on broken things and broken friendships (Content box 2, page 293–4) and how these might or might not be mended. Explore with the children how they and other people feel if one of their special belongings is spoiled, broken or used by someone else. How hurt would they feel? Ask them to think about the difference between being hurt by falling down, and having their feelings hurt.

Hurt knees and hurt feelings

me with my knee hurt
I am bleeding and crying.
I want a plaster and a
wash to make me better
and a cuddle

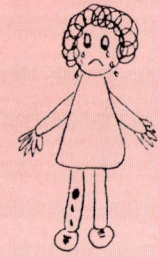

Sherina

me and my feelings
hurt no blood no dirt
I am crying. A plaster
isnt any good.
I want someone to
make me better

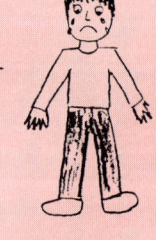

Timmy

Discuss what we can do when we feel hurt, for example, finding someone to tell, or doing something else with a friend. Who could they tell? What would they say? Help the children to role-play some situations in which they can be the comforter, the person who is hurt or the person saying 'I'm sorry'.

This is an opportunity to include some early discussion on first aid.

Talk with the children about how they might help a friend whose feelings had been hurt. What could they say or do?

Activity 3 ● ***What can I remember?***

- Talking together. Recall. Organising memories. Presenting information.
- Class or group and individual activities.

Ask the children to talk about the times they remember most. What can they remember about being a baby, or a toddler, or starting school? Ask them to bring to school photographs of themselves, or they could draw pictures to help them remember. What are the happiest, funniest, noisiest or saddest times they remember? When were they most suprised, angry, disappointed or jealous?

Help them to make individual books, or a class book or wall chart to display their memories and help them to share their personal experiences. **Family work**: invite the children's family network to contribute. What do they most remember about the child, the birth, the worrying and happy times, the funny and sad times?

The sharing of memories is an important aspect of relationships and self-esteem, and can be reinforced through **family** involvement.

My mum remembers me being born. Sherina

I remember running off with no clothes on. Josh

I remember when we had our new baby. Terri

My dad remembers when I got lost. Andy

I remember starting school. Tom

We all remember when our cat died. Even my dad cried. Ranjit

My sister remembers me being a pest. Sharon

Invite the children to return to their network charts (Content boxes 1 and 2, pages 286–7, 291–2) and pick out the people who have known them for a long time, the people with whom they share school memories, and the people who have joined recently.

Content box 5 Focus on special places

What makes some places special to me? What makes our classroom special? How do we keep it looking and feeling good? What spoils it? How do we feel if places are dirty or broken up? Where do I feel happy and safe? Which are the places I wouldn't go to? Which places are special to other people, or our pets? What can we do to keep their places happy for them?

Activity 1   *What makes some places special to me?*

- Talking together. Presenting information. Drawing. Painting. Model-making.

- Class and group activities.

Cross-curricular links: the work in this area could be linked with topic work which explores the immediate locality, and with visits to places of interest.

Talk with the children about the places in and around the school which are special to them and to people they know. Help them to make an illustrated chart which can be added to over time.

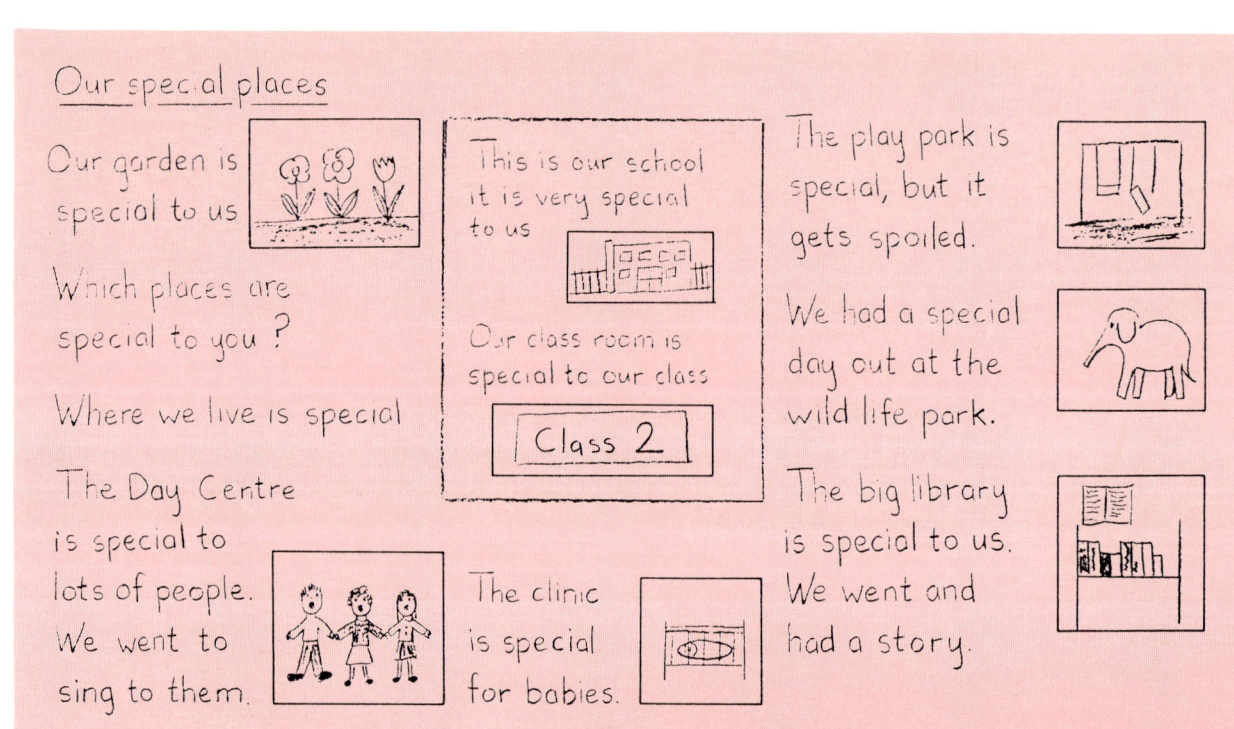

Encourage the children to look at their classroom. If they were showing visitors around what would they want to show them? How would the visitors know the room was special? What would the visitors see or not see? Who keeps the classroom happy, looking good and special? What do they do? Who brings things to school? What spoils it? Who spoils it? What can we do about it? Extend the work to look in the same way at the school, the playground and other places which the children think are special. How do they feel when these places are happy and well cared for? How do they feel when these places are dirty, broken up or spoiled?

There are opportunities here to look with the children at places in the locality which people are making special efforts to improve, or where there are particular problems relating to litter or vandalism.

Ask the children to describe the places which are special to them within the school environment, for example, the places where they and their friends like to talk, play, share things or hide from others.

Ask the children to work in groups and use drawing or painting, model-making and writing to describe and explore these places. Can they say which places are small and quiet and can be used to retreat to? Which places are used for imaginative play and physical activity? Are any of these places dangerous or secret? How do they take care of these special places? How do they feel if people spoil them?

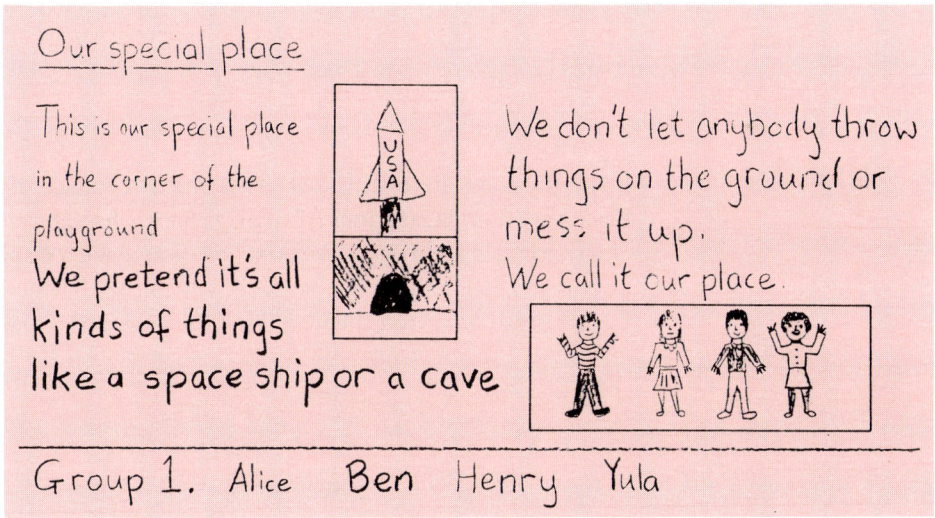

Activity 2

Places I wouldn't go to. Other people's special places.

- Using literature. Talking together. Collage. Drawing. Writing.

- Class or group activities.

Using children's literature which deals with imaginary fantasy worlds could be a starting point for exploring places which the children might see as frightening, dangerous or spoiled in some way. This would provide additional opportunities to reinforce keeping safe messages and warnings about potentially dangerous places in the locality.

Ask the children to think about the special places which pets choose for themselves, especially the places where they sleep or escape from people. What makes these places special for each pet? How do pets behave if they can't have their special places, or if someone disturbs them or spoils their special place? How do the children feel when someone takes over or spoils their special places, or makes them feel unsafe there? Encourage them to take this further and look at how other people might feel if their special places are spoilt, invaded or changed.

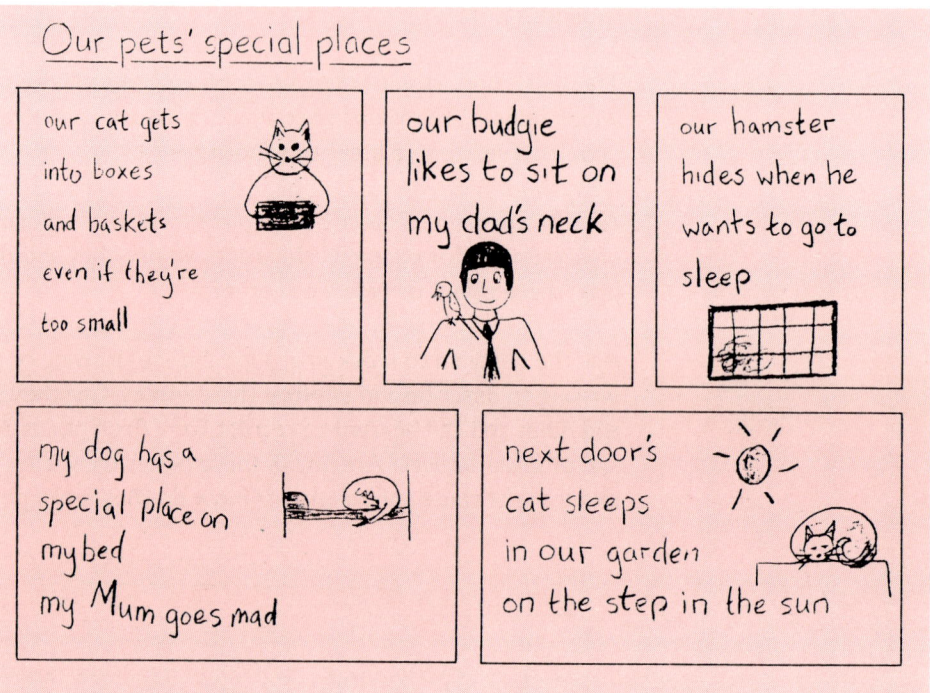

Invite the children to share in the making of a collage of happy places. Help them to bring together illustrations from magazines, photographs and their own drawings and writing. In addition they could help you make a display of books, stories, poems and songs about happy places which they have enjoyed. Conclude this work by looking at what the children think they can do to make places happy or happier.

8 & 9

Action Planner
Me and My Relationships

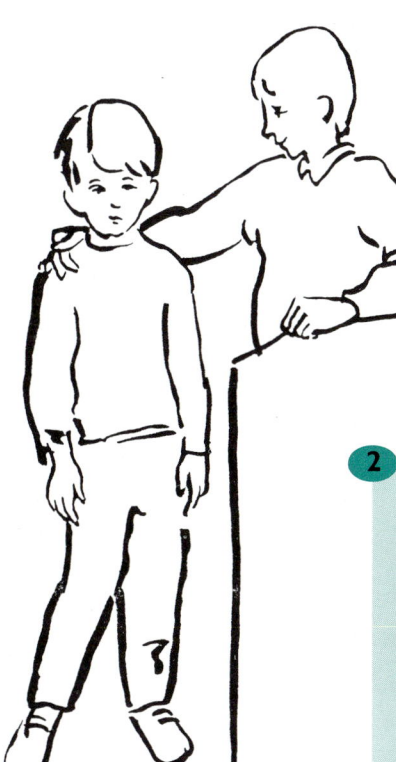

2 **Focus on friends and friendship**

How do I choose my friends now? What is the best way to make friends? What can break friendships? Are there rules about being friends? Do friends share secrets? Do I have to keep dangerous secrets? Or secrets about bodies and babies? Or grown-ups' secrets? Who can I ask for advice? How can I recognise dangerous people? What is the best way to say 'No'? Who is the leader of 'our gang'? What should I do if my gang doesn't make me feel safe?

4 **Focus on memories and growing up**

What are my best memories? Can I remember being born? What can I find out from these memories about myself? What will people remember about the person I am now? How do animals and people show their feelings? How do some animals help people with special needs? How do I explain dying? Why don't some people want to see us being sad? When have I helped someone who was sad?

1 **Focus on special people**

How has my network of special people changed? Do all my special people know each other? Which people did I choose? Is my network like other people's? How have my views on what people do to make me happy changed? What do I do to make them happy? What kinds of problems do we have? When am I expected to be grown-up? Should people expect different things from girls and from boys? How do I feel when I, or people around me, quarrel? Does sharing our feelings help? How can I work things out?

3 **Focus on feelings**

What do people mean when they talk about love and liking? How do we care about people? How can we help people with special needs? What kinds of feelings and moods do I have? What do people mean when they say 'I'm bored'? How important is sharing? What if I don't want to share or I feel jealous? How can I deal with these feelings?

5 **Focus on special places**

What do we think makes a healthy neighbourhood? What would we encourage or ban? What rules would we have? Who would be in charge? What could we do about vandals, noise and dogs? Are the places around here healthy and happy? Who could show us how to improve them? Where is my pet's special place? How do I feel if someone spoils my special place? Where can little children, old people or disabled people go?

Classroom Strategies and Activities for Ages 8 and 9

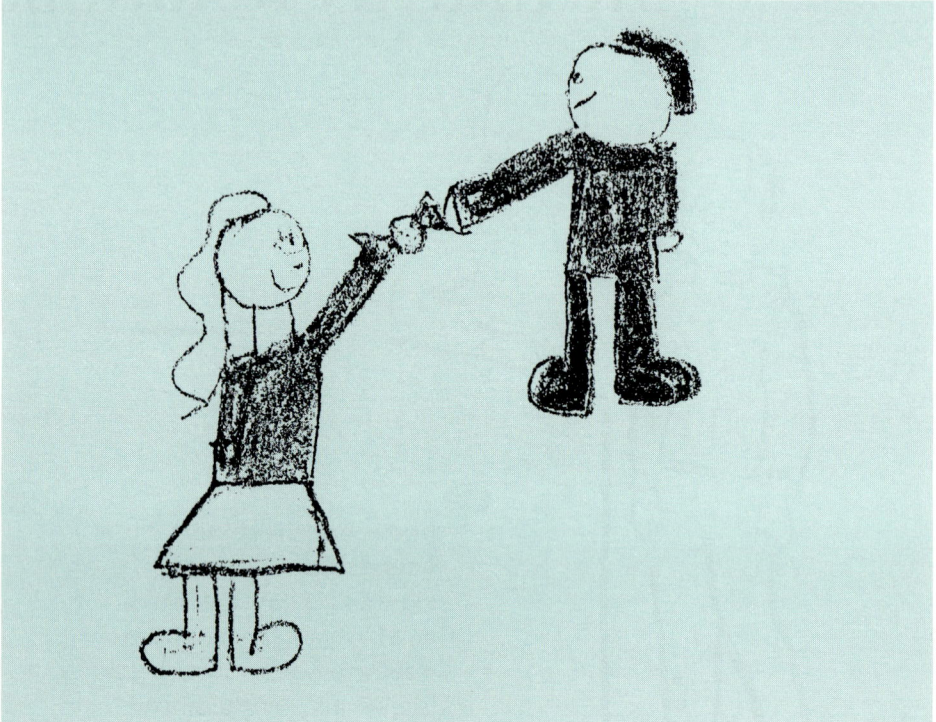

Key messages ●

Learn:

- to talk about your feelings.

- who it is safe to talk to and confide in.

- that in a dangerous situation it is best to just tell someone about it rather than to threaten to tell.

- the difference between good secrets which make people happy and bad secrets which hurt or frighten people.

- all you can about how your body works, and how it will change as you grow up.

- that different groups of people have different ways of living, learn about them and try to stop others from picking on them.

Understand:

- that your network of people is growing and changing, you are important to all of them, but in different ways.

- that if there is a sudden change in your network, for example, if someone goes away or dies, it is not your fault.

- that your special people want you to make your own choices but they stop you from doing things sometimes because they worry about you.

- that the best friends are the loyal people you value and enjoy being with – friendship cannot only be measured in gifts.

- that it is best to tell someone about friends who try to persuade you to do something stupid or unkind.

- that sometimes grown-ups cover up their feelings. It may be because they don't want to worry you, but if it frightens you tell someone about it.

- you don't have to keep secrets.

Practise:

- thinking for yourself.

- keeping safe.

- respecting other people and their possessions as if they were your own.

- telling safe people about your worries and fears.

Content box 1   Focus on special people

How has my network of special people changed? Do all my special people know each other? Which people did I choose? Is my network like other people's? How have my views on what people do to make me happy changed? What do I do to make them happy? What kinds of problems do we have? When am I expected to be grown-up? Should people expect different things from girls and from boys? How do I feel when I, or people around me, quarrel? Does sharing our feelings help? How can I work things out?

Activity 1   *How has my network of special people changed?*

- Talking together. Illustrating relationships in diagram form. Writing. Drawing.
- Class or group and individual activities.

Invite each of the children to draw and label a network of their special people, with themselves at the centre. They could include people at school, out of school, their families and extended families, pets and special adults outside the family relationship. The children's families could be invited to help by providing photographs, memories, and 'portraits' which they have drawn.

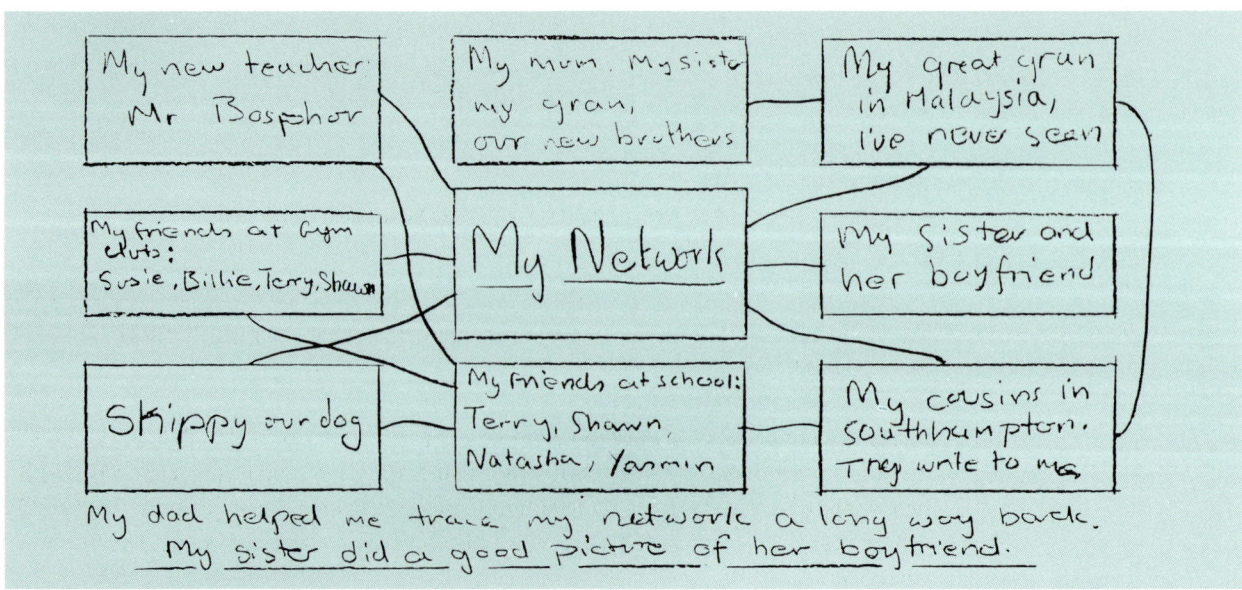

Ask the children to pick out those who have recently joined the network or left it for some reason, and to talk and write about them. This could be a good time for the children to share their work, to look at other children's networks, especially those which extend into other towns, countries, cultures and other patterns of family life.

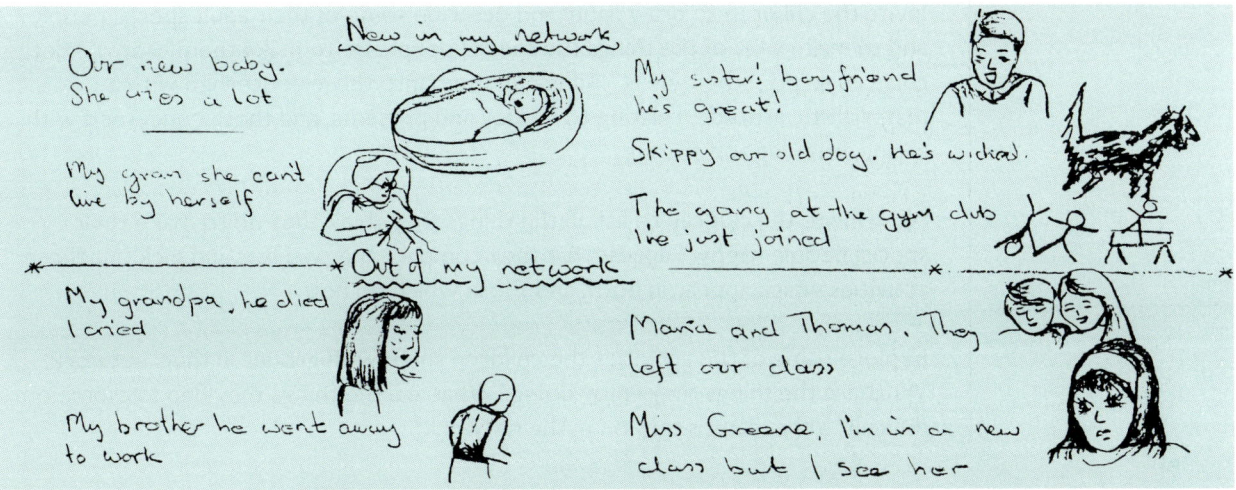

There are opportunities for children to talk about how they feel when people leave for different reasons, which could include family break-up or death.

Talk with them about new people coming into their networks and the reorganisation required to make room for them. Children may need to talk about being expected to adjust to new people joining their networks, their need for time to get used to this and the possible difficulties in the early stages.

This could be a good opportunity to introduce some early sex education in the context of the family.

Suggest to the children that they look at the groups in their network and pick out the different ways in which they are connected. You could start by asking them questions like these:

- Is there one person who is known by everybody?

- Which groups meet?

- Which groups never meet?

- Which people have been chosen by you as your special people?

- Which people were chosen for you?

The children could draw lines across their network charts to show these connections.

Invite the children to share their network charts in pairs or in small groups, and to identify for each other those people with whom they get on easily and those with whom they have difficulties sometimes. Can any of the children join their network charts together because they meet out of school or because their families know each other?

Activity 2 ● *How do we make each other happy?*

- Describing. Drawing. Categorising. Presenting information.
- Class or group and individual activities.

Invite the children to draw, label and describe some of their adult special people and to make a list of the things the special people do to make them happy. Ask the children to pool their ideas, and group them into those concerned with a materialistic attitude, relating to money and presents, and those concerned with caring, listening and sharing.

Now invite the chidren to list all the things they think they do to make their special people happy. Suggest that they compare the two lists and pick out those activities which appear in both, and those which do not.

Explore some of the activities the children share with groups in their network. What are the things they enjoy doing? What are the things they find tiresome or difficult? What causes tension in the network?

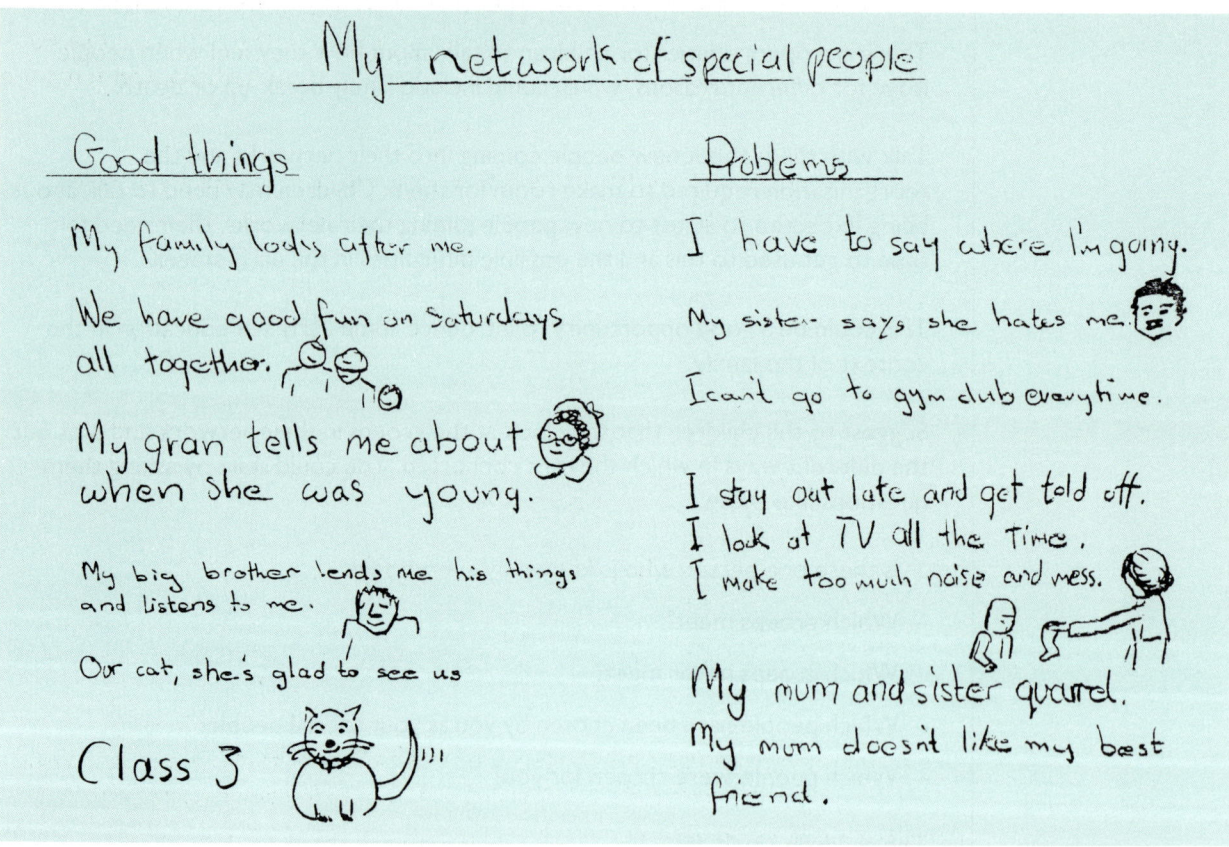

This activity could be extended to explore the questions: How do my special people make me feel grown-up? babyish? clever? stupid? proud? good at things? not good at things?

There are opportunities here to talk about how the children feel when they are expected to be grown-up at some times but not others, and to discuss stereotyped sex roles, gender attitudes and discrimination.

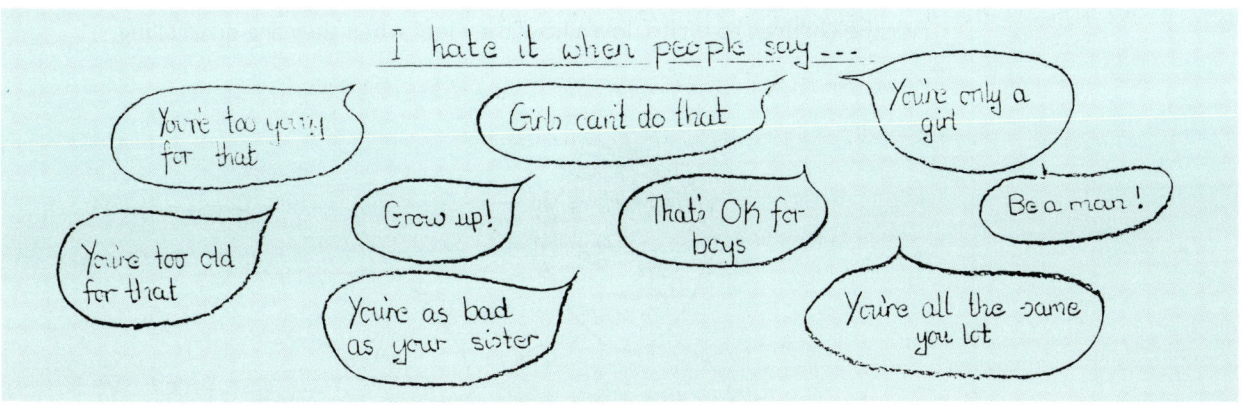

Activity 3 ● ***How do I feel when people quarrel?***

- Role-play. Talking together. Writing.

- Class or group and individual activities.

Role-play or talk with the children about a situation in which two friends are quarrelling, both claiming the same person as a best friend. Say to them: 'You can hear them, you know they are quarrelling about you. How do you feel? What do you want to do? What do you want them to do?' Ask them to share their ideas and feelings.

Explore with the children how it feels when they see and hear adults in their network quarrelling.

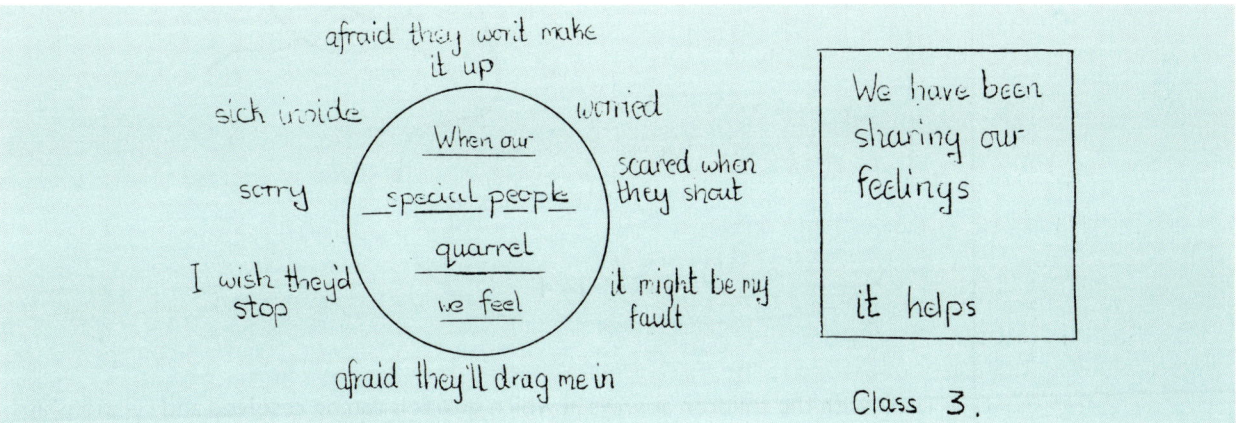

Ask the children to recall times when they had quarrels with other people. What did they quarrel about? Collect and group together their reasons for quarrels, using headings such as:

- Ownership.

- Breaking the rules.

- Breaking promises.

- Breaking a bargain.

- Being blamed for something.

Ask the children to write down how they feel when they are quarrelling:

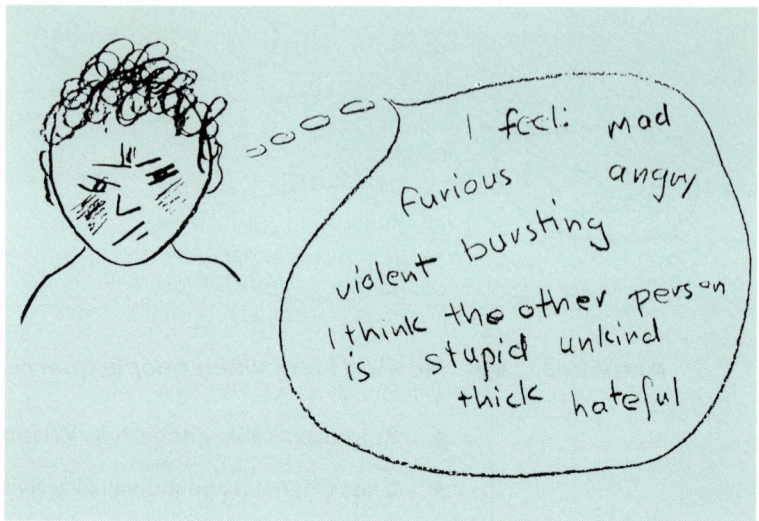

and when the quarrel is over:

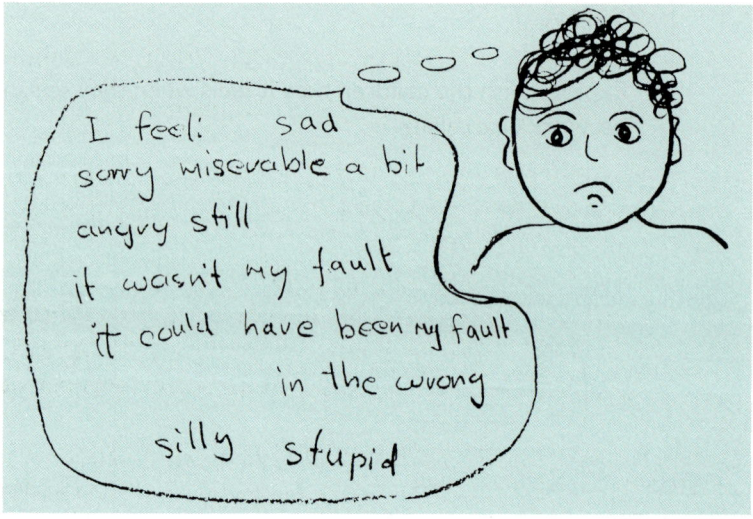

Look with the children at ways in which quarrels can be resolved and relationships restored.

Content box 2   Focus on friends and friendship

How do I choose my friends now? What is the best way to make friends? What can break friendships? Are there rules about being friends? Do friends share secrets? Do I have to keep dangerous secrets? Or secrets about bodies and babies? Or grown-ups' secrets? Who can I ask for advice? How can I recognise dangerous people? What is the best way to say 'No'? Who is the leader of 'our gang'? What should I do if my gang doesn't make me feel safe?

Activity 1

What do I like about my friends? What do they like about me?

- Categorising. Talking together. Writing. Drawing.
- Class or group and individual activities.

Invite the children to write and/or draw all the things they like about their best friends *without* mentioning names. Ask them to share their responses, in groups or as a class.

Help them to group their responses using categories such as: appearance, personality, the things we do together, etc. Take this further and discuss the importance of mutual trust and support, shared interests and concerns.

This can be a materialistic stage of development in the understanding of relationships, the children may respond with reasons for friendship such as: 'He is good looking', 'She wears fashionable clothes', 'He has a bicycle', 'She gives me money', etc. But it is also a time when children are becoming aware of and becoming able to put into words characteristics such as loyalty, trustworthiness and sympathy as the ingredients of good friendships. Similarly they are becoming increasingly aware of differences in people's personalities and their own friendship preferences.

This is a time when children often choose single sex peer groups for play and work. It could be valuable to explore with the children why this is so. Ask them to recall what they did when they were younger, when they were under 5, or in the Infant School. Did they prefer to play with younger or older children? Did they play in single or mixed sex groups? How, and why, have they changed? Do they think their views will change again later on?

Invite the children to repeat the previous writing and drawing activity, this time exploring what they think their friends like about them. Ask them to help analyse their responses as before and invite them to share their positive feelings about themselves (you could add your positive view of each child). Emphasise that it is what people *are* rather than what they *have* or own, which is important.

Activity 2 ● ***Making friends***

●   Devising advertisements. Making rules. Presentation. Writing. Drawing.

●   Class or group and individual activities.

Ask the children to make a note of the three or four most important things they would look for when choosing and making friends.

WANTED

a friend aged 9, girl or boy.
Must like running, fishing
and playing with models.
Must be kind to animals.

Must stay friends. and
not fall out too much.

Give full details.

REPLY

to

Box 41

care of

Mr Bosphor

Class 3.

Invite them to write and design an advertisement for the 'Wanted column' of a friendship page in a class, school or club magazine, using a box number rather than a name. Invite children to display and share their advertisements and talk about the ones they might like to respond to.

Suggest to the class that they start a friendship club for people who are wanting to make new friends or more friends. The children could devise a club name, badge and slogan, and think of a meeting place. Ask them to write the 'Club rules' in a way which would make people feel welcome. The children could draw up a contract to be signed by club members.

Club Eight to Ten

CLUB RULES:
○ Everybody can join.
○ We make everybody welcome.
○ We don't make up our minds about people just by looking at them.
○ We try to do one friendly thing every day or more.

Friend club

8 – 10

Activity 3 ● *Making and breaking friendship links*

- ● Discussion. Generalising. Writing. Drawing.

- ● Class or group and individual activities.

Take with the children about the kinds of things friends do for each other. What do they say to each other when things are going well? What do they say when things are going badly? How can they tell their friends how much they value them?

Suggest to the children that they think of friendship as a chain linking two people. What kinds of things link people together? For example, liking the same things, living near to each other, etc. Ask the children to think and write about their friendship links. Were they made quickly or slowly?

Our Friendship Links

Nazim and me were new on the same day. We were both a bit shy. We sat together. We made friends that day. We were only 5. Now we are 8 and we are still best friends. We made a good chain.

Lonny

Ask the children to think about friendship chains between themselves and other people. What makes the chain stronger, so that problems and quarrels don't break it for ever? For example:

– doing things together.

– keeping promises.

– saying nice things about them.

– being loyal.

– not being selfish.

– sharing.

– helping each other.

– getting on with your family.

Children could work in friendship groups to talk about this. Ask them to explain it in writing and drawings.

Next, ask the groups to look at the types of activities which could cause a friendship chain to break. Ask them to pool their ideas. For example:

— criticising them behind their back.

— breaking their trust.

— wanting everything your own way.

— only liking them for their money.

— going off with other people.

This work could be extended to help the children explore their relationships with adults, particularly those in their family networks.

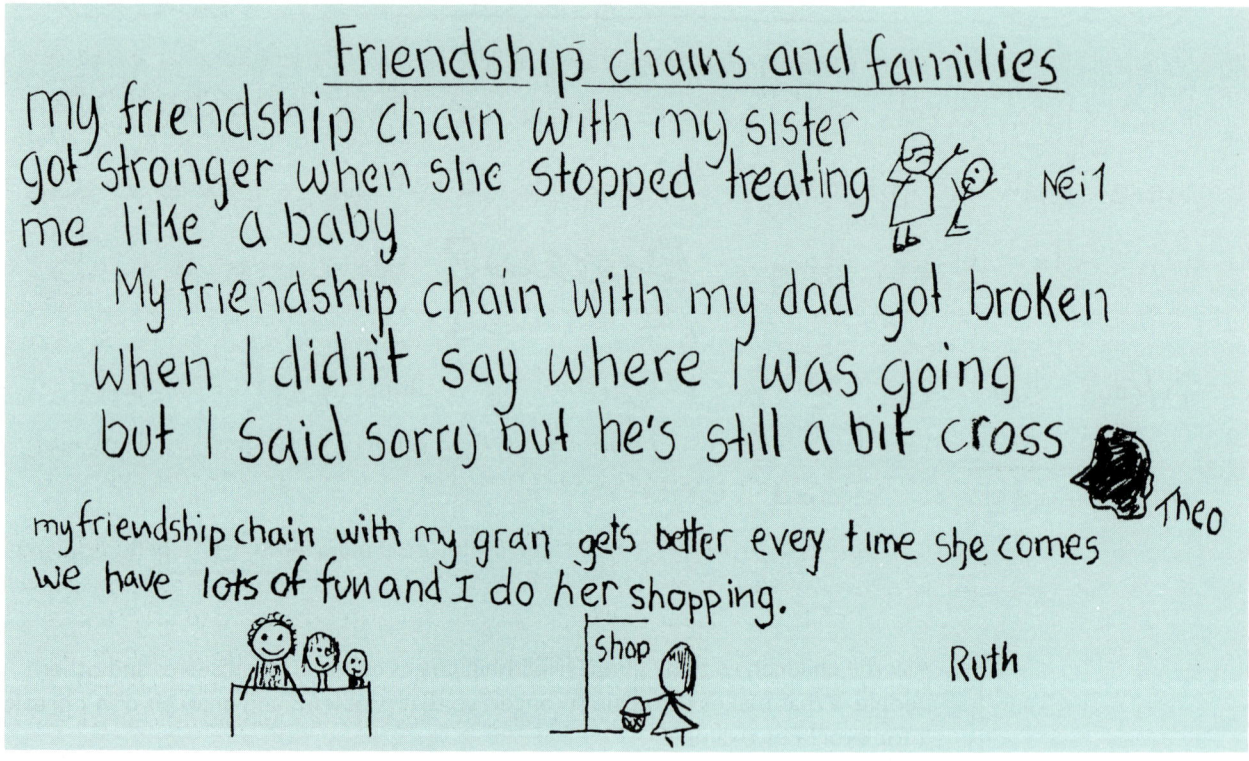

Friendship chains and families

My friendship chain with my sister got stronger when she stopped treating me like a baby   Neil

My friendship chain with my dad got broken When I didn't say where I was going but I said sorry but he's still a bit cross   Theo

my friendship chain with my gran gets better every time she comes we have lots of fun and I do her shopping.

Shop   Ruth

Activity 4 ● *Keeping the rules*

● Analysing the rules of a game. Discussion. Role-play. Describing. Drawing. Generalisation.

● Class or group activities.

Explain to the children the rules of the game 'Simon Says'. Ask the children what they would do if Simon told them to do something unkind, for example, to mock, or pick on a person, or to do something dangerous to themselves or others. How would they respond? Ask the children to role-play these situations and report back. How did they say 'No'? How did they tell Simon that he was being unkind, dangerous, racist or sexist? For example:

— 'That's unkind.'

— 'That's a stupid idea.'

— 'That's dangerous.'

— 'That's not fair to girls.'

— 'We don't do what you say, we think first.'

— 'We want to make up our own minds.'

Ask the children to think about what they would say, or do, if there were a lot of Simons and they were on their own? How would they deal with that kind of pressure? Explore the strategies they think they might use, for example, running away, giving in, asking someone else for help, etc. Ask the children to decide which would be the most successful strategy for them.

Talk with the children about the importance of keeping secrets, an aspect of friendship viewed as very important by this age group. How do they feel when someone says 'I'll tell you a secret – promise not to tell'? For example: Do they feel:

— special?

— important?

— pleased?

— scared?

How would they feel if the secret was about something dangerous or frightening? What would they say or do? Would they keep the secret or tell someone?

It is possible that the children, when talking about secrets they have been told, may include some about sex, reproduction and the human anatomy. Some may include secrets which have racial undertones, or which relate to other people's physical appearance or disabilities. This could be a time when children might want to be able to reveal some of their concerns and fears. It could also be an appropriate time to reinforce previous learning about secrets which adults might try to force them to keep. This might include secrets about being hurt or abused in some way. Teachers will need to be particularly alert to this and the ways which it can be effectively dealt with through school and social work channels. Most LEAs will have clear guidelines for such eventualities, the first step being to alert the head teacher.

Encourage the children to recall the secrets which they have shared with grown-ups. Emphasise the secrets which were good, fun and exciting. Invite them to remember the difficulty of keeping the secret, the surprise on the face of the person when the secret was shared, the good feelings among the people involved. Contrast these with the 'bad' feelings generated by secrets which are unkind or frightening. This is an opportunity to emphasise the importance of finding someone to trust and tell about these things, and to 'practise' explaining problems.

Activity 5 ● *How can I recognise dangerous people?*

- Role-play. Talking together. Drawing.

- Class or group and individual activities.

Teachers may wish at this time to incorporate materials specifically devised to prevent child abuse. (See Appendix 2, page 424–6.) Some of this material may focus on the dangers of talking to strangers, and a useful starting point may be to explore with the children their perceptions of strangers.

Invite the children to role-play, or to talk about, situations in which they are the strangers, for example:

— being a new member of a class.

— joining a club.

— going to another school, another town or country.

How does it feel to be the stranger? What helps them to feel at home?

Ask the children how they would help a visitor find the school secretary or the head teacher. Remind the children that strangers in these cases are not necessarily dangerous but will feel out of place and lost.

It is important that children see the differences between people being strangers in the sense of being newly arrived, and needing help, and people being strangers in the sense of being dangerous people who may approach and confront the children or attempt to take them away. The children may believe that they can recognise dangerous strangers from their appearance. Encourage them to draw pictures of strangers, to describe and share their illustrations. Emphasise that many such 'strangers' cannot be picked out by their *appearance* and do not carry 'warning signs'. They may well look and sound like ordinary everyday people and it is more important to look for danger signals in what they ask or say and how they behave.

The children need to practise recognising some opening gambits which might be used in potentially dangerous situations. For example, offers of rides, sweets and presents, requests for help; messages said to come from the child's home, etc. They need to learn that these are danger signals and will need to practise ways of saying 'No' and finding a safe place to go, or a safe person to tell. This may also be an appropriate time to explain to the children that sometimes people known to them can behave in a strange and dangerous way and that it is important to find someone to tell and to go on telling until help is provided.

Teachers will find themselves faced with the task of both protecting and reassuring the children. The support of families and others in the community is critical if the teacher is to balance these activities, and use specific material about child abuse.

Activity 6 ● *Who is the leader of our gang?*

● Language work. Writing. Talking together.

● Class or group and individual activities.

Invite the children to think of and write down all the different words and phrases which describe groups of children, organised or not, containing two children or more. For example:

– pair.	– trio.	– squad.
– couple.	– foursome.	– mob.
– duo.	– team.	– crowd.
– doubles.	– class.	– several.
– partners.	– gang.	– lots.

Talk with the children about leaders. How can you tell who is the leader in these different groups? What do leaders do and say? Is there always a leader? Remind the children of the game Simon Says. Would the children *always* do what the leader said? What might happen if quarrels started in the group?

Ask the children to think how they would feel if they were in a dangerous place and they were alone. Would they feel safer if they were in a group with a leader, or in a group without a leader?

Opportunities may develop for children to talk in their own way about group behaviour, peer pressure and team spirit. How would they feel if the group or the crowd they were part of behaved in an unkind or dangerous way? What if it bullied people or caused damage? Would they be able to stand alone and say they thought it was wrong?

Content box 3   Focus on feelings

What do people mean when they talk about love and liking? How do we care about people? How can we help people with special needs? What kinds of feelings and moods do I have? What do people mean when they say 'I'm bored'? How important is sharing? What if I don't want to share or I feel jealous? How can I deal with these feelings?

Activity 1   *Liking and loving*

- Talking together. Writing. Categorising. Presenting information. Drawing. Role-play.

- Class and group and individual activities.

Hold a brainstorming session with the children. Ask them to call out all the things they love, or hear people say they love. For example, 'I love my Mum', 'I love chips,' 'I love your dress' etc. Ask them to write down as many of these items or activities as they can.

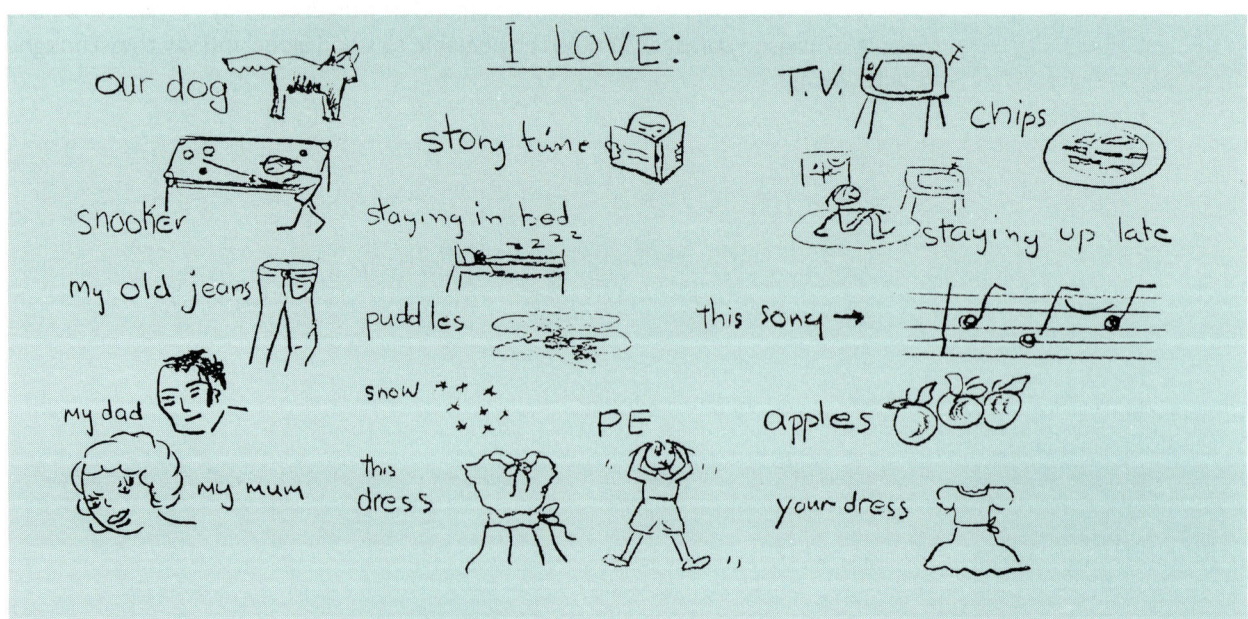

Invite the children to group these items into two categories: 'like' and 'love'. What do the children think is the difference between 'love' and 'like'? Talk with them about the things and people they like all the time, and the things and people they like some of the time. Do they still love people even when things go wrong?

Invite the children to work in friendship groups to make charts or large-scale books which show the range of people, places, activities and things they like.

In addition you could ask them to make books or charts about the people who like them, the people who love them some of the time, and the people who love them most or all of the time.

Pose this question: 'Your friend wants to let you know she or he really likes you. What does your friend do and say?' You could ask the children to respond to this through group discussion, through drawing and writing or role-play.

Explore the responses. How many of the children have a materialistic attitude? For example, 'He would give me money, or a present'. Encourage them to look at a wider range of responses. Ask them how it feels when someone lets them know that they are liked, even though it may be embarrassing at first and emphasise how important it is to thank them.

Suggest to the children that they make a contract with themselves to make a friend feel good that day, at school or at home. Ask the children to illustrate and write about how they felt when people have shown them that they love them.

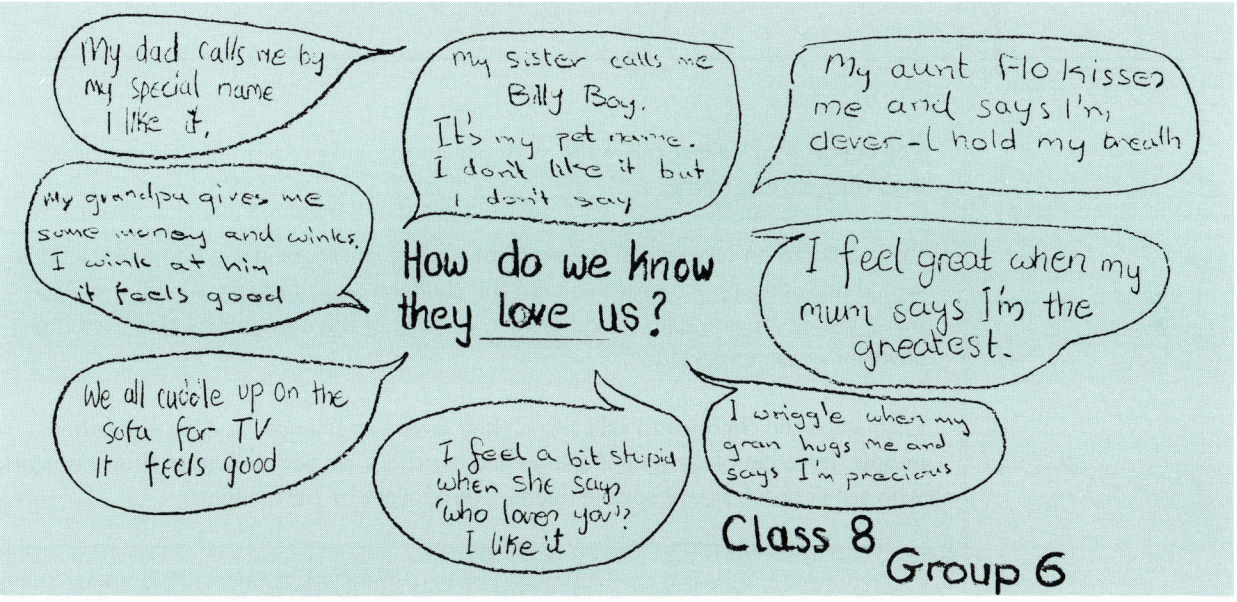

Activity 2 ● ***How do we care for people?***

- Collecting pictures. Library skills. Survey work. Talking together. Visits and visitors. Project work.

- Class or group activities.

Make a collection of pictures of pets, including the children's own paintings, pictures from newspapers, magazines, picture postcards and posters. Ask the children to look through the classroom library to find books about domestic and unusual pets. Ask them to include reference books and stories and poems about real, mythical and imaginary pets.

Explore with the children how the different pets would need caring for and who would do it. Encourage them to think about the need for regular care, a commitment on the part of the carer, and what this means in day-to-day terms.

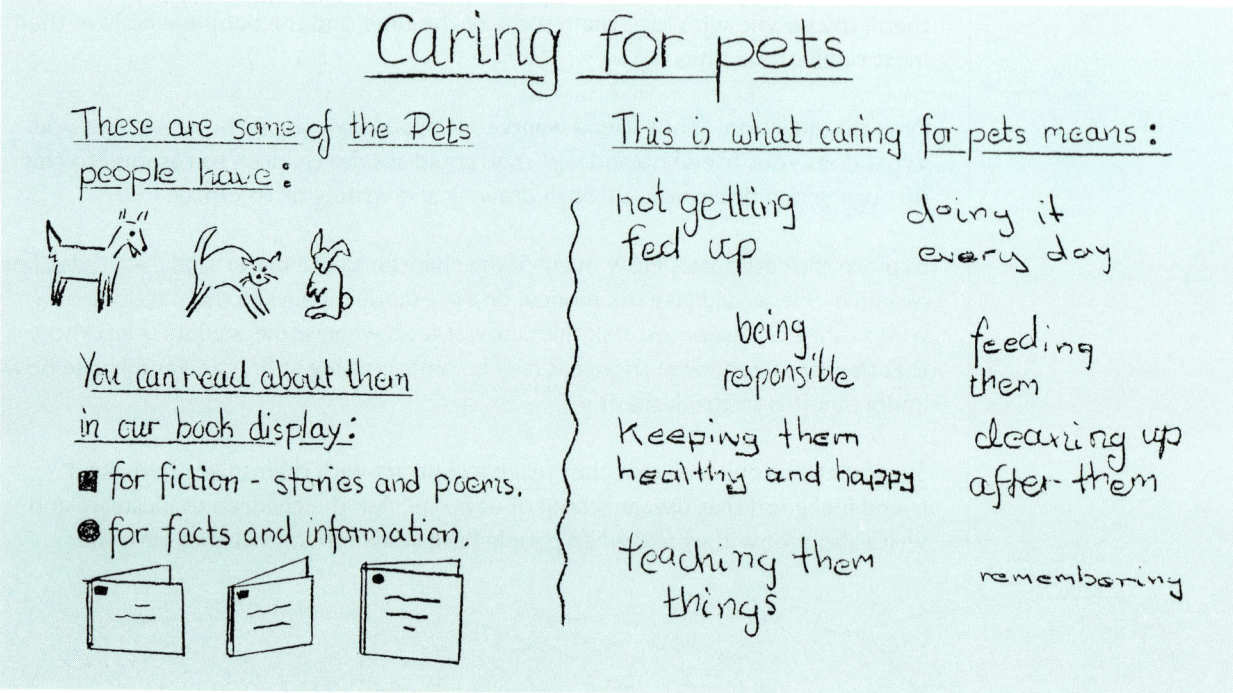

The children could link this work with organising and presenting a survey of the pets they have at home.

You could go on to explore the work of a range of carers in the community. This would provide opportunities to take the children on out of school visits, and to invite visitors to the school, and bring the work of the community closer to the children's own experience.

Encourage the children to talk about their own experiences as carers of other people, for example, younger sisters and brothers, or people within their network who are ill or who have special needs – temporary or permanent.

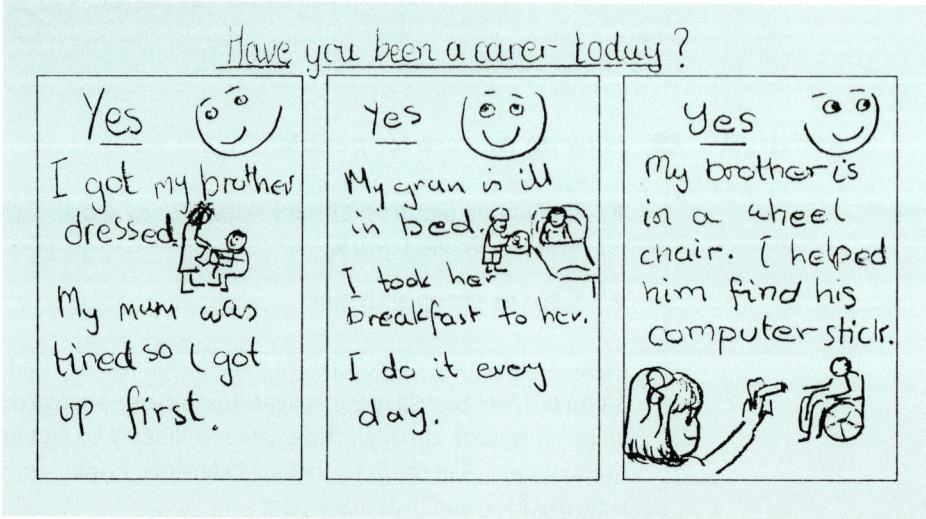

There are **cross-curricular links** with social studies, geography and project work here.

Invite the children to extend their work on caring to look at ways in which they can care about people they do not know, but whose problems or handicaps they are beginning to understand. There will be opportunities to focus on people with disabilities, on poverty, disease, famine and the work of community and national charities. Help the children to distinguish between their day-to-day caring activities, and caring groups in the wider world.

<u>We care about these people, but we don't know all their names.</u>

Children who are blind,
old people who get cold in winter,
Children starving,
people who haven't anywhere to live

We had a fun run to get some cash.

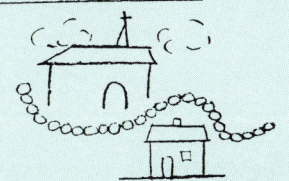

We had a big jumble sale.

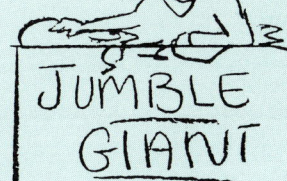

We helped make a mile of pennies in the town.

We found out a lot about them ....

We asked them to come to our concert.

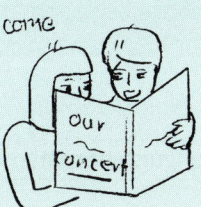

A lady showed us a dog she was training to help someone who was blind.

Activity 3 ● *Fancy that!*

- Talking together. Writing. Drawing. Language work.

- Class or group and individual activities.

The word 'fancy' has changed its meaning and is now commonly used to imply some kind of real or imagined physical attraction between two people. Children of this age may be hearing it used in this and other contexts, to imply caring for or loving. It could be important for them to explore and clarify the range of meanings of this word.

Ask the children to plan a party or celebration for an imaginary occasion or a local or national religious festival. Begin to plan the food with them, asking the question: 'What kind of food do you fancy for the event?' The children could make a list of foods and plan and illustrate a menu.

There are **cross-curricular links** with language work here.

Explore with them the many meanings of the word 'fancy', collecting up phrases and sentences in which it occurs.

FANCY THAT!

What do you fancy for tea? **Means:** What do you think you would like?

Do you fancy going for a walk? **Means:** would you like to?

I fancy beans on toast **Means:** I think I would like beans.

Fancy Pants **means:** Showing off your new clothes.

I fancy that person as a friend **Means:** I think I would like the person, but I'm not sure

Fancy that! **means:** That's surprising

Fancy cakes **means:** pretty ones.

Fancy dress **means:** You're pretending to be someone else.

Some children may be ready to try to distinguish between 'liking', 'loving', 'caring for', 'caring about' and 'fancying'.

Activity 4 ● *Feelings, moods and boredom*

- Exploring personal feelings through drawing, writing, language work and presentation.
- Class or group and individual activities.

Invite the children to make a series of quick sketches of themselves showing in each a different emotion, for example, happy, sad, worried, excited, disappointed, relieved, angry or cared for. The drawings could be presented in comic strip form or as a 'flick book'.

There are **cross-curricular links** with language work here.

This is a good opportunity to extend the children's vocabulary including words such as confident, shy and determined. Ask the children to help you make a collage of pictures cut from magazines showing a wide range of feelings and write around it the vocabulary the children have explored.

Ask the children to share with each other some of the times when they have experienced these feelings. Encourage them to think about whether the feeling was caused by something they did, or something someone else did. How did they cope? When was it easy, or difficult?

Talk with the children about what they and other people mean when they say 'I'm in a bad mood', 'I'm in a good mood', 'She's in a funny mood, or 'He's moody.' Ask them to think of times when they were in a good mood. What made them feel that way? Was it because of something someone else had done? Was it because of something they themselves had done? Explore how it feels to be in a good mood or in a bad mood. The children could share, and illustrate, their views in small groups.

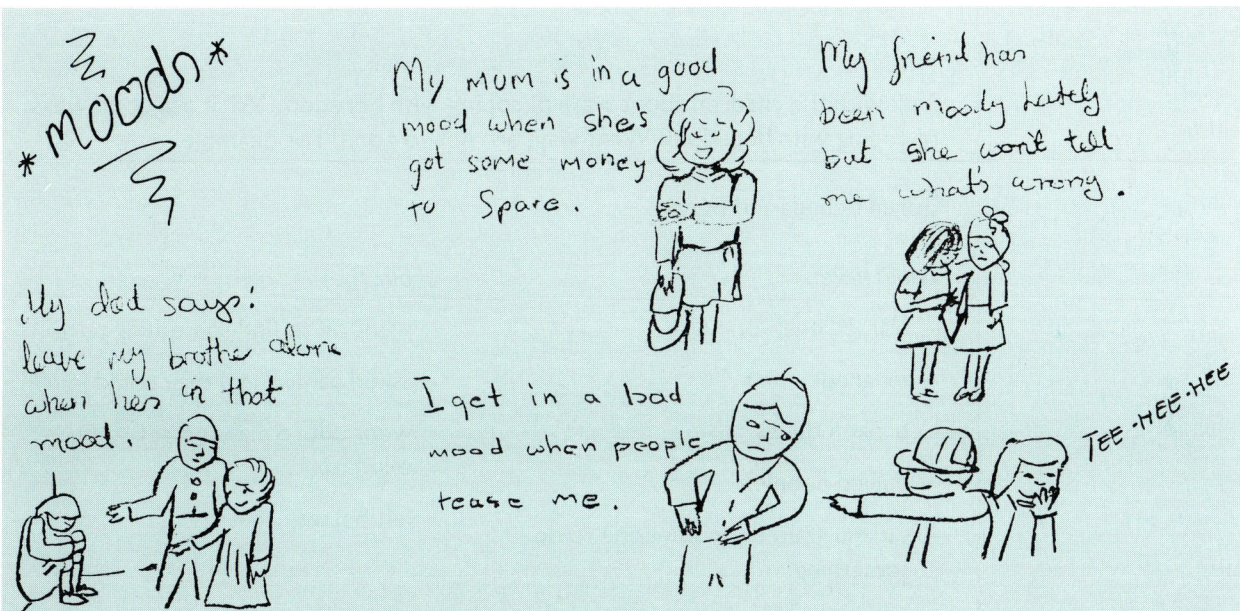

Explore with the children what they can do to help other people who are having a bad mood. What makes it better? What makes it worse?

Explore what the children think they can do to help themselves when they are in a bad mood, for example, tell someone about it, try to forget about it, do some exercise, or stay away from people.

These activities can help children develop a greater awareness of the way different moods affect them and other people.

Invite the children to invent, name and illustrate a character who is always bored, and always saying 'I'm bored'. Ask the children to think about the statements: 'I'm bored', and 'It's boring'. Invite the children to recall times when they have heard people say things like this. What do they *really* mean? Ask them to write about, and illustrate this.

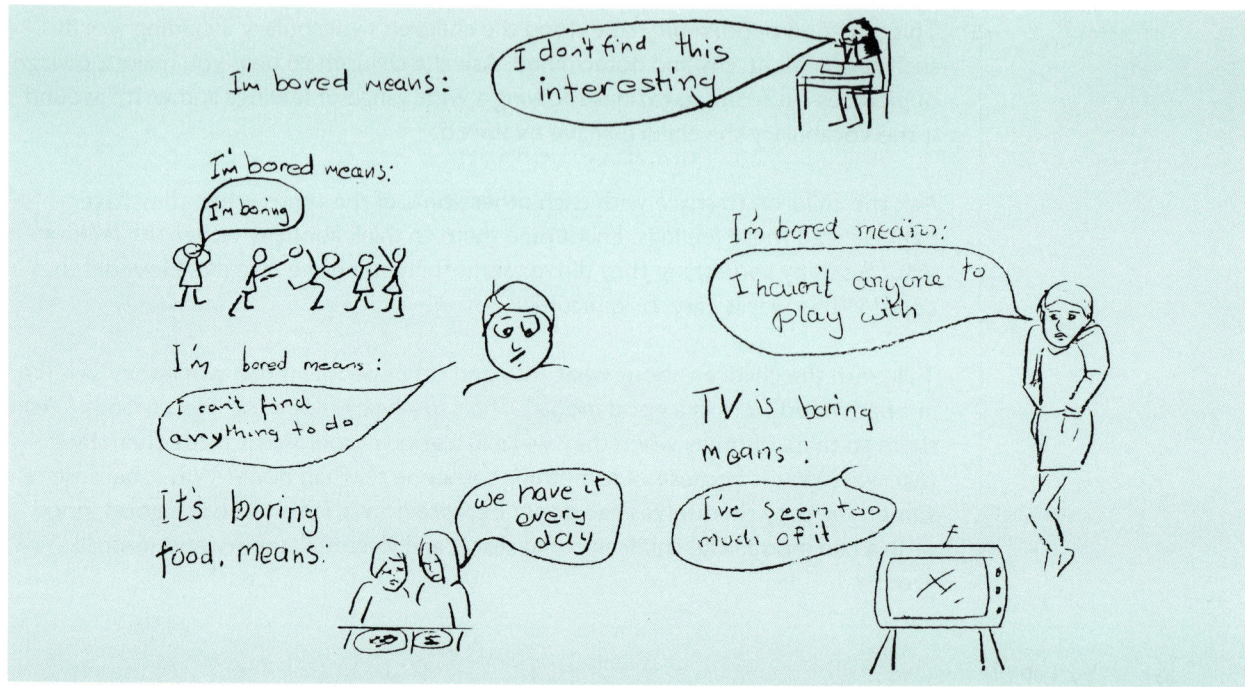

Talk with the children about ways of coping with boredom. What are good ways of coping with boredom? What ways are not so good? For example:

Bored Belinda and Benjie –

could have:

— blamed everyone else

— moaned.

— broken things.

— bullied people.

— sat and waited for someone to do something.

— felt worse than ever.

but they:

— went off to find something to do.

— asked someone if they could join in.

— went out to play and get some exercise.

— felt better.

Ask the children to think up some messages for people who say they are bored or that things are boring. For example:

— find a job to do.

— help someone.

— don't just sit there – do something.

— it's not boring – it's you.

— join something.

— get some exercise – you'll feel better.

— try again.

— get a friend to help.

Activity 5 ● *Sharing*

- Play-making. Drawing. Role-play. Discussion.

- Class or group and individual activities.

Ask the children to write a play with illustrations on the theme Saving Up For Something Very Special, for example, a bicycle. Afterwards, help some of the children to present the play to the rest of the class.

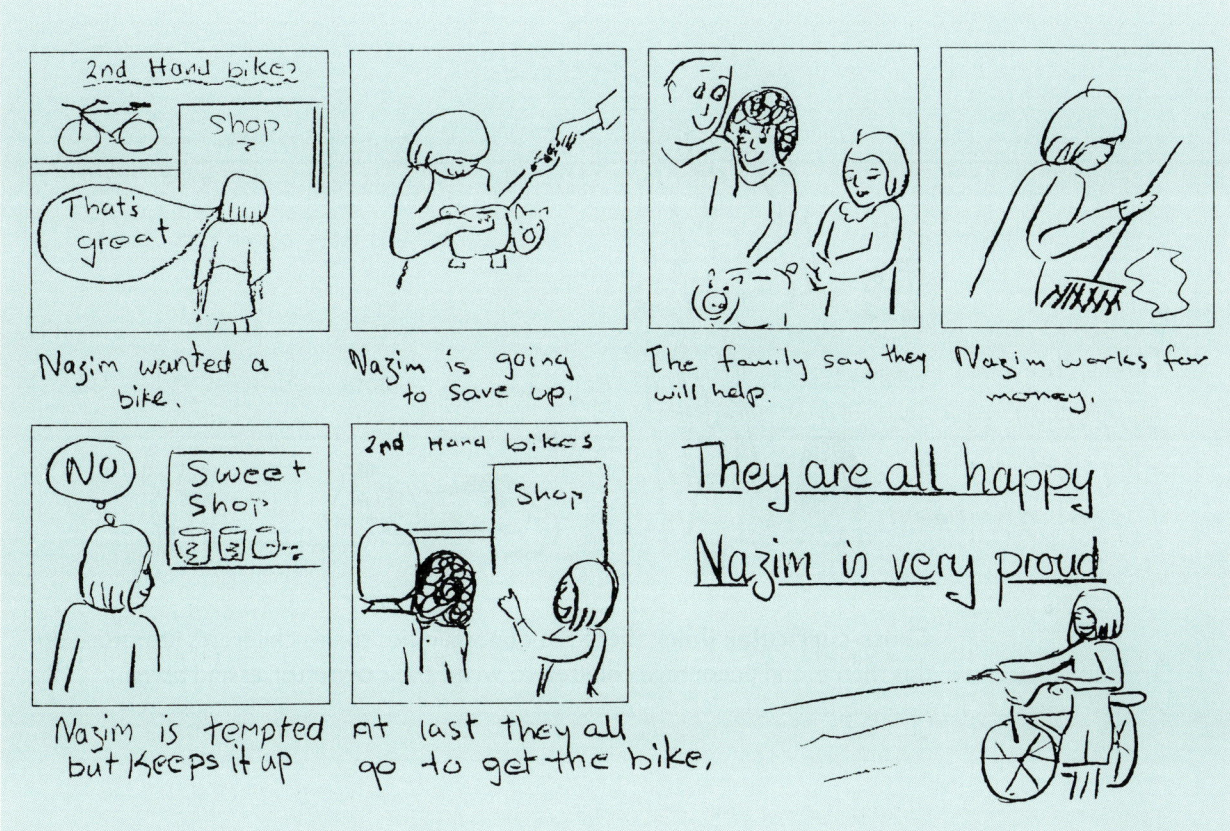

Nazim wanted a bike.

Nazim is going to save up.

The family say they will help.

Nazim works for money.

Nazim is tempted but keeps it up

At last they all go to get the bike.

They are all happy Nazim is very proud

Ask the children to think about the new bike. Would Nazim lend it to anyone? How would she feel if someone used it without asking her? Ask the children how they feel about their special things. Do they like people using them without asking? Do they feel happier if people ask their permission before touching them? How do they cope with this problem? Do they:

— get upset or cross if people touch their things?

— hide their special things?

— label them with their name?

— tell someone about it?

— feel happy when people ask, and thank them afterwards?

Explain to the children that people should respect their things, and that they have a right to say 'No', 'Don't touch', etc. and that it is important to tell someone if people do not co-operate.

Some children may be able to draw comparisons between their feelings of ownership and their feelings of possessiveness towards friends or relatives. Is having a special person different from having a bicycle? Are there times when they want to keep their special people to themselves and not share them with others? Do they sometimes feel jealous because their friend has her or his own network?

Jealous feelings can be very strong at this age and children may find sharing their experiences helpful. Ask them to talk about, and illustrate, occasions when they felt jealous. It is important that they realise that adults too feel like this.

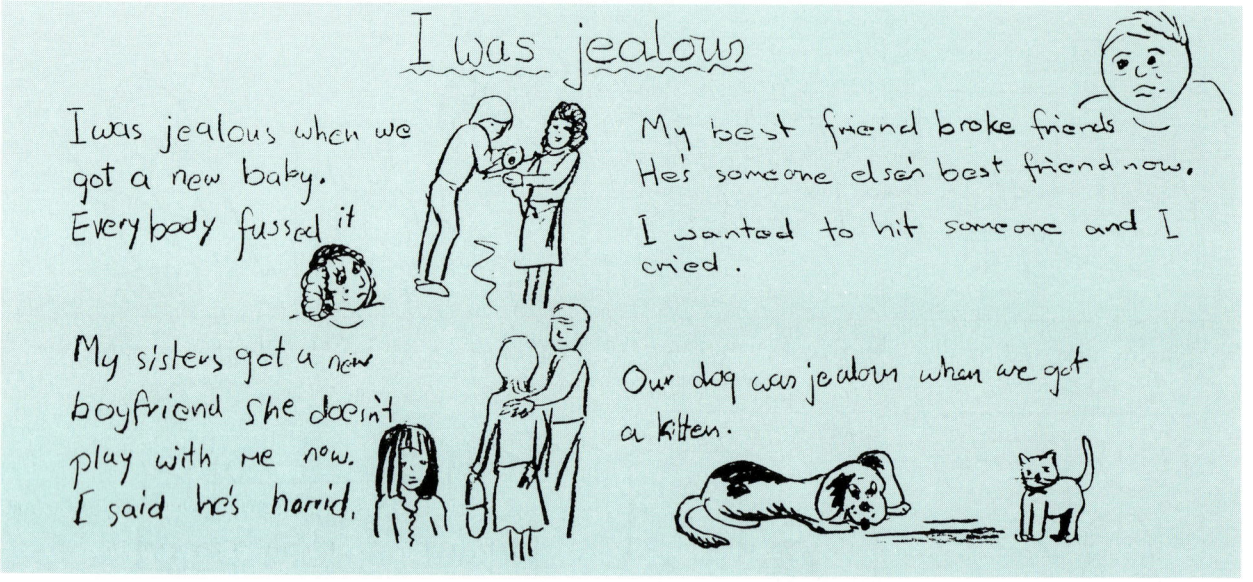

Cross-curricular links: there are opportunities to use children's literature on this theme, and encourage children to write their own stories and plays.

Content box 4   Focus on memories and growing up

What are my best memories? Can I remember being born? What can I find out from these memories about myself? What will people remember about the person I am now? How do animals and people show their feelings? How do some animals help people with special needs? How do I explain dying? Why don't some people want to see us being sad? When have I helped someone who was sad?

Activity 1   *Memories*

- Talking together. Drawing. Writing. Project work.

- Class or group and individual activities.

It is important that children begin to be aware of the unique role memories play in people's relationships. What a person remembers, and what other people remember about that person, is unique.

There are **cross-curricular links** with local and family history here.

The work in this section could develop into project work which explores the lives and experiences of older people in the community and in the children's family networks. It could encourage the children to value these people and to see how their past experiences contribute to life today. It could also provide a starting point for children to explore family roots in distant places.

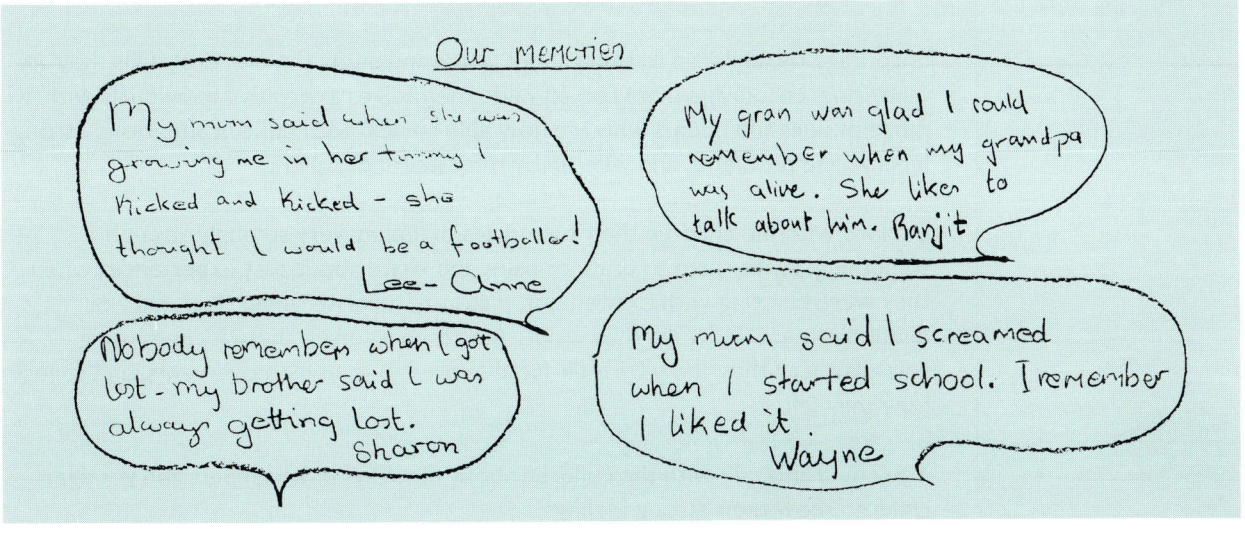

Our memories

My mum said when she was growing me in her tummy I kicked and kicked - she thought I would be a footballer!
Lee-Anne

My gran was glad I could remember when my grandpa was alive. She likes to talk about him. Ranjit

Nobody remembers when I got lost - my brother said I was always getting lost.
Sharon

My mum said I screamed when I started school. I remember I liked it.
Wayne

Although some of the children will have had similar experiences, they will discover that there were also differences in outcomes or feelings, and these can be shared. They will also begin to realise that these memories are part of how they relate to their special people.

The children could ask some members of their family networks to remember what they (the children) were like when they were very young: their birth, infancy and early childhood. It can be revealing to the children to discover that the occasions they thought were important landmarks may be thought insignificant by their relatives, or may have been forgotten by them, or remembered differently.

Ask the children to think, draw and write about themselves as they are now at the age of 8 or 9. What do they think people will remember about them as they are now? For example,

- I think my family will remember I got my swimming certificate.

- I think they will remember all my front teeth growing.

- My friend will remember we broke friends and made up.

- I think my Mum will remember the good salads I made.

- My Dad says he will remember me because I've learned to ride my bike properly.

- Mr Harpin will remember me. I'm the class bookworm.

Ask the children to think, draw and write about what they will want to remember about themselves at this age. For example,

- Swimming a length. I nearly gave up.

- Having to wear specs.

- Not being scared of the dark, not so much anyway.

- Using the word processor – it's great.

- Going to camp without my family.

- Getting better at doing things on my own.

Encourage the children to think about, value and enjoy the practical skills they are mastering. Encourage them too to value themselves as positive individuals with a range of skills and talents who are now able to deal with difficult situations, strong feelings and problems, and who enjoy the esteem of others.

Explore with the children their memories of feeling very strongly about something. Invite them to draw or paint and write about past experiences when they were bursting with excitement, pleasure, surprise, anger, fear, hate or disappointment. How did they react? Ask them to enact these feelings using role-play. Can they show by their facial expressions, body movements, and speech how they felt?

You could also talk with the children about the ways in which pets and younger children show their strong feelings.

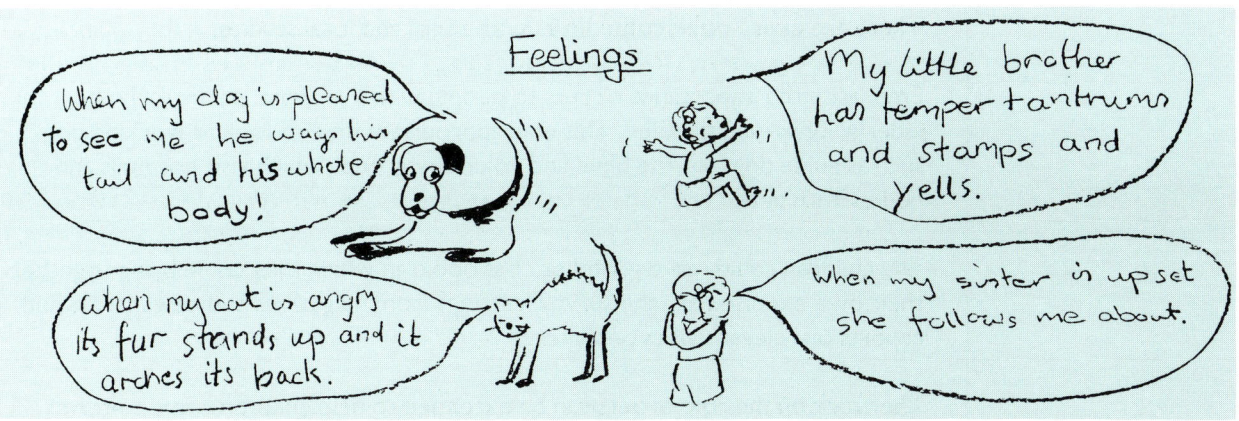

Feelings

When my dog is pleased to see me he wags his tail and his whole body!

My little brother has temper tantrums and stamps and yells.

When my cat is angry its fur stands up and it arches its back.

When my sister is upset she follows me about.

Activity 2 ● ***Our pets***

- Survey work. Drawing and writing. Presenting information. Exploring feelings. Visits. Visitors. Talking together. Using literature.

- Class or group activities.

Remind the children of the work they did in Content box 3 (page 322) when they looked at the needs of pets. The importance of relationships with pets in people's lives is well documented and you can explore this with the children. Remind children of the survey they did on pets. Now ask them to carry out a survey on *why* people have pets.

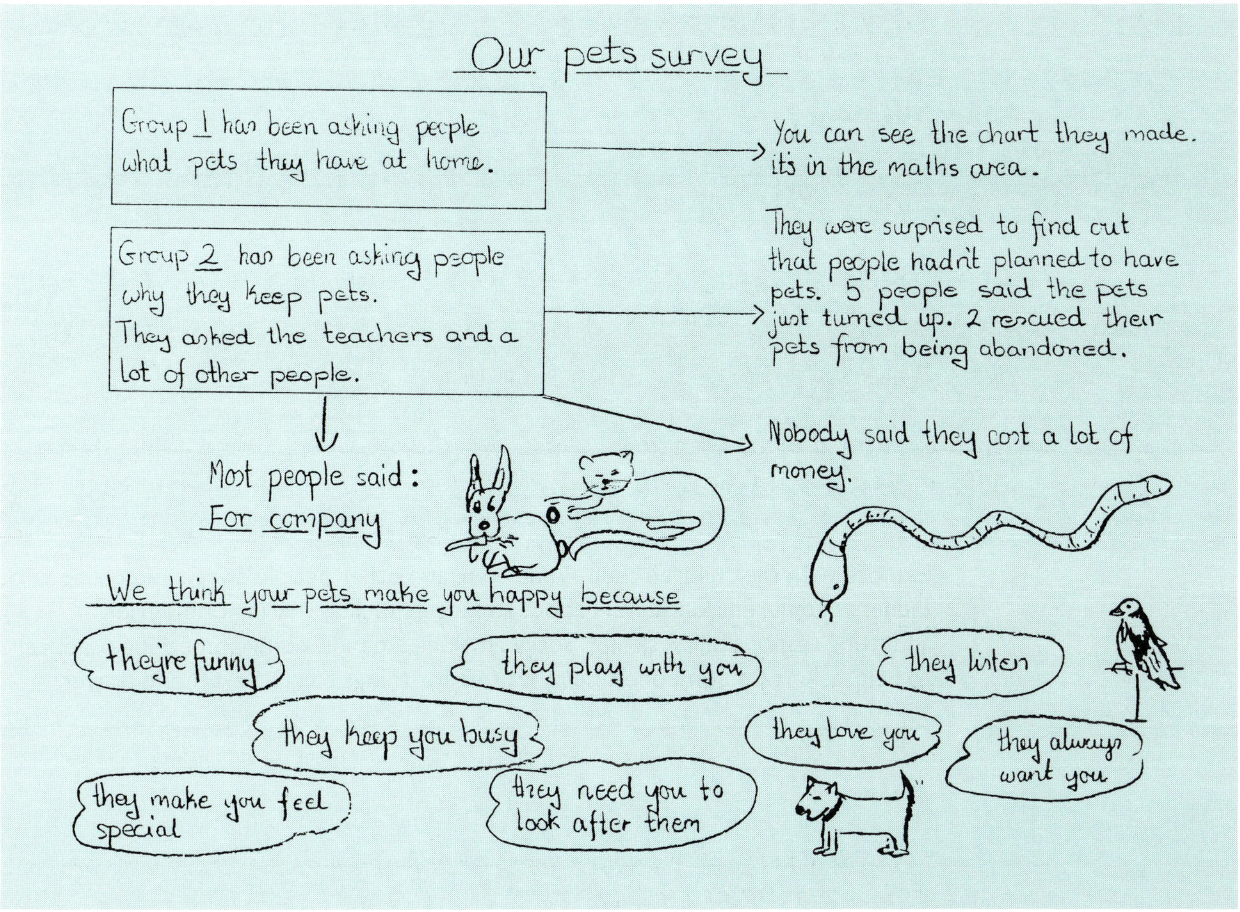

Our pets survey

Group 1 has been asking people what pets they have at home.

You can see the chart they made. It's in the maths area.

Group 2 has been asking people why they keep pets.
They asked the teachers and a lot of other people.

They were surprised to find out that people hadn't planned to have pets. 5 people said the pets just turned up. 2 rescued their pets from being abandoned.

Nobody said they cost a lot of money.

Most people said:
For company

We think your pets make you happy because

they're funny

they play with you

they listen

they keep you busy

they love you

they always want you

they make you feel special

they need you to look after them

There are **cross-curricular links** with social and local studies.

Emphasise the importance of pets to people who live alone, particularly the elderly, infirm and disabled. This is an appropriate time to look at working dogs such as guide dogs for the blind and voluntary groups which visit hospitals and homes with pets.

The children could make group or class books in which they could bring together their own experiences, the survey, cuttings from magazines and newspapers and reports on relevant visits or visitors.

The work on the role of pets can be extended to help children come to terms with aspects of separation, loss and death. Many children will have experienced concern when a pet is missing, delight when it returns, sadness when it fails to return, and grief if it dies. Sharing these experiences and finding the words which pin down their feelings can be very helpful.

Explore with them the word 'sad', which many children use to describe a whole range of feelings. How many different kinds of sad feelings can they find? **Cross-curricular links**: literature, particularly poetry, and music may be helpful here.

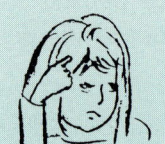

All Kinds of sad

We thought about all kinds of feeling sad

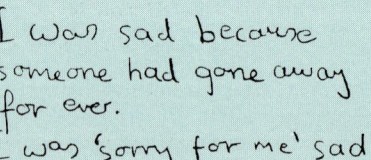

I was sad because someone had gone away for ever.
I was 'sorry for me' sad.

I was sad because someone had been horrid to me.
I was 'hurt feelings' sad

I was sad because my dog was dead.
I was sad for him and me.

I was sad about the starving children.
I was 'sorry for them' sad.

I was sad because I'd been horrid. I was 'sorry about it' sad.

Explore with the children their, your own, and other people's ways of dealing with sadness of different kinds. Talk about strategies such as sharing one's grief, admitting responsibility, saying 'Sorry', making amends, doing something practical to help, asking for someone's help, waiting for things to get better and prayer.

Content box 5   Focus on special places

What do we think makes a healthy neighbourhood? What would we encourage or ban? What rules would we have? Who would be in charge? What could we do about vandals, noise and dogs? Are the places around here healthy and happy? Who could show us how to improve them? Where is my pet's special place? How do I feel if someone spoils my special place? Where can little children, old people or disabled people go?

Activity 1   ● ***What makes a happy, healthy neighbourhood?***

- Planning. Model-making. Talking together. Evaluation. Generalising.

- Class and group activities.

Cross-curricular links with environmental studies: the work in this content area could provide starting points and opportunities to explore aspects of environmental health, such as pollution of different kinds including noise pollution, and the care of children's play areas.

Ask the children to work in groups and make a plan or model of a 'super-healthy' town, district or village. Suggest they begin by holding a brainstorming session to think of ideas on what they would include or forbid. What notices and warning signs would they need to make? What facilities would they provide especially for children? Who would be in charge of keeping different places healthy? What would their jobs involve? What would everybody in the model town have to do to keep it healthy? How could they prevent people from spoiling the place by, for example, vandalism, or the exercising of their dogs in the wrong places, etc?

Encourage the children to design posters and rule books. What new officials might they recruit? Ask them to illustrate aspects of life in their healthy model town.

Encourage the children to explore and evaluate their neighbourhood, starting with their school, to see how healthy it is. How does it rate on a scale of 1 to 10? Is there something which they could do immediately to improve the rating? Is there something they could plan for which would improve things more slowly? Who could help them in their campaign to make the neighbourhood more healthy?

Activity 2 ● *My special place – your special place?*

- Using poetry. Talking together. Writing. Drawing. Collage-making.

- Class or group and individual activities.

Remind the children of the work they did relating to the importance and care of pets for Content boxes 3 and 4. Ask them which of their pets has its own special place? Which is happy anywhere? Read them *Cats Sleep Anywhere*, by Eleanor Farjeon. (See Appendix 2, page 428.) How do pets feel if they are moved from their special places or if the places are spoiled, moved or taken over? What do they do? Ask the children how they feel if someone takes over or spoils their special places either in the classroom or at home. How do their relatives feel if the same thing is done to them? Talk about their responses. For example:

— 'Our cat likes to sleep on the window sill in the sun. In winter it sleeps on the boiler. It hates it when you move it.'

— 'I like to read in the book corner. I hate it when people keep pestering me or play about and make a noise.'

— 'My sister likes her bedroom best. It's full of pop star pictures. She makes us all knock on the door. I forget and she gets so cross. I think it's daft.'

— 'My Great-Gran sleeps in her chair in the afternoon. She gets upset if you wake her up. But she says she wasn't really asleep.'

Talk about how other people might feel in similar circumstances and emphasise that people need respect and privacy. Discuss the feelings of older people, the ill, the handicapped or disabled, younger children and others whose feelings might be ignored by helpers with 'good intentions'.

Encourage the children to observe and record in some way the positive contributions of people who have special needs but who have been able to work towards a positive place in life.

Conclude this activity by inviting the children to make a collage of happy places, particularly places which have been made happier and healthier by people's efforts. The collage could incorporate photographs from magazine and newspaper reports of local improvements such as new buildings and new or proposed new amenities as well as the children's own drawings and writing. The collage could also act as a backcloth to the children's models.

10&11

Action Planner
Me and My Relationships

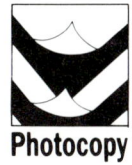

Photocopy

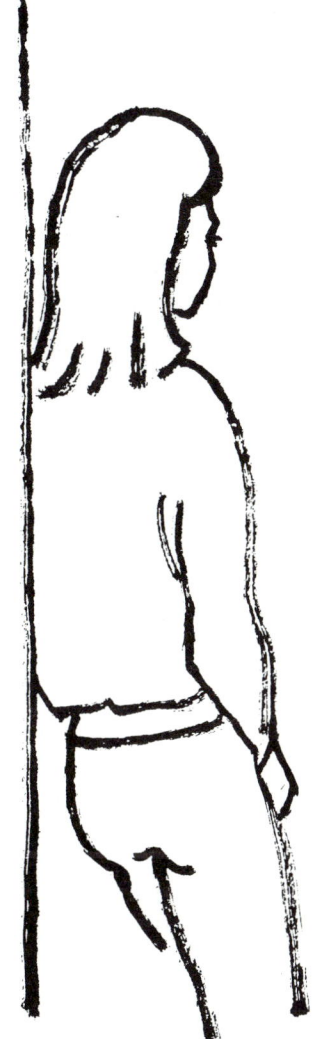

2

Focus on friends and friendships

What is a friend? What do I mean by a best friend? a girl friend? a boy friend? What do other people mean? What do we mean by couple, mates, parents, family, relatives, wife, husband, lover? How do I cope with my new feelings about girls and boys and body changes? How can I cope when I feel left out? How do I cope when people comment on my race, my sex, my body, my accent or my family? What do good leaders do? How do I cope with group pressures, secrets and promises? What kinds of people do I choose as friends? Am I easily persuaded?

4

Focus on memories and growing up

Have I ever felt bursting with feelings? Did I show, or disguise them? How do I feel if someone important stops loving me, goes away or dies? What do I mean by falling in love, falling out of love and fancying someone? How much is it to do with sex? How do we make relationships grow and last? How do I leave a sad relationship behind? What are the happiest and saddest days I can remember? What memories do I share with my friends? How important are memories?

3

Focus on feelings

How do I react to day-to-day demands? Does it depend on the mood I'm in? How can I learn to cope with my moods and feelings? How can I become sensitive to other people's moods? What am I looking forward to about being grown-up? How many of my worries about the future are about sex, disease or drugs? What can I do about this? How do I think I have changed? How do girls' and boys' bodies change as they become women and men? Who do I admire now? Can I put myself in someone else's shoes?

5

Focus on special places

What makes some places special? Where do I go to be alone? Are these places safe? How do I feel when people invade my special places or misunderstand my reasons for going there? How do people feel when they have no special place? Where do I go when I want company and fun? Are these places safe? Which places do I want to forget? Can I work out the network of places I visit? Do I care for these places? Do they make me feel good and confident? How would I organise my special places if I could? What is a vandal? Why do I think they do it?

1

Focus on special people

How has my network of special relationships changed? How much do my special people like each other? How do I feel about being in the middle? How do they treat me? Who chooses these people? How do I think people learn to get on with each other? What are the rules? How can you recognise the group I belong to? How do we treat people? What's good about being one of a group?

Classroom Strategies and Activities for Ages 10 and 11

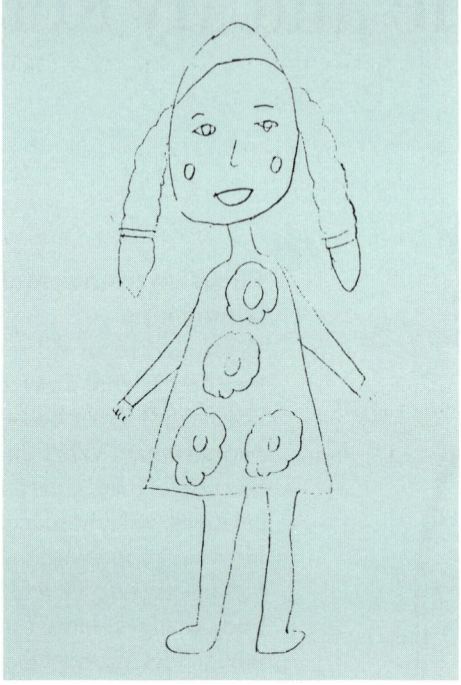

Key messages ●

Learn:

- who you are.

- what you are good at.

- why people like you.

- what upsets or hurts you.

- to cope with your own and other people's moods and feelings.

- the difference between best friends, boyfriends and girlfriends.

- that there are different rules for different kinds of relationships.

- who you can talk to and how to ask them to listen.

- how you should behave towards girls, boys, people who are different, old people and people with special needs. Learn more about them.

- how men and women make babies and how they look after them.

- about falling in love, and falling out of love and what this means to different people and to you.

Understand:

- that your network of people is growing and changing but your family is always special.

- how people feel. Think about why they say and do things.

- that although you want to choose your own friends and act independently your family may not agree because they worry about you.

- that your friends have their own networks and that you have to share them with others.

- that sometimes people have their own problems with relationships and although you may feel hurt, left out, or afraid that it could be your fault, it isn't. Talk to them about it.

- that when you are sad and upset about something it helps to share your feelings with somebody.

- that we all grow at different rates so do not worry if you seem different from your friends.

Practise:

- talking about problems with people you trust.

- thinking for yourself and making up your own mind.

- saying 'No' to friends sometimes. It is not always easy.

Content box 1   Focus on special people

How has my network of special relationships changed? How much do my special people like each other? How do I feel about being in the middle? How do they treat me? Who chooses these people? How do I think people learn to get on with each other? What are the rules? How can you recognise the group I belong to? How do we treat people? What's good about being one of a group?

Activity I   ● ***How has my network changed?***

- Talking together. Writing. Drawing. Assessment. Evaluation.
- Class or group and individual activities.

Ask the children to think back to the network of special people they had when they were babies or toddlers. How have these networks grown and changed? Ask them to chart the changes in three or four stages using writing and drawing.

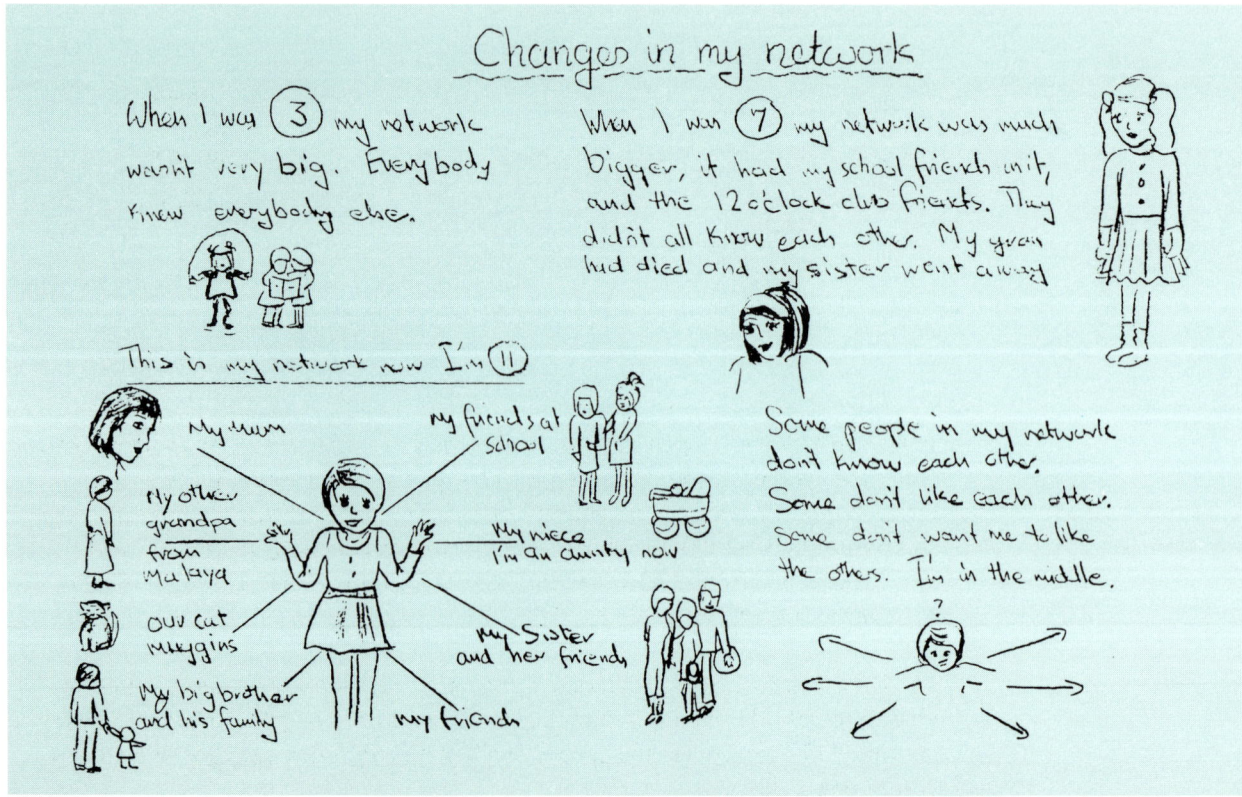

There is an opportunity here for the children to talk about the tensions which arise within their current network of relationships and to share with others the feeling of being 'in the middle'.

Ask the children to use the term 'relationship' when they mean the way they relate to or get on with, other people. Invite them to consider the different relationships between people within their networks. Which relationships are always good? Which relationships vary? Which relationships are difficult?

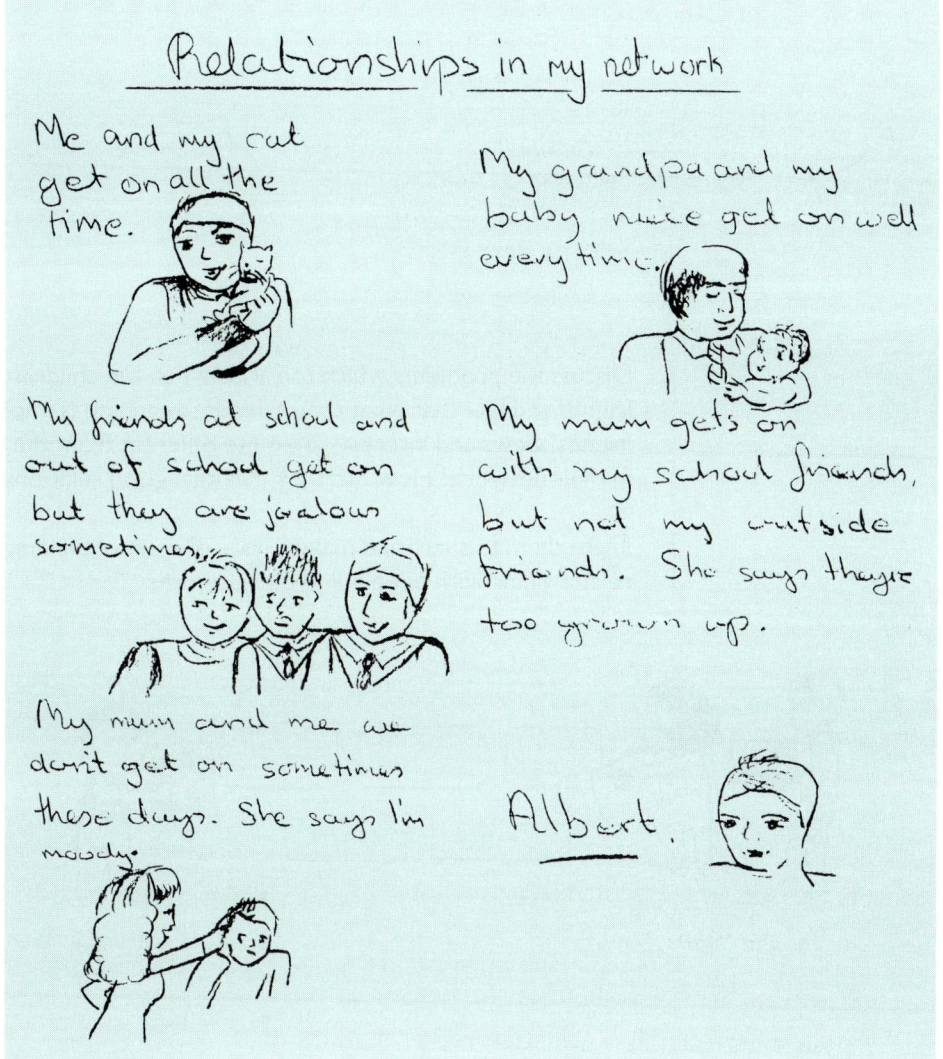

Invite the children to look at how people treat them. How has this changed from when they were 7 years old? Are they now given more responsibility, independence, choice and freedom? In which situations? When and why are they still treated as young children? How might they convince the people in their networks that they are growing more responsible and more capable of making their own choices?

Ask the children to look again at the people in their networks. Can the children identify which of the people there were chosen *by them* and which were chosen *for them*? (This might be an appropriate time to talk about adoption as a special way of being chosen.)

Choosing

These are the people in our network chosen for us:

- Real mums and dads, sisters and brothers;
- new mums, dads, sisters and brothers;
- relations;
- our teachers.

You have to learn to get on with them. Sometimes it's not easy, you fall out but you make up.

These are the people we choose for ourselves:

- Our friends at school;
- our friends out of school;
- grown ups who aren't family.

Sometimes we think these are the most important.

Discuss the problems which can arise when the children want to choose their own friends and feel that what their friends say and do is important. What if their friends' views and interests are quite different from the views of the other people in their network? How can they maintain good relationships with everyone?

Invite them to share and make a note of ways of building up better or stronger relationships with people in their networks.

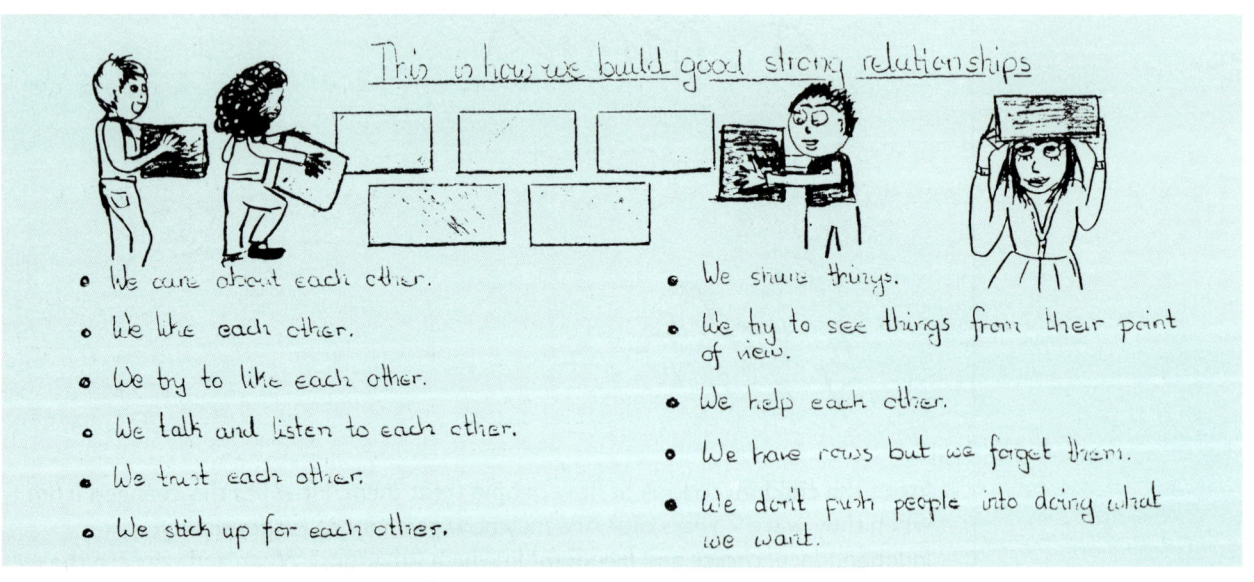

This is how we build good strong relationships

- We care about each other.
- We like each other.
- We try to like each other.
- We talk and listen to each other.
- We trust each other.
- We stick up for each other.

- We share things.
- We try to see things from their point of view.
- We help each other.
- We have rows but we forget them.
- We don't push people into doing what we want.

Activity 2 ● *Learning to get along with one other*

- Talking together. Writing. Exploring the rules of relationships.
- Class or group and individual activities.

Invite the children to think of ways in which personal relationships in the classroom could be improved. Ask each child to think of something he or she could do to contribute to these better relationships within the next day or two, and to make a confidential contract with herself or himself. Ask the children to consider how they will tell if they have been successful.

Repeat this activity, but this time ask the children to think of ways in which relationships with people out of school might be improved.

By this stage, the children will have begun to be aware that the different relationships they are exploring appear to have different sets of rules. Encourage the children to try to think about and write down these rules. Who devised them? How important it is to keep them? What rules do best friends, couples, sisters etc. have? For example, these could be the rules for Pen Friends:

- Take it in turns to write.

- Do your best writing.

- Keep on writing.

- Ask them about themselves.

- Tell them about yourself.

- Don't criticise their lifestyles.

Activity 3 ●   *My friends*

- Talking together. Evaluation. Presenting information.

- Class or group and individual activities.

Ask the children how they feel about their network of friends. Is it too big or too small? Help them to explore their networks of close friends. Ask them to summarise the nature of this network in writing and drawing, using a coding system to show 'school' and 'out of school' friends, and friends who are older or younger than they are.

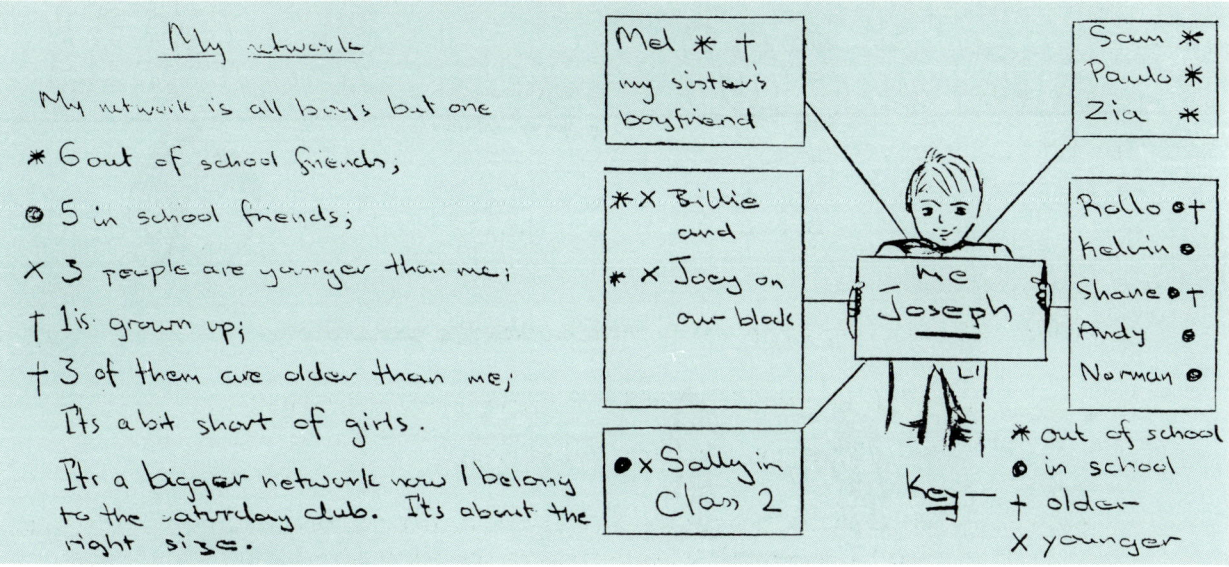

Encourage the children to talk about the changes in the balance of in-school and out-of-school friends, boy and girl friendships, older and younger friendships and friendships with adults within their networks. Some children may find that their networks have grown, others may find that their networks have become smaller and more focused for specific reasons.

There are **cross-curricular links** with language work here.

Ask the children to think of words and phrases which describe groups of people for example:

— a family.

— a club.

— a group.

— a band.

— a choir.

— an orchestra.

— a team.

— a society.

— a union.

Which words would they use to describe *their* friendship groups, for example, 'our crowd', 'our gang', etc., and *other people's* friendships, for example, 'your lot', 'your set'.

How would a stranger know which children belonged to which group? Would they be recognised by what they wear, or say? Or would they be recognised by what they laugh at, read, play, like or hate?

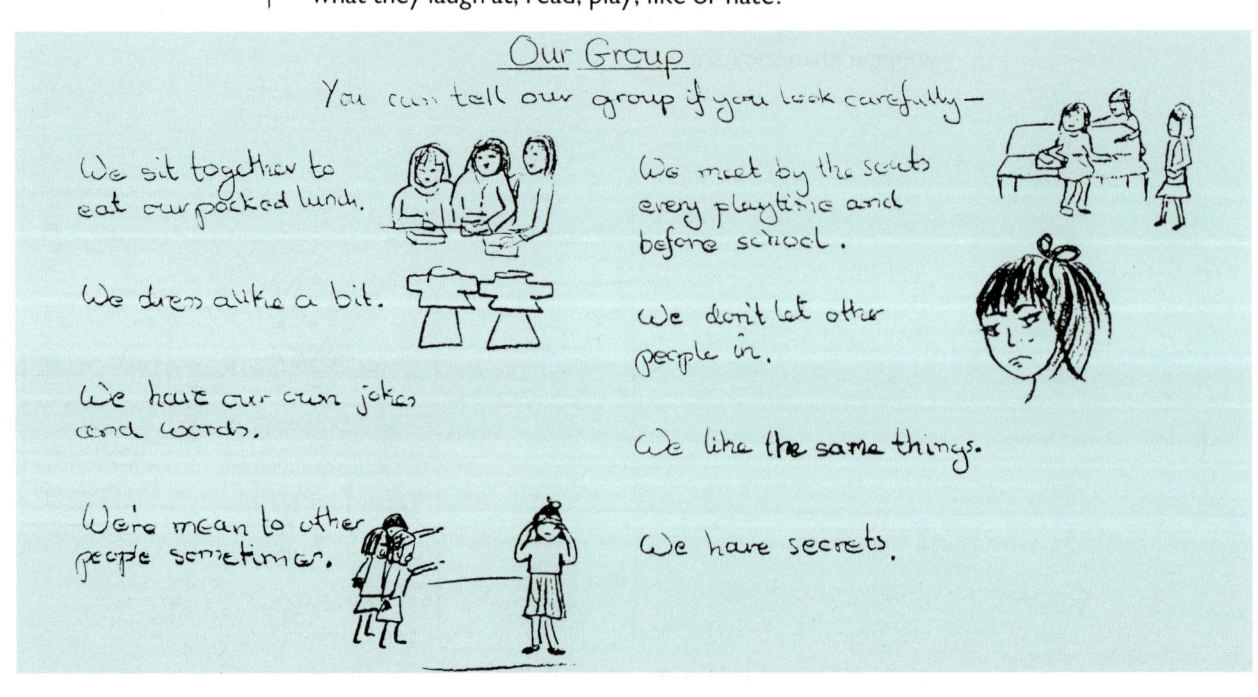

Our Group

You can tell our group if you look carefully —

We sit together to eat our packed lunch.

We dress alike a bit.

We have our own jokes and words.

We're mean to other people sometimes.

We meet by the seats every playtime and before school.

We don't let other people in.

We like the same things.

We have secrets.

Content box 2 Focus on friends and friendships

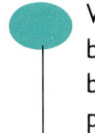

What is a friend? What do I mean by a best friend? a girl friend? a boy friend? What do other people mean? What do we mean by couple, mates, parents, family, relatives, wife, husband, lover? How do I cope with my new feelings about girls and boys and body changes? How can I cope when I feel left out? How do I cope when people comment on my race, my sex, my body, my accent or my family? What do good leaders do? How do I cope with group pressures, secrets and promises? What kinds of people do I choose as friends? Am I easily persuaded?

Activity I ● ***What is a friend?***

- Discussion. Description. Evaulation. Vocabulary work.

- Class or group and individual activities.

Invite the children to complete the statement: A friend is . . . You could hold a group brainstorming session, or ask them to work individually, writing and illustrating their responses and sharing them with others.

Talk with the children about their views on what a friend is and does, about the relationship between friends, and how it feels to be a friend.

There are **cross-curricular links** with language work here.

Draw a word box, and write in it words and phrases which include 'friend'. Help the children to define some of these words and phrases.

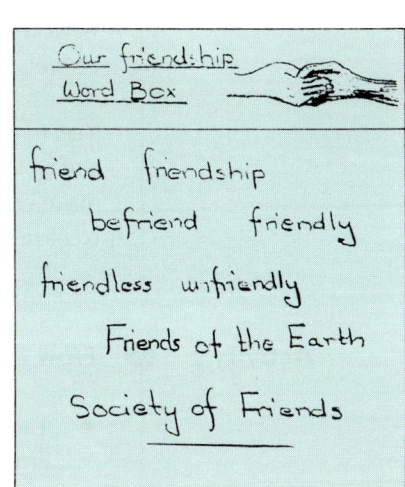

Invite the children to try to pin down what they mean when they use or hear phrases such as 'a best friend', 'an old friend', 'a new friend', 'a Pen Friend', 'a boyfriend' or 'a girlfriend'. Encourage them to share their views.

Extend the work to look at words and phrases which describe a relationship between two people, for example:

– a pair.

– a couple.

– partners.

– pals.

– twosome.

– mates.

– grandparents.

– aunt and uncle.

– wife and husband.

– lovers.

There may be local phrases to add to this list.

Talk to the children about the way these phrases are used to describe two people of the same sex, two people of the opposite sex, two people of the same age, etc. (Sensitive issues may arise in the course of this discussion.)

Some of the children will already have their own views on what is involved in these relationships, and may be seeking answers to a range of personal questions, or reassurance. Some may be basing their views on first-hand experience within their networks or in the wider groups with which they may now be mixing. Many will have based their perceptions and understanding on what they see and hear on the television, in newspapers and teenage magazines etc. Some may see themselves on the brink of some kind of special relationship. Some may be looking for ways of coping with new feelings. It is important that these children have the time to share what they are experiencing, to be able to use their personal private language and to feel at ease with public language.

You may find opportunities to explore group pressure on children to conform, and to look at when this can be a help and when it can be a problem. You can also make children more aware of others outside the group, especially those who seem to have few friends.

Activity 2 ● *How can I cope when I feel left out?*

- Talking together. Describing situations and feelings. Vocabulary work. Empathy.

- Class or group and individual activities.

Invite the children to explore how it might feel to be standing outside, looking through a window at people enjoying some celebration. **Cross-curricular link**: you may wish to use starting points for this from children's literature.

Write and draw a 'circle of feelings' to describe that experience in words and phrases. Next, ask the children to think about how it might feel to be involved in such a celebration. Write and draw a 'circle of feelings' to describe that experience. Talk about how it feels to be part of a friendship group, and how it helps in different situations.

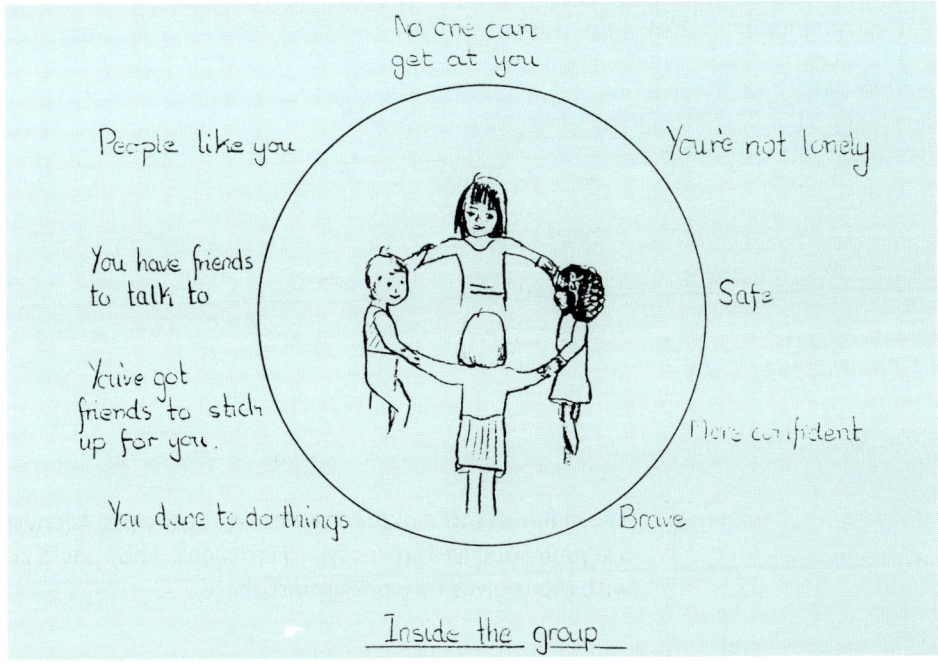

Inside the group

Explore with the children how it feels to be outside a group wanting to get in. The theme of being an outsider is one which is frequently explored in children's literature and this can provide starting points for this work.

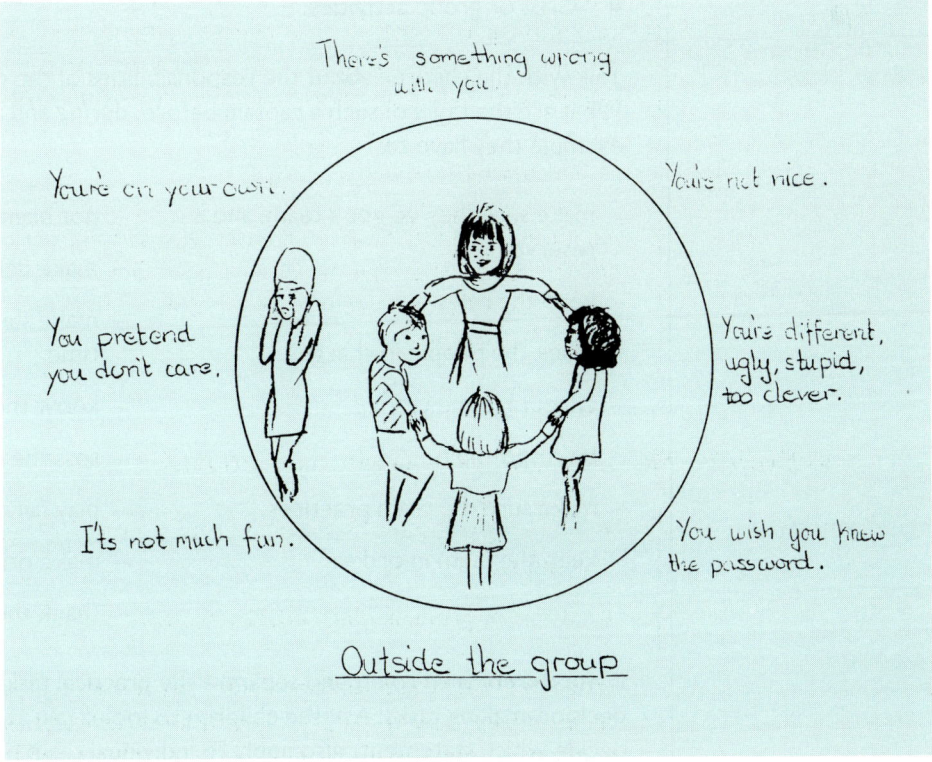

Outside the group

Hold a brainstorming session to help the children think of the strategies they might use to cope with being left out or being unable to break into a group. Which strategies are the best? Ask them to write them down.

Coping with feeling left out

Our Group thinks:

Good ways
Look for friends of your own. ✓
Don't let them see it matters. ✓
Get on with something else. ✓
Show them what you're good at. ✓
Be friendly and helpful and they might ask. ✓

Bad ways
Hanging around them. ✗
Showing off in front of them. ✗
Saying you don't care. ✗
Trying to babe your way in. ✗
Getting a grown-up to make them let you in. ✗
Calling them names ✗

The children could extend their investigation of friendship and look at discrimination and stereotyped attitudes. They could go on to make 'contracts' with themselves to work against these.

Activity 3 ● *What do leaders do?*

- Talking together. Generalising. Writing. Evaluation.
- Class or group activities.

Talk with the children about the responsibilities of the captain of a sports team. What are the tasks of such a captain before, during and after the event? For example they have to:

- make sure they've got a team, and a reserve.
- keep the rules.
- thank the people in charge.
- encourage the team.
- be responsible.
- make sure the team practices.
- keep the team in order.
- not blame the team if it loses.
- make decisions.
- make sure everybody turns up on time.
- know the rules of the game.
- toss the coin.
- play fair.
- make others play fair.
- thank the other team afterwards.

Invite the children to try and separate the practical tasks from the attitudinal, decision-making tasks. Ask the children to look again at what they have said and decide which statements also apply to individual team members.

Talk with the children about the occasions in school when they work in groups. Do they have, or need to have, captains, team leaders or group leaders? Ask the children to write down the responsibilities and jobs which group leaders have. How many of the group leader's tasks are practical ones and how many involve personal skills? For example, a group leader should:

- be sensible.

- not be bossy.

- not lose things.

- write properly.

- not have favourites.

- be organised.

- give everyone a turn

- do her share.

- settle rows.

- listen.

- set a good example.

Invite the children to look at their own friendship groups in the same way. Is there a leader? Who is it? Is it always the same person? How is the leader chosen? What kind of example does the leader set?

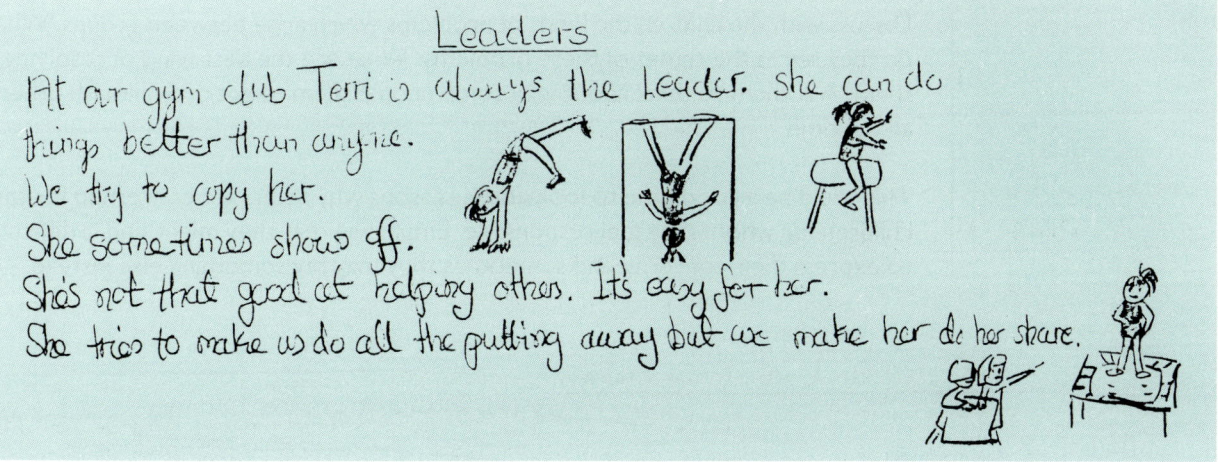

Leaders

At our gym club Terri is always the leader. She can do things better than anyone.
We try to copy her.
She sometimes shows off.
She's not that good at helping others. It's easy for her.
She tries to make us do all the putting away but we make her do her share.

Activity 4 ● ***How can I cope with group pressure?***

- Group discussion. Presentation. Categorising.

- Class or group and individual activities.

Ask the children to draw a network chart around their friendship group to show their relationships with other groups.

Encourage the children to talk about the people in these groups. How well do they get on with each group? Encourage them to use categories such as:

- we get on well all the time.

- we get on well some of the time.

- we have some problems.

- we have lots of problems.

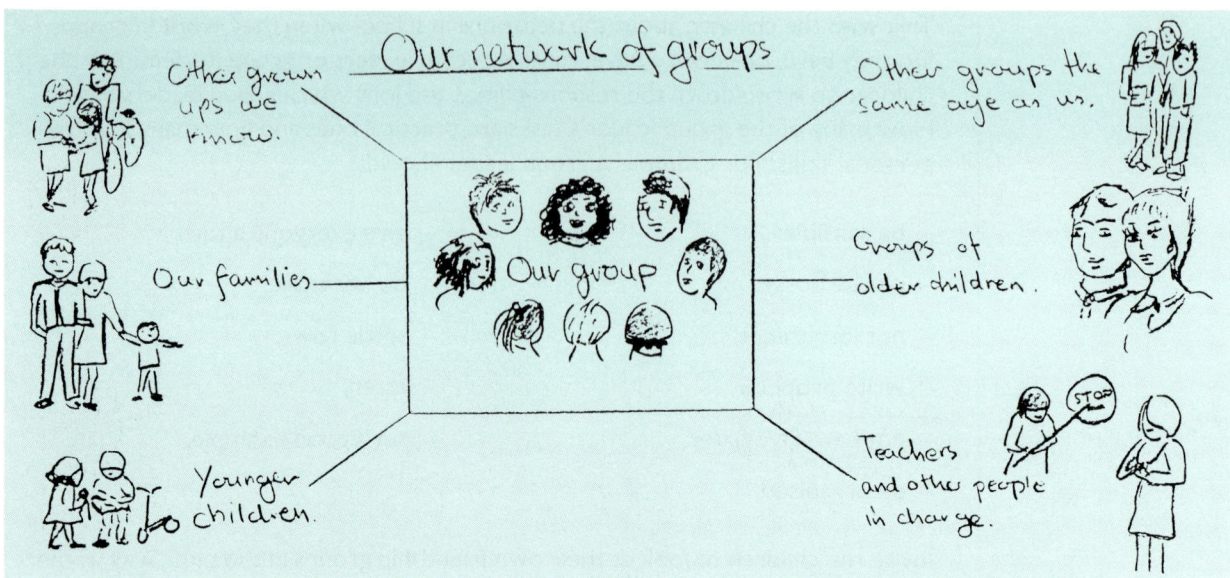

Ask them to colour code their network drawings appropriately.

Discuss with the chidren the kinds of problems which arise between groups. What do they see as the causes of these problems? What are the best ways of resolving them? Ask them to think about why some people seem to get on well with others all the time.

This could be a good time to look at the reasons why adults are concerned for the children for whom they feel responsible. Emphasise that they might find it difficult to express their concerns, and sometimes they may say something else instead.

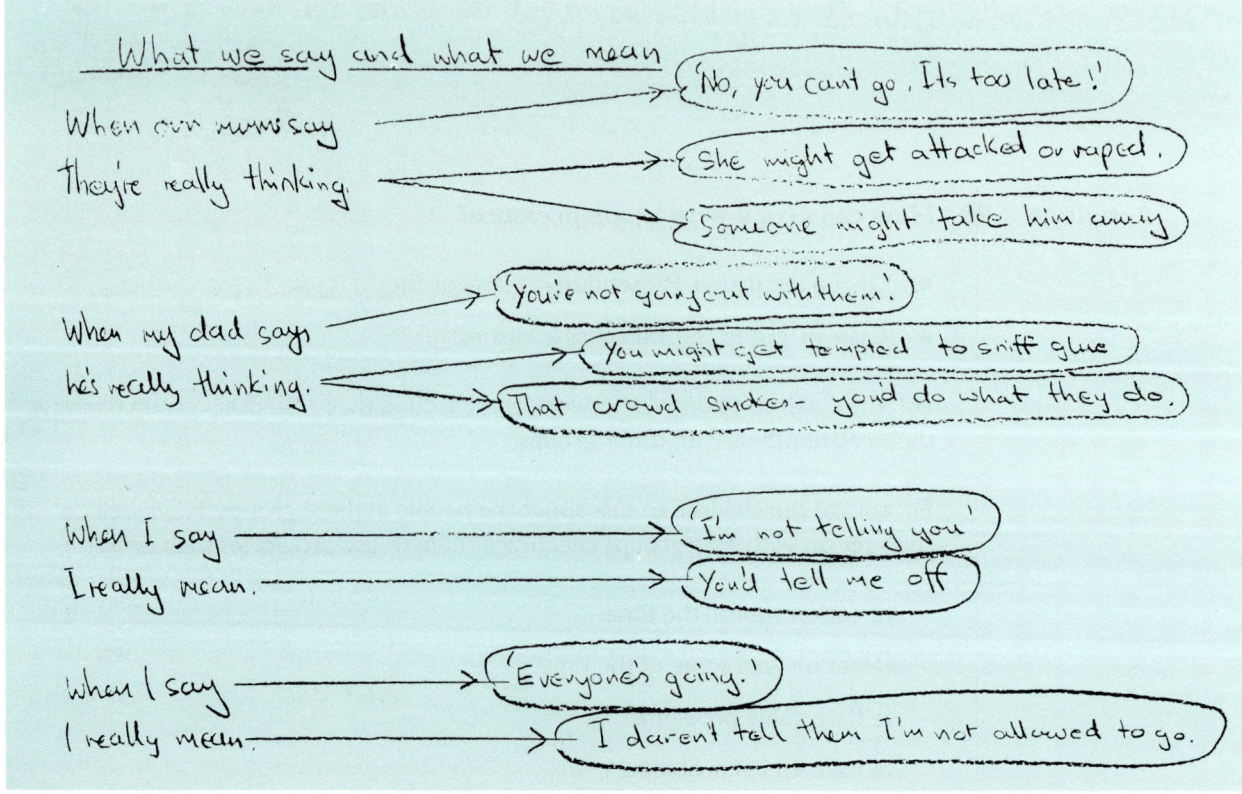

Ask the children to look again at their group networks and to talk about the groups with whom they share secrets. What kind of secrets do they share? Which secrets do they keep within their groups and why?

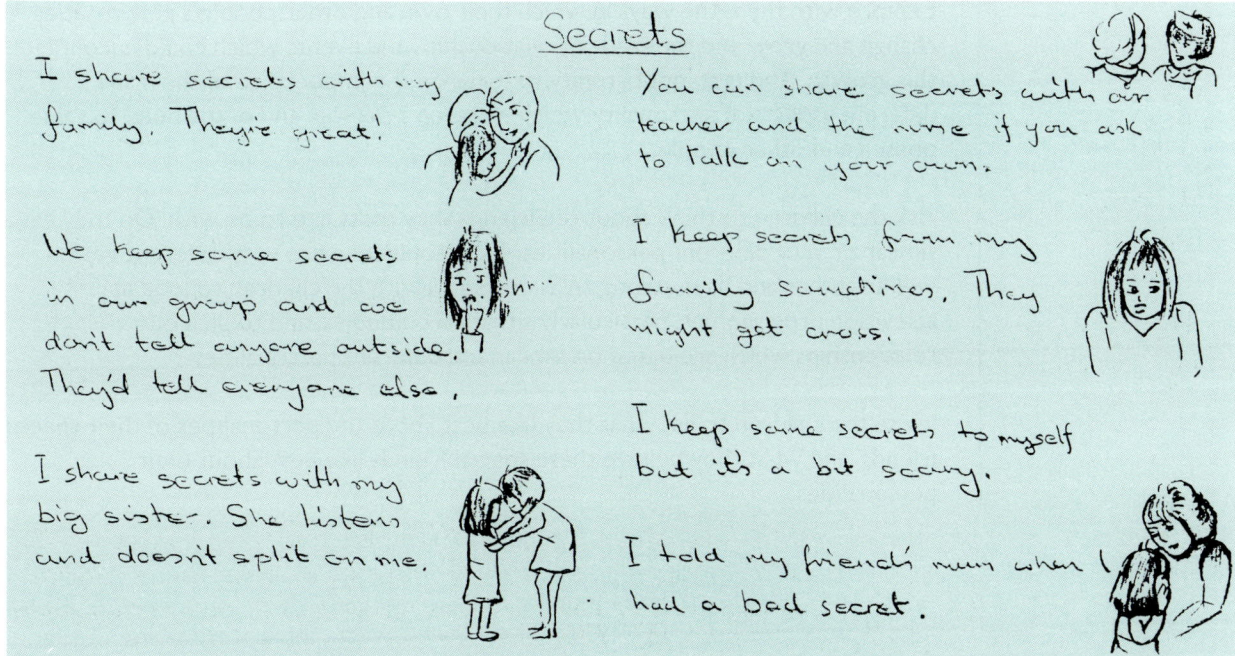

Secrets

I share secrets with my family. They're great!

We keep some secrets in our group and we don't tell anyone outside. They'd tell everyone else.

I share secrets with my big sister. She listens and doesn't split on me.

You can share secrets with our teacher and the nurse if you ask to talk on your own.

I keep secrets from my family sometimes. They might get cross.

I keep some secrets to myself but it's a bit scary.

I told my friend's mum when I had a bad secret.

There are opportunities here for children to reveal a whole range of personal feelings and concerns about their physical growth, their sexuality, their feelings and relationships. Teachers will need to be aware of and prepared to deal with the issues and questions which may arise.

Activity 5 ● ***What kinds of people do I choose as friends?***

- Talking together. Writing. Describing. Summarising. Generalising. Using television programmes.
- Class or group and individual activities.

Ask the children how they describe people. For example, do they describe their appearance, their jobs or their personalities?

Ask the children to think about different kinds of personalities. Ask them to complete the phrase 'People can be . . .'. For example:

– quiet.	– lively.	– confident.	– shy.
– thoughtful.	– noisy.	– brave.	– nervous.
– loners.	– fun.	– not easily upset.	– easily upset.
– gentle.	– one of the crowd.	– aggressive.	– bossy.
– grown-up for their age.	– young for their age.		

Cross-curricular links: the children could make use of this type of vocabulary to describe people they know personally, people they know through the media or through history and literature.

Explore with them the ways in which their own and other people's personalities change and grow and the kinds of relationships and events which could encourage this growth. This is an opportunity to focus on the importance of the many different aspects of personality which make up a person, and of the need to value oneself and other people.

Ask the children to think about the friends they most like to be with. Do they have similar or very different personalities? Do people who are very different get on well together and have strong relationships? Invite the children to look at television programmes, particularly situation comedies, and to pick out relationships which are based on similar and different personalities.

Invite the children to list what they like best about the personalities of their special friends, and what they believe these special friends like best about their personalities.

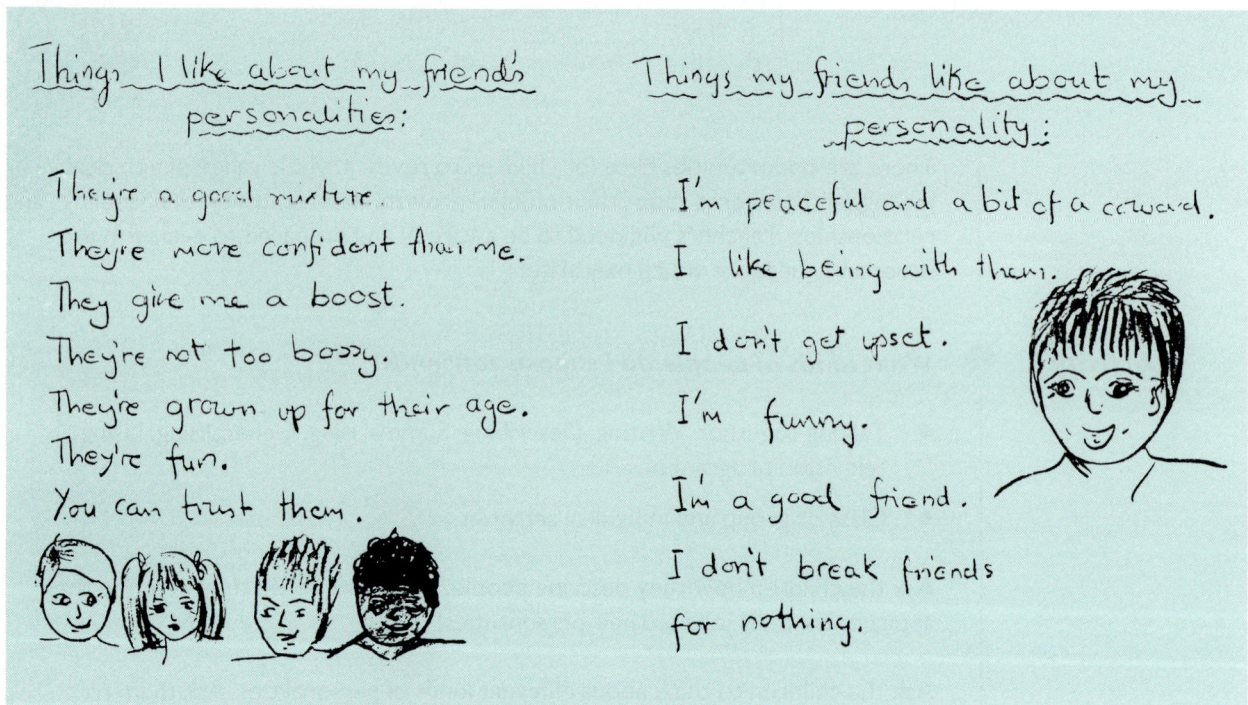

Things I like about my friend's personalities:

They're a good mixture.
They're more confident than me.
They give me a boost.
They're not too bossy.
They're grown up for their age.
They're fun.
You can trust them.

Things my friends like about my personality:

I'm peaceful and a bit of a coward.
I like being with them.
I don't get upset.
I'm funny.
I'm a good friend.
I don't break friends for nothing.

The children will have opportunities to talk about how and why they choose their friends and how and why their friends choose them, and to learn to value many different aspects of their own and other's personalities.

Ask the children to try to recall occasions when they were persuaded by a friend, or a group of friends, to do something. Was it something they didn't want to do, or were unsure about? Were they easily persuaded? Were they glad they had been persuaded? Were they sorry? Ask the children if it is more difficult to resist persuasion from special friends or from a larger friendship group. Ask the children to take a vote and write about it.

Class 5 are investigating persuaders.

This week people have tried to persuade us:

1. to help
2. to keep secrets
3. to lie
4. to do something risky
5. to listen to their problems
6. to smoke
7. to lend them money
8. to swap something
9. to do their work for them
10. to break the rules

Is it easier or harder to resist persuasion if your best friend is trying to persuade you?

This is how they tried to do it:

- saying "I know you won't tell."
- pleading
- bullying
- asking
- saying "you're chicken".
- saying "be a pal."
- saying "It's grown up"
- saying "If you don't I will do something terrible."

We took a vote
16 said "yes it is harder."
13 said "no it's not, it's easier."

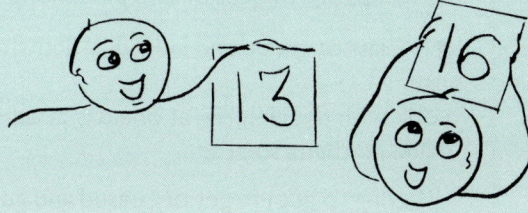

Content box 3   Focus on feelings

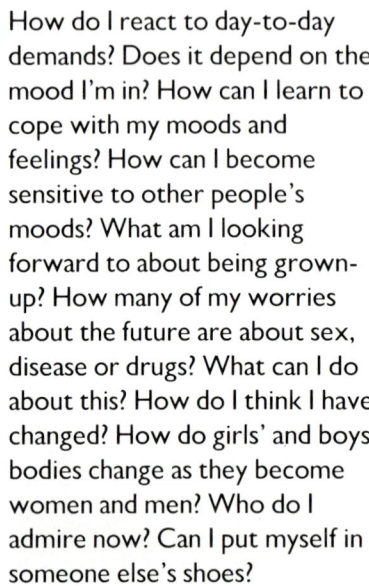

How do I react to day-to-day demands? Does it depend on the mood I'm in? How can I learn to cope with my moods and feelings? How can I become sensitive to other people's moods? What am I looking forward to about being grown-up? How many of my worries about the future are about sex, disease or drugs? What can I do about this? How do I think I have changed? How do girls' and boys' bodies change as they become women and men? Who do I admire now? Can I put myself in someone else's shoes?

Activity 1   *Day-to-day demands and my moods.*

- Exploring personal feelings through talking together, writing, drawing, empathy, evaluation and presenting information.

- Class or group and individual activities.

Look with the children at one day at school and the different demands that are made on them, such as:

— having to get up, get organised and get to school at the right time, with the right things.

— having to wait in the playground, line up to come in, be quiet and hang up one's coat etc.

— having to be physically active in one lesson and quiet in the next, or being artistic in one lesson and then having to carry out investigations and write reports in the next.

— having to work alone, in pairs, groups and teams, having to be leaders and be led, having to be competitive and non-competitive.

Ask them to write their own versions of the day you have discussed.

Talk about the children's reactions to the demands of the day. Do they always feel like being energetic, friendly, co-operative, quiet, a listener, or a leader? Does it depend on how they are feeling? How do they behave if they are in a good mood? How do they behave if they are in a bad, irritable or worried mood? Discuss their responses, which might include:

— join in, you might find it's OK.

- refuse to do any work.

- join in but grumble or sulk.

- laugh it off.

- pretend to enjoy it.

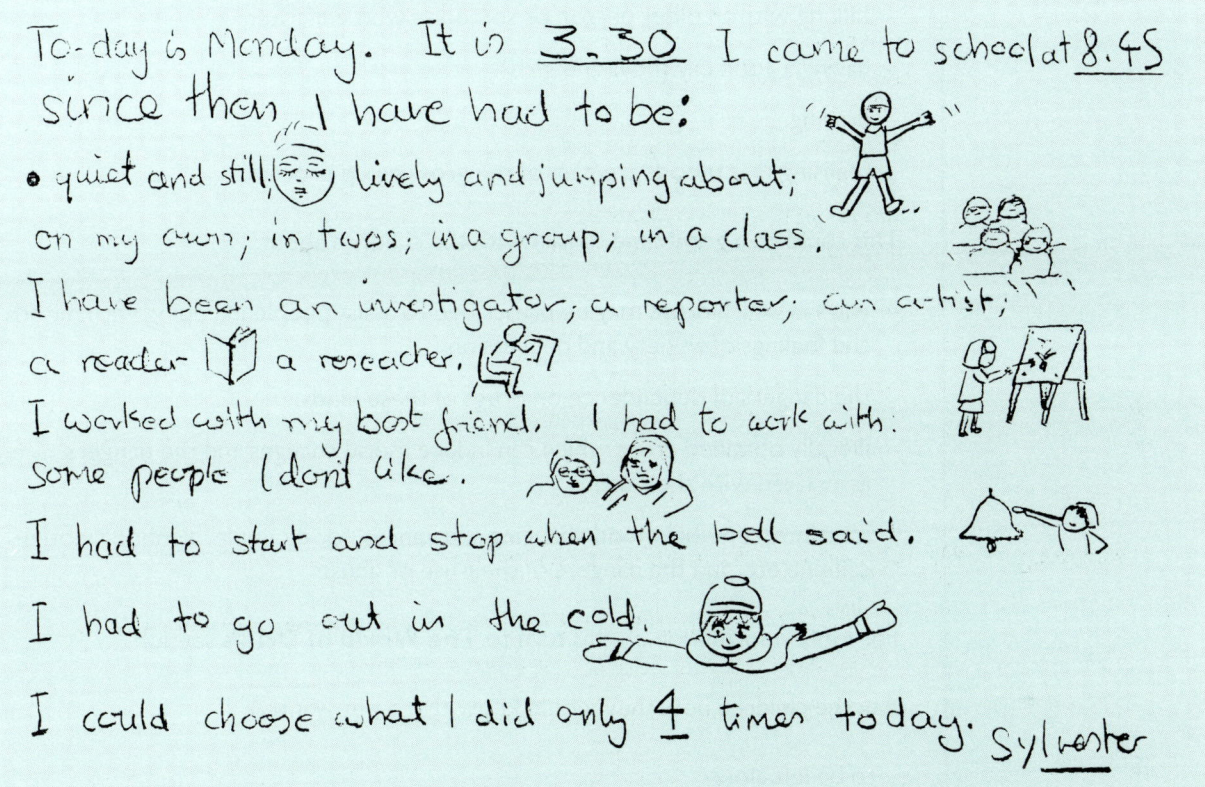

To-day is Monday. It is **3.30** I came to school at **8.45** since then I have had to be:
- quiet and still; lively and jumping about; on my own; in twos; in a group; in a class.
I have been an investigator; a reporter; an artist; a reader a researcher.
I worked with my best friend. I had to work with: some people I don't like.

I had to start and stop when the bell said.

I had to go out in the cold.

I could choose what I did only **4** times today. Sylvester

Ask the children if they remember days when they weren't in the mood to do anything. Have there been other times when they felt happy enough to try anything? Were there times when nothing seemed to go right, or when they could have exploded with anger or wept? Ask them what they think causes these changes in mood?

This could be a good time to link the discussion to the physical changes of early adolescence, the different speeds at which these changes happen, and their impact on emotions. Ask them if they think there are differences in the ways girls and boys change and react.

Ask the children if they can remember times when they were in a mood, for example, a teasing mood, a mood in which they want to be alone, etc. Can they remember a time when their moods changed rapidly? Encourage them to talk about mood swings, how surprising they can be, and how difficult it can be to explain or cope with them. Talk with them about the coping strategies they might try to use, such as:

- talking with friends, and possibly finding they have the same feelings.

- relaxing until the mood begins to change.

– changing one's activity, particularly taking exercise.

– fantasising about an 'ideal' holiday for yourself or something which you want to do.

– shouting into an empty room.

– treating the mood like a monster that must be got rid of.

– talking with an older person or someone who will listen.

– having a good cry (boys and girls).

– praying.

– realising that moods are part of the growing up process.

This could be a good time to talk with the children about:

– ways in which drugs may be prescribed to assist people in coping with moods and feelings of anxiety and depression.

– the dangers of dependence on drugs of these kinds.

– illegally obtained drugs which can induce mood changes and the dangers associated with their use.

– socially acceptable mood changing substances, for example, alcohol, nicotine, caffeine etc, and the dangers of their use or abuse.

For more information on this turn to **The World of Drugs** section.

Ask the children how they would know that a pet wanted:

– to be left alone.

– to be played with.

– to be comforted.

How would they know that a friend was:

– excited?   – angry?

– wanted to be left alone?   – in a bad mood?

– in trouble?   – feeling down?

– upset?

How much would their friend communicate about his or her mood by body language, or tone of voice, or by what he or she said and did? Ask the children to explore through talking, movement or role-play:

– ways of helping the friend cope with their mood.

– 'catching' the friend's mood as if it was an infectious disease.

– ways in which they could resist 'catching' the mood.

This activity could provide an opening for talking about the way in which the strong emotions and moods of others, particularly friends, can sweep children into difficult situations. You could then encourage them to practise coping strategies, for example, saying 'No', 'I need time', 'I need to ask about that', 'Don't pressure me', etc.

Activity 2 ● *What am I looking forward to about being grown-up?*

- Talking together. Writing. Evaluating change. Presenting information.
- Class or group and individual activities.

Explore with the children some of their feelings about growing up. Emphasise the different rates of both physical and emotional growth and development. Remind the children of their individual 'time clocks'.

Talk about the ways in which we can help our bodies to grow strong, although we cannot force change. Look at how learning to manage some of our feelings can help the growing up process.

Invite the children, working in pairs, to talk about and list some of their feelings about growing up. Suggest they use headings such as:

'We are looking forward to . . .'
'We are worried about . . .'

Ask them to share what they feel with other children. Are there differences between what the girls and boys think? Can they say why feelings about growing up differ?

Invite the children to think about their present lives and lifestyles. Can they think of two or more things they would miss if they were suddenly grown-up?

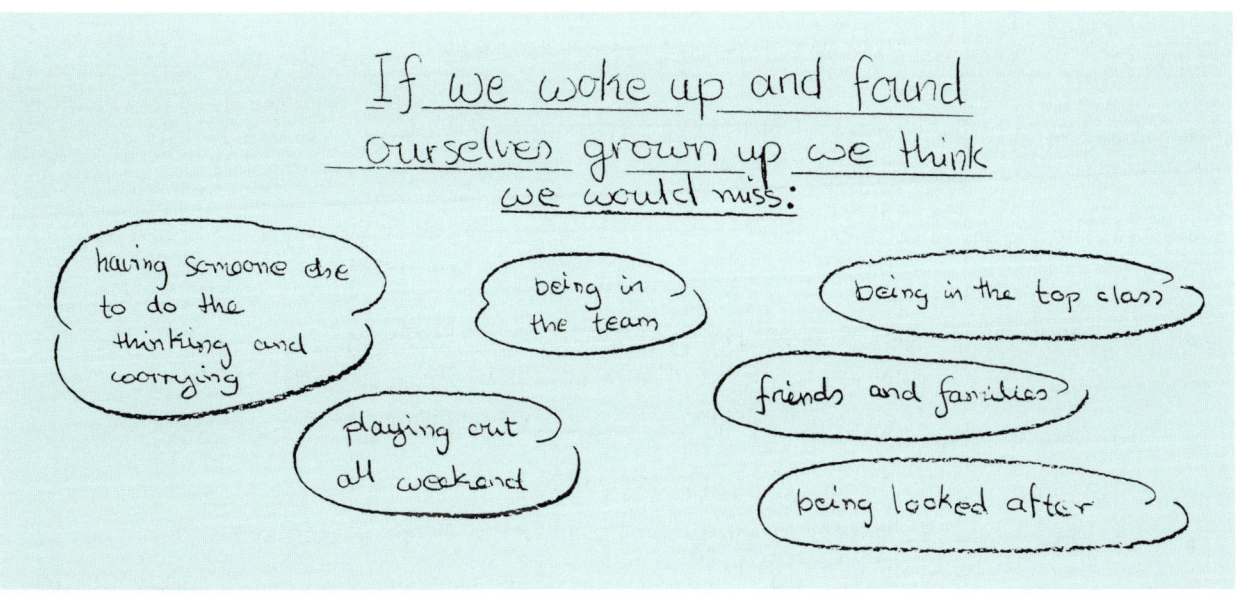

If we woke up and found ourselves grown up we think we would miss:

having someone else to do the thinking and worrying

being in the team

being in the top class

playing out all weekend

friends and families

being looked after

Activity 3 ● *How are we changing?*

- Talking together. Categorising. Writing. Drawing.
- Class or group and individual activities.

Hold a brainstorming session, inviting the children to think of all the ways in which they have changed in the last three years. Ask them to organise their responses into three categories: *appearance*, *personality* and *relationships*. For example:

Appearance:	Personality:	Relationships:
– I look more grown up.	– I don't cry so much.	– I'm not scared to say No.
– You can tell I'm a girl.	– I don't scream for my Mum.	– I can say I'm sorry.
– I'm taller.	– I'm more moody.	– I can put myself in someone else's shoes.
– My hair is darker.	– My feelings go up and down.	– I worry about people more.
– I haven't got gaps in my teeth.	– I don't tell people things.	– I know when people are pretending.
– I don't bite my nails.	– I worry about myself and things.	– I stay friends with people.
– I'm more clumsy.	– I'm not so scared.	– I choose my friends.
– My voice is different.		
– I'm not so energetic.		

Ask the children to suggest changes which they would like to make now. Ask them to look for one change which realistically could be made and to talk about how this might be done. What help might they need at school? Or at home? Some children may like to make contracts with themselves. Encourage them to write these and sign them.

What I'd like to change about me.	What can I do about it?
• I'd like to be taller.	→ Nothing.
• I'd like to be more energetic.	→ Get a friend to join and keep me going.
• I'd like to stop my voice going funny.	→ Nothing.
• I'd like to stop blushing all the time.	→ Not worry so much.
• I'd like to be better at saying no to persuaders and dangers.	→ Keep practising.

Namo Smith.

This could be a good time to introduce or revise specific sex education material, using body changes as a starting point. Invite the children to think of changes they have noticed in people around them.

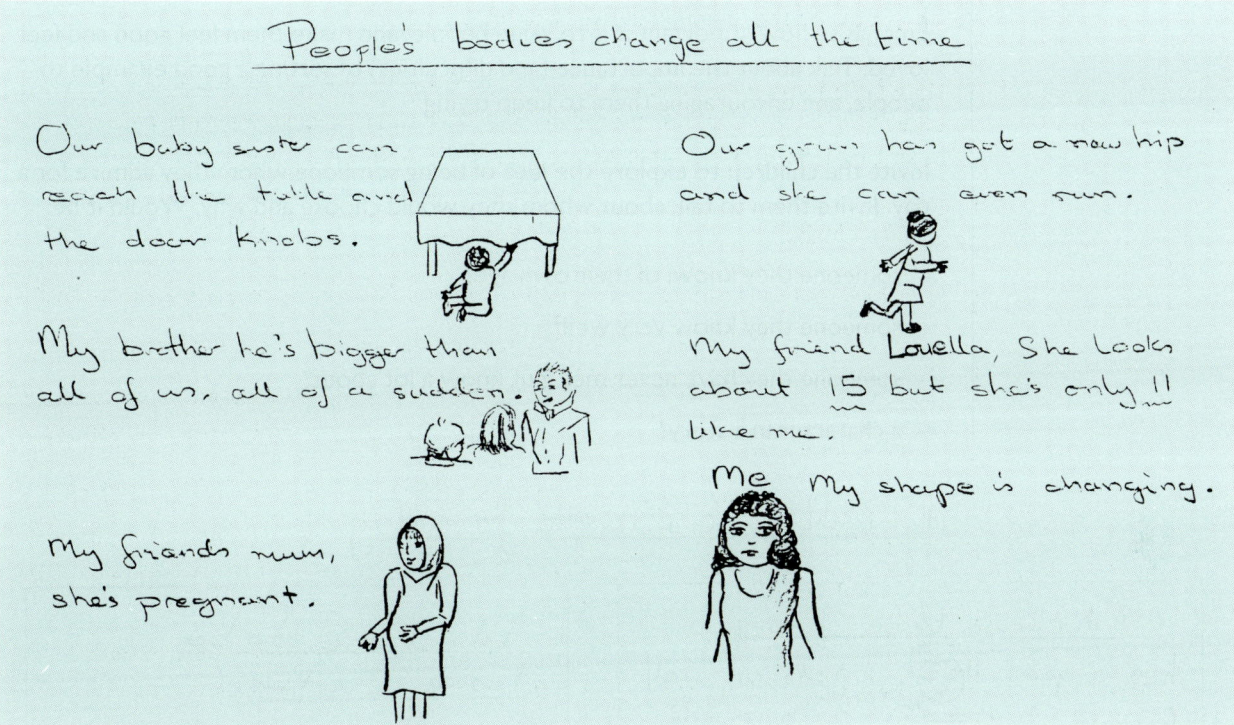

People's bodies change all the time

Our baby sister can reach the table and the door knobs.

My brother he's bigger than all of us, all of a sudden.

My friends mum, she's pregnant.

Our gran has got a new hip and she can even run.

My friend Louella, She looks about 15 but she's only 11 like me.

Me My shape is changing.

Activity 4 ● ***Who and what do I admire?***

- Talking together.
- Class or group and individual activities.

Ask the children to imagine that they are grown-up and have children of their own. What would they want *their* children to be like? Hold a brainstorming session and ask the children to group their responses under headings such as: *looks*, *health* and *personality*. For example:

Looks:	*Health:*	*Personality:*
– good looking.	– fit.	– happy.
– not too fat.	– non-smokers.	– clever.
– not too thin.	– non-drug users.	– sensible.
– happy looking.	– good teeth.	– honest.
– not clumsy.	– strong heart.	– capable.
– beautiful.	– energetic.	– loving.
– graceful.	– clean.	– well-behaved.
		– friendly.
		– resilient.

Ask the children to think about their responses. Could they help their children to be like this? How would they help them? Which of these things cannot be developed through parental help?

Emphasise how important it is to value people, and make them feel good and feel loved. Talk about the importance (and difficulties) of setting a good example to people, and encouraging them to keep trying.

Invite the children to explore the idea of being someone whom they admire for a day. Invite them to talk about whom they would choose and why. Would it be:

— someone they know, of their own age?

— someone they know very well?

— someone they have never met, but know a lot about?

— a character in a story?

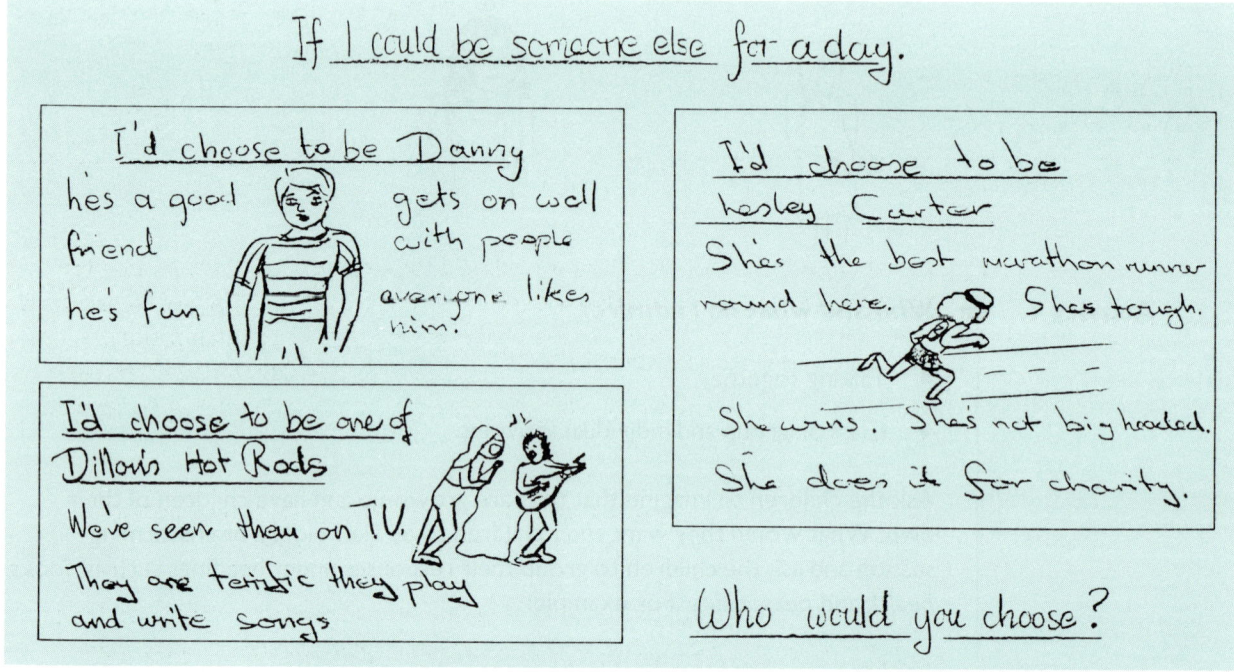

Ask the children to write about what it is they admire about their chosen person. Children may find it difficult at first to differentiate between a person's personality and the type of lifestyle that person has, and may need help to do this. Ask them to share their work with each other.

Activity 5 ● *Putting myself in someone else's shoes*

- Talking. Writing. Drawing. Collage-making. Empathising. Role-play.

- Class or group and individual activities.

Ask the children to write an advertisement in which they invite people to take over their person and personality for a day. (You could contribute your own advertisement.)

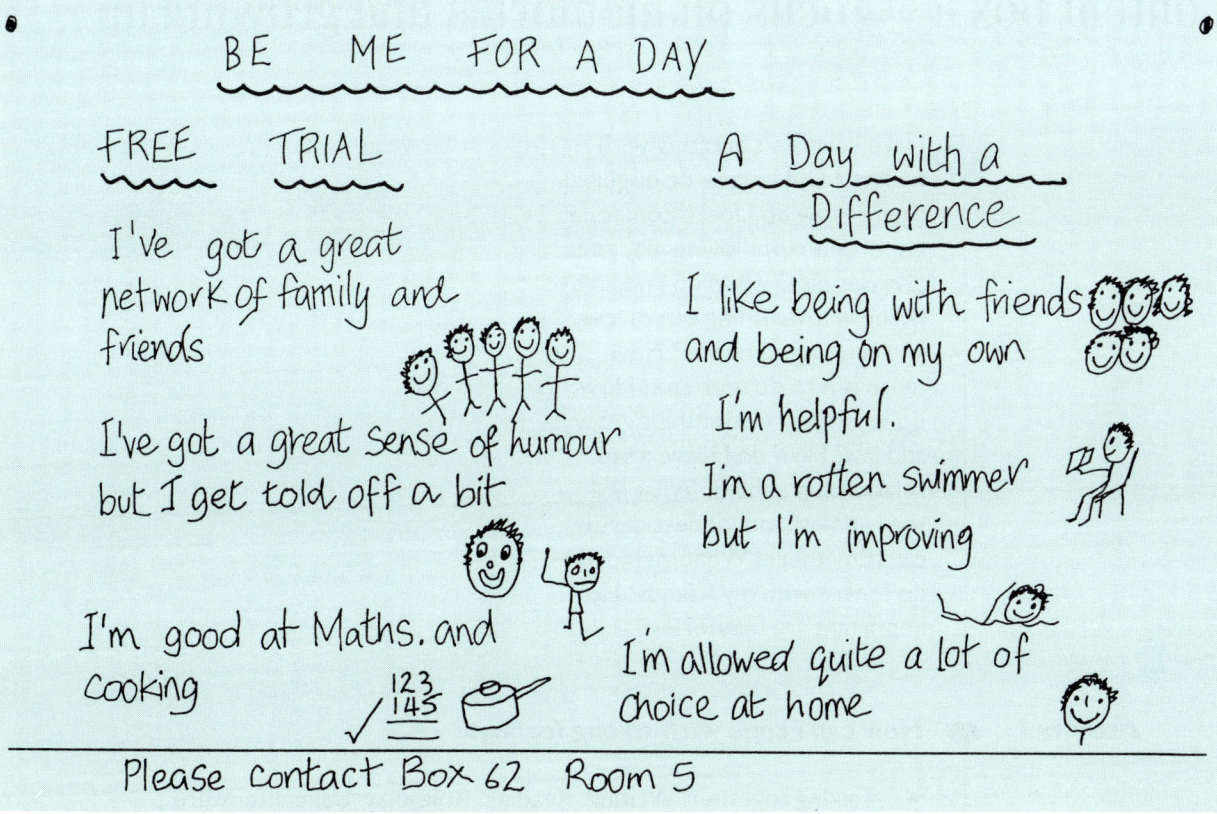

BE ME FOR A DAY

FREE TRIAL

I've got a great network of family and friends

I've got a great sense of humour but I get told off a bit

I'm good at Maths. and cooking

A Day with a Difference

I like being with friends and being on my own

I'm helpful.

I'm a rotten swimmer but I'm improving

I'm allowed quite a lot of choice at home

Please contact Box 62 Room 5

Ask the children to draw different kinds of footwear, especially those used for specific jobs and activities. Alternatively, they could make a collage of pictures cut from magazines. They could include shoes worn by dancers, athletes, skaters, skiers, climbers, farmers, fishermen, deep sea divers, fire fighters and gymnasts. They could also include shoes which are made to help people cope with physical needs or disabilities.

Ask the children to choose one type of footwear and say how they imagine it would feel to wear it. How would they walk or run in them?

Talk about the meaning of the saying 'Put yourself in someone else's shoes' as a way of trying to see things from another person's point of view. You and the children could invent role-play situations in which:

— adults face the problem of explaining their own strong feelings.

— children are receiving conflicting messages from peers and adults.

For example:

— Two adults are talking heatedly when a child comes in and demands to know what is wrong. Do the adults pretend nothing is wrong, or risk upsetting the child by telling her the truth?

— A child is asking his parents for permission to go out with friends that evening. He says everyone is going, but has been sworn to secrecy about where they are planning to go and will not say where he is going. Do the adults immediately forbid him to go out, or is there some way of negotiating the situation?

Content box 4   Focus on memories and growing up

Have I ever felt bursting with feelings? Did I show, or disguise them? How do I feel if someone important stops loving me, goes away or dies? What do I mean by falling in love, falling out of love and fancying someone? How much is it to do with sex? How do we make relationships grow and last? How do I leave a sad relationship behind? What are the happiest and saddest days I can remember? What memories do I share with my friends? How important are memories?

Activity 1   *How can I cope with strong feelings?*

- Talking together. Writing. Reading. Role-play. Using literature.
- Class or group and individual activities.

Invite the children to recall times when they felt very disappointed about someone or something. Can they describe the feeling? Can they enact the body language associated with it? How strong a feeling was it? How did they cope with their feelings? How long did they last?

Ask the children to draw a 'circle of strong feelings' which they have experienced, or have been aware of other people experiencing.

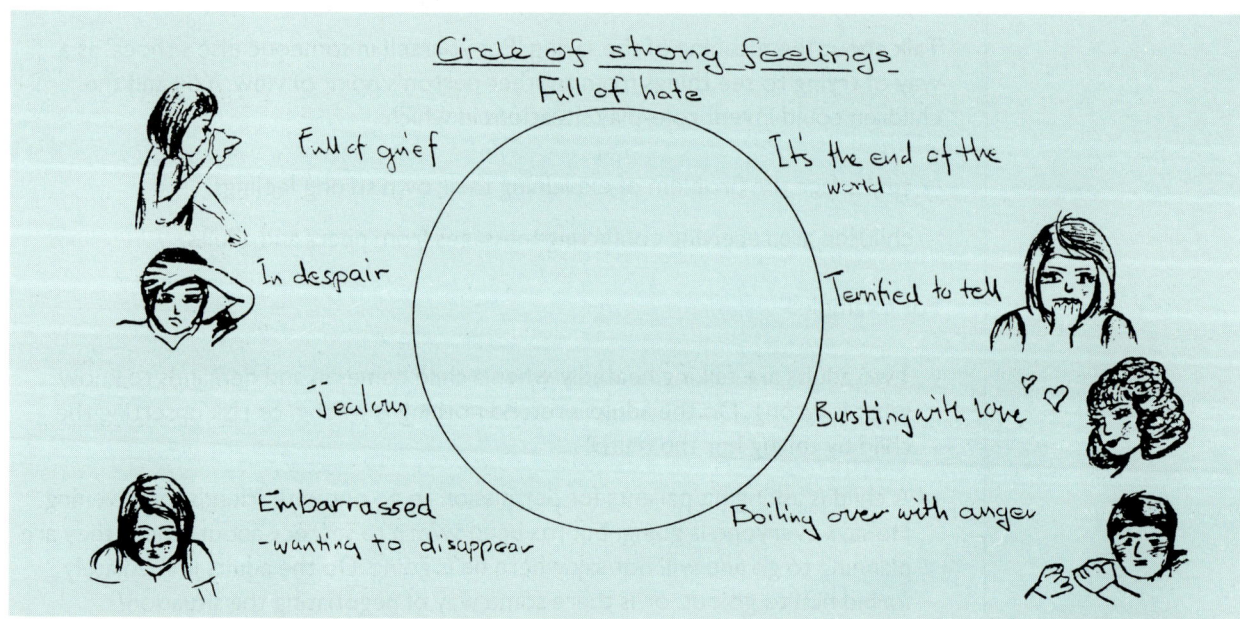

Cross-curricular links: explore these feelings with the children through role-play, writing, creative activities, poems, stories, drama, and television programmes. How do fictitious characters deal with their strong feelings? Do they show them, disguise them, give in to them, pretend to forget them, tell everyone, keep silent or ask for help?

Ask the children to look at their own experiences when strong feelings were aroused. How did they deal with their feelings? Did the adults around them help or not? Did the adults understand, listen and accept that the children had these feelings? Or did they ignore them? Did they try to protect the children?

This could be a good time to discuss with the children how they would react to other people's strong feelings. Ask the children to role-play or talk about being in a situation in which a small child in their care:

— has a temper tantrum or a nightmare.

— loses a precious toy.

— learns that their pet has died.

— has to go into hospital and is frightened.

What would they say? How would they cope with the child's feelings? How could they help?

Ask the children to recall situations in which they have had to deal with an adult's strong feelings.

My gran died.
My dad cried, but he didn't
want us to see him.
I gave him a big hug.

My sister got engaged.
She was so excited, she
couldn't stop talking.
I laughed but she didn't
mind.

My mum and dad
broke up. They
kept pretending when
I was there.
I cried at night.

What would
you have
done?

My mum got in a rage
I stayed out and didn't say where
I was going. She thought I'd
been killed or something.
I said I was sorry.
I can see now how bad it was.

My brother has to go for
a big operation. He's
scared stiff. I didn't
know what to say to
help.

Group 2   Class 5
How we coped with other people's
strong feelings.

Children's literature provides many examples of people's strong feelings which are dealt with in different ways. You can use contemporary stories, myths and traditional tales from other countries and cultures.

Strong feelings

> In the story 'Comfort Herself' the grown ups got very worked up. Comfort spoke out about how she felt and they listened.
> Douglas

> Narcissus was a drip. He just sat and moaned and did nothing and died
> Thelma

Activity 2 ● *Loss and separation*

- Talking together. Drawing. Writing. Presenting information. Extending vocabulary. Role-play.

- Class or group activities.

Explore with the children how it feels to lose something important, such as a pet, an important item at school, an important souvenir or present. Ask the children to work in two's or small groups to make picture charts showing the feelings of one child in the group throughout the day when he or she lost something.

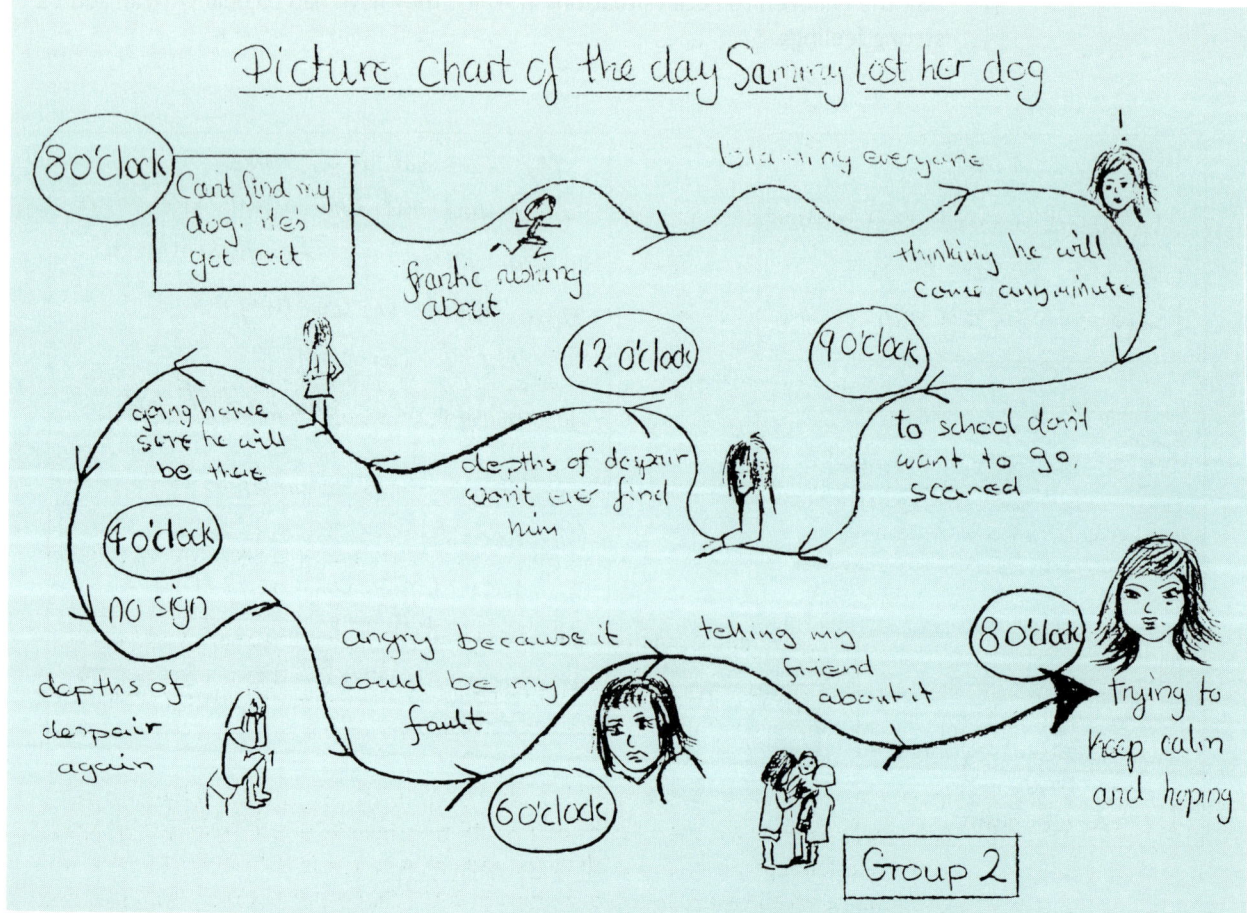

Picture chart of the day Sammy lost her dog

8 o'clock — Can't find my dog. it's got out

frantic rushing about

blaming everyone

thinking he will come any minute

12 o'clock

9 o'clock — to school don't want to go, scared

going home sure he will be there

depths of despair won't ever find him

4 o'clock — no sign

depths of despair again

angry because it could be my fault

6 o'clock

telling my friend about it

8 o'clock — trying to keep calm and hoping

Group 2

Ask them to come together to share their charts. Do people tend to feel the same way about this? Are the same phrases used by several people to describe how they felt?

This could be a good time to look at the strong feelings which arise when people are involved in separation (temporary and permanent), loss, death and grief. In the course of our research children indicated that they wanted to talk about painful feelings. Group work can provide opportunities for this, but it is important that group work skills are introduced and practised previously so that children can develop their own rules of confidentiality and respect. Other children may benefit from opportunities to talk in a one-to-one way with a supportive adult.

Invite the children to role-play or talk through situations in which adults and children are involved, for example:

— Two adults have just heard that a member of the family has died. The child of the family comes in. What do they do or say? What does the child ask, do or say?

— Two adults are talking about separation (temporary or permanent), when their child comes in. What does each of them say, do and feel?

Activity 3 ● *What do I mean when I talk about 'love'?*

● Writing. Drawing. Talking together. Exploring language and meanings. Presentation.

● Class or group and individual activities.

Ask the children to write about, or draw and label:

— one thing they love and care about.

— someone they love and care about.

— someone who loves and cares about them.

Encourage them to share and think about what they have written, and to think about the difference between loving a thing or an activity, and loving a person.

This provides an opportunity for you and the children to talk about:

— the way loving relationships can grow and change, particularly at the adolescent stage.

— their views on falling in love, its meaning and how sex is connected to love.

— what is meant when someone says 'I fancy him' or 'I fancy her' as a way of saying 'I think or imagine I could like or love that person'.

Invite the children to illustrate falling down, falling off, falling into, falling out of, falling over, falling through, falling among thieves, free falling, falling sick, falling on your feet, falling ill, falling flat, falling behind, falling out and falling into line. Which of these phrases actually involves a physical fall? What do the other phrases mean?

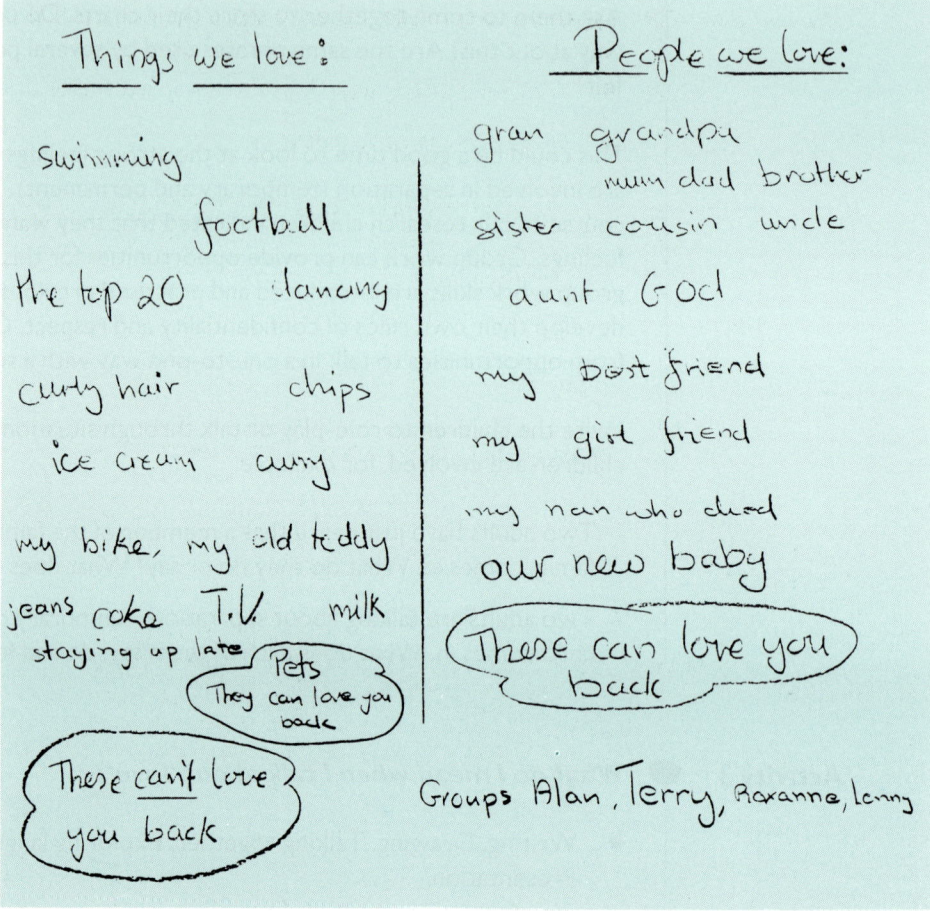

Things we love:

swimming

football

the top 20   dancing

curly hair   chips

ice cream   curry

my bike, my old teddy

jeans coke T.V   milk
staying up late

Pets
They can love you back

These can't love you back

People we love:

gran   grandpa
       mum dad brother
sister cousin uncle

aunt God

my best friend

my girl friend

my nan who died
our new baby

These can love you back

Groups Alan, Terry, Roxanne, Lenny

Ask the children to explain their perceptions of 'falling for someone', 'loving someone' and 'falling out of love'.

Falling for someone

- You're finding out you like them.

- They're attractive.

- You want to be with them a lot.

- You think you could love them.

- You want to get to know them better.

Loving someone

- Wanting to stay with them.

- Caring about them.

- Sharing things: work, worries, feelings, money.

- Wanting to look after them.

- Putting up with them in bad moods.

- Being faithful.

Falling out of love

- You still like them but you don't love them anymore.

- You don't get on together anymore and aren't happy.

- You love somebody else.

Children may use this discussion of the different aspects of love to talk about problems which exist within their own family networks. They may also use it to ask questions about their own and others' sexuality, body changes and functions, child abuse and AIDS. It could be an appropriate time to incorporate into your programme material which is specifically designed to tackle these issues.

Activity 4 ● *How can we make relationships grow and last?*

- Writing. Talking together. Drawing. Evaluating. Extending vocabulary.
- Group and pair activities.

Ask the class to work in groups to list the daily needs of:

— indoor plants.

— pets.

— people.

What do all these things need to grow strong?

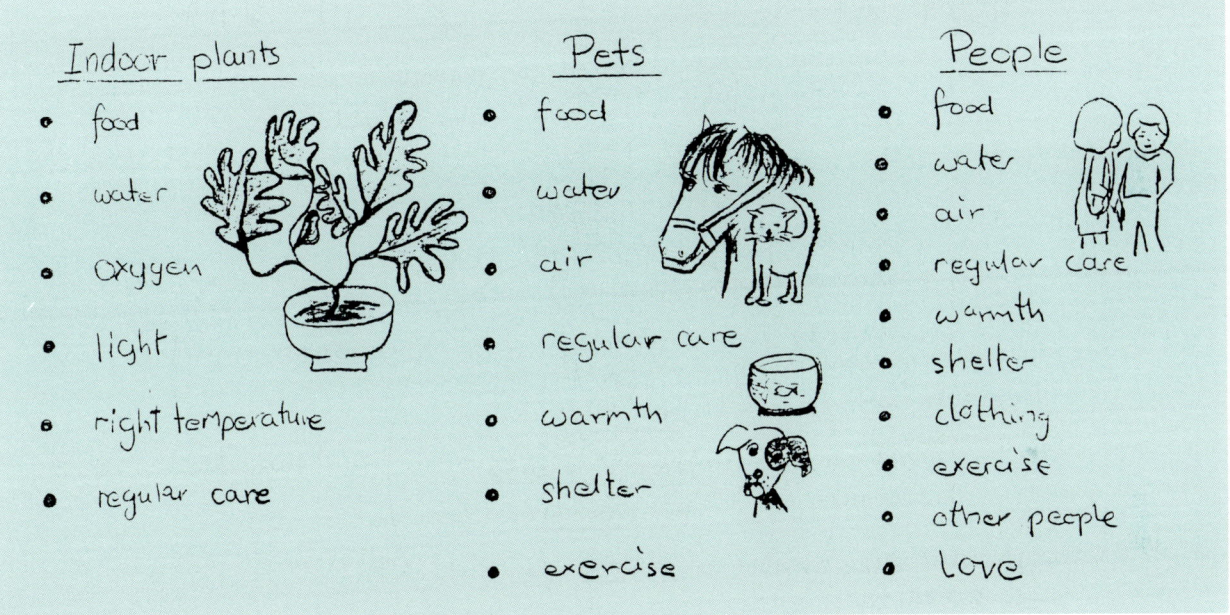

Indoor plants
- food
- water
- oxygen
- light
- right temperature
- regular care

Pets
- food
- water
- air
- regular care
- warmth
- shelter
- exercise

People
- food
- water
- air
- regular care
- warmth
- shelter
- clothing
- exercise
- other people
- love

Talk with the children about how people need to be cared for. Ask them to add a relationships column to their lists and to think about how relationships are 'fed' and made stronger.

Talk about the kinds of things which stop growth – in plants, pets, people and relationships.

Ask the children to talk in pairs about how they feel when a friendship breaks up. Can it be a friendly break or must someone always feel hurt? Ask the children to draw two 'circles of feelings' to describe (1) the feelings involved when they break off a friendship with someone, and (2) the feelings involved when a friend of theirs breaks off a friendship with them.

Ask the children to share their feelings and to explore the positive as well as the negative ones. This would be a good opportunity to:

— move on to look at other relationships, including any which cause the children concern, or which they would like to end or need support in coping with.

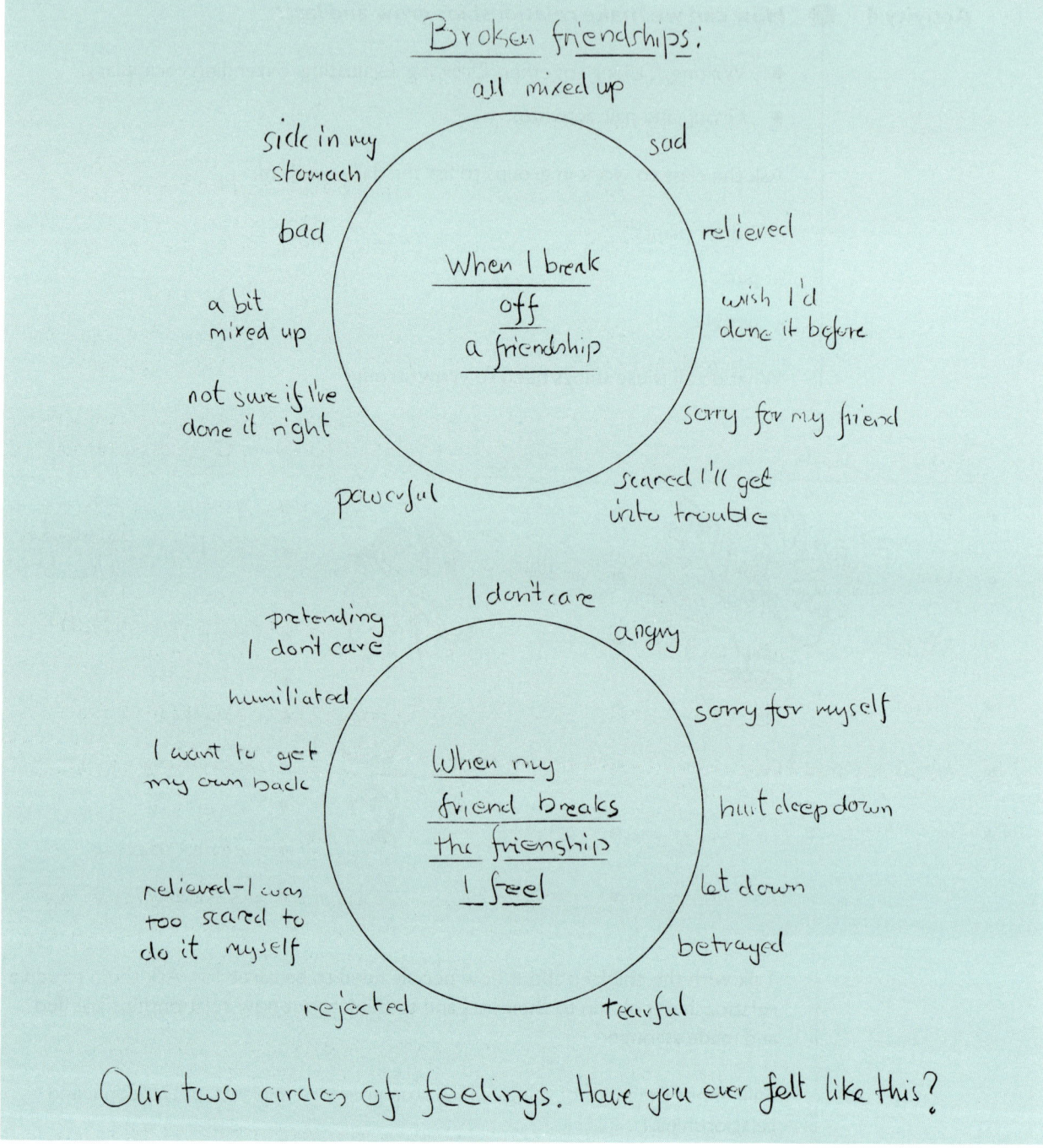

Broken friendships:

all mixed up

sick in my stomach

sad

bad

relieved

a bit mixed up

When I break **off** a friendship

wish I'd done it before

not sure if I've done it right

sorry for my friend

powerful

scared I'll get into trouble

I don't care

pretending I don't care

angry

humiliated

sorry for myself

I want to get my own back

When my friend breaks the friendship **I feel**

hurt deep down

let down

relieved–I was too scared to do it myself

betrayed

rejected

tearful

Our two circles of feelings. Have you ever felt like this?

- reinforce children's understanding that their bodies belong to them, and that no relationship should require that they submit to being touched, or used, in ways which confuse, frighten and hurt them.

- practice strategies for saying 'No', and telling people to stop and listen and help.

The children will begin to be aware that sometimes they and the people they have relationships with may feel hurt, but recovery is quick, while at other times the hurt goes very deep and recovery takes a long time.

One way in which children can reflect on their own strong feelings is to keep a personal, private note book in which they can record them in their own way.

Activity 5 ● *Memories*

- Talking together. Drawing. Writing. Sharing experiences. Empathy.

- Class, group and pair activities.

Ask the children to think about the happiest times they remember and to talk together in groups to share their experiences. Invite them to choose their own way of recording their memories, using drawing and/or writing, and to appoint someone to report back to other groups.

Invite them to contribute to a collage of pictures and quotations which describe their own happy experiences or illustrated stories and poems on this theme.

Invite the children to repeat these activities, this time looking at the saddest times they remember. This could provide further opportunities to share feelings of loss, separation, and grief and bereavement. It is possible that some children remember feeling that they were responsible for the loss, or being excluded or protected from grief, or that the adults were pretending that everything was as before. Ask the children how they and the adults around them reacted.

Some children may find it helpful to write down what they felt, or said, or did, while for others, talking about their feelings may be all that is needed.

You could draw the discussion together by asking the children to think about:

— how they might have felt, and what they might have done, in other children's situations.

— what they have learned by listening to other children's experiences.

Invite the children to work in pairs and talk about and record in their own way their funniest, most frightening, exciting and strangest memories. Ask them to share their memories with other pairs. Do they have many in common?

Ask the children to tell you their earliest memory. (You could make your own contribution here.) When and where was it? What could have made this event stick in their memory? Who or what has reminded them of it?

Invite the children to ask some of the people in their family or friendship networks questions such as:

'What is your earliest memory of me?'
'What is your funniest, saddest and most frightening memory of me?'
'What are your own earliest memories?'

Ask the children to imagine that they woke up one morning to find they had completely lost their memories. They did not know who they were, where they lived, what day it was, what school they went to, who lived with them etc.

Ask them how they would feel? How might other people treat them if they had to ask questions such as: 'Where am I please?', 'Do I know you', 'How do you get dressed?' etc. What kind of response from people would help? What would make them feel worse?

This would provide an opportunity to look at the importance of memory to everyone, and the need to know about the past. Encourage the children to talk about the adults and older people in their family networks. Do they talk about the past? Do they sometimes tell the same story several times? Emphasise the difficulties and confusions of the very elderly, and the importance of sympathetic listening and help.

Content box 5   Focus on special places

What makes some places special? Where do I go to be alone? Are these places safe? How do I feel when people invade my special places or misunderstand my reasons for going there? How do people feel when they have no special place? Where do I go when I want company and fun? Are these places safe? Which places do I want to forget? Can I work out the network of places I visit? Do I care for these places? Do they make me feel good and confident? How would I organise my special places if I could? What is a vandal? Why do I think they do it?

Activity I ● ***What makes some places special?***

- Talking together. Writing. Describing places. Exploring feelings.

- Class and group activities.

Ask the children to recall the places which they remember as being special. Encourage them to imagine these places and to describe or illustrate them. They can include places they have visited or places where they have previously lived. Can they isolate any particular spot which they recall as 'theirs'?

Places we remember

I remember a seaside place but I've forgotten its name. We went there for day trips lots of times. I made them always go to the same bit by the old sea wall a long way away. My special bit was the rock pools. I didn't want anyone to help, I was always in the pool it was an ace place.

Eugene

My special place was at my great grans house, in her big old chair. I always played in it on my own. She gave me an old table cloth and I played lots of pretend games. I can still remember the special smell of the house and cloth it makes me a bit sad

Norie

The idea of a relationship between people and places can be explored by asking the children to think about what makes their memories of these places so special. Was it because the places themselves were different, beautiful or exciting? Was it because of something the children did there, or something that happened? How did the places make them feel? Can the children find the words to express some of the good feelings they had, and still have, about these places?

Invite the children to hold brainstorming sessions in small groups to think of some of these feelings. Help them incorporate their responses into a 'circle of feelings'.

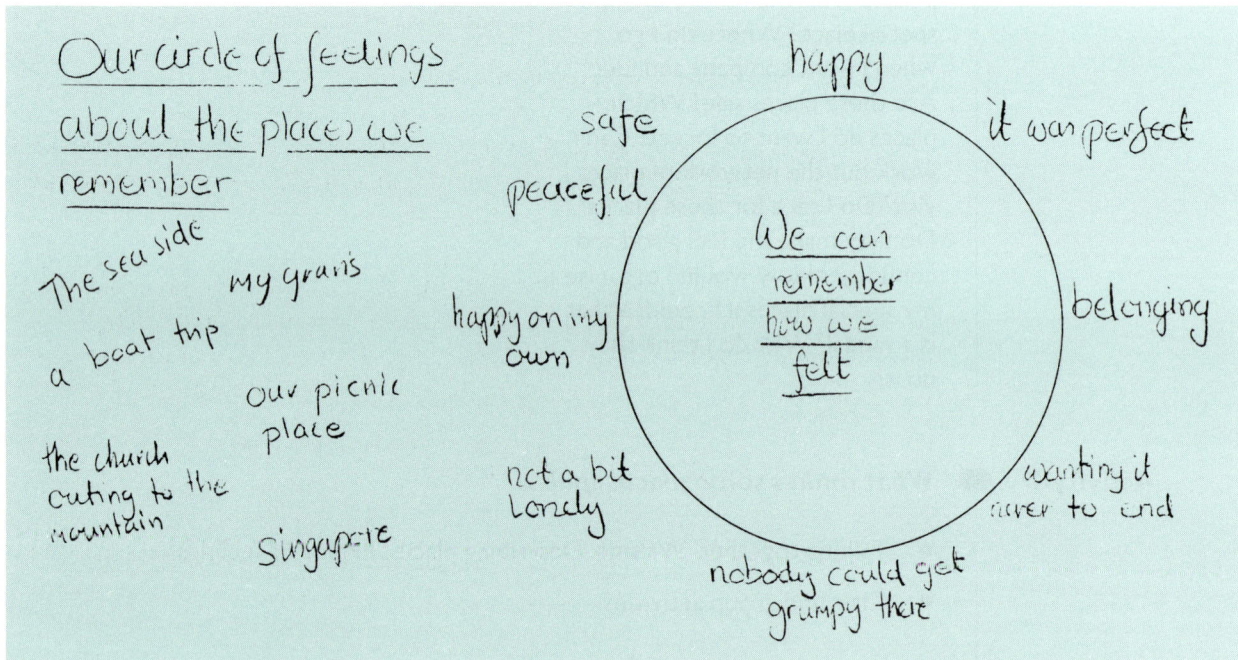

Our circle of feelings about the places we remember

The sea side my grans a boat trip our picnic place the church Outing to the mountain Singapore

happy
safe
peaceful
it was perfect
happy on my own
We can remember how we felt
belonging
not a bit lonely
wanting it never to end
nobody could get grumpy there

Activity 2 ● *Where do I go to be alone? Where do I go for company?*

- Talking together. Drawing. Writing. Describing. Empathy.

- Class and pair activities.

Invite the children to work in pairs to describe, write about or illustrate the places at home, at school and in the neighbourhood where they go when they want to be away from other people and to do what they want. Ask them to pick out the places which they consider safe, risky or potentially dangerous, and ask them to say why they think this. Some children may find these places within their home or friendship networks, others may not. Some schools are able to provide the children with places where they can be alone.

Invite the children to share their work and to explore how they feel when:

– they find a special place and make it their own.

– their privacy is threatened or misinterpreted by others.

– they are unable to find any such place.

– they disturb other people's privacy.

Discuss with them the need for people to have privacy, and the strong, lasting relationships people build with these special places and how it feels to leave them.

There are opportunities here to talk about the children's feelings and attitudes to:

- people coming to this country from abroad.

- people who may appear different in some way.

- people with special needs or disabilities which confine them to a limited range of places.

- old people and their need for special places.

- people who are homeless or in inadequate, crowded homes.

The children could then repeat these activities and look at the places they go to find company, fun, excitement, to find friends and to test their skills and abilities against others.

Ask the children to say which of these places they see as safe, risky, or dangerous, and to say why. This is a good opportunity to look at aspects of risk taking, particularly those involving the mastering of specific skills, such as road user skills and sports skills, and to revise previous work on personal safety skills.

Activity 3   ●   *How do we feel about different places?*

- Talking together. Drawing. Creative activities. Writing. Language work. Role-play. Empathy.

- Class or group and individual activities.

Ask the children if they can remember visits they have made where they failed to make a good relationship with the place. Ask them to share their experiences with a friend or small group and to discover what made the memory of the place less than happy.

Invite the children to work together to draw and describe the network of places where each of them goes, using home and school as starting points. They could present the network as:

- a model with background pictures.

- a wall story or collage of pictures, diagrams and writing.

- a class or group set of books.

Ask the children to list all the places they visit and show by colour coding those they visit occasionally and those they visit regularly. They could include places they or their families have lived in previously. Ask them to identify also:

- places with which they feel they have a good relationship, places they care for and which make them feel good.

- places where they feel confident enough to go alone.

– places where they would go only with friends or with a known responsible adult, or where they know they would find a responsible adult.

– places they would avoid.

Emphasise with the children the importance of finding out from responsible sources as much as they can about any new places they plan to go to, or places that they are pressured into going to. Make it clear that it is still important to tell parents or family where they are going, and to know some emergency tactics.

Invite the children to talk about, describe through writing, and/or drawing, a place (real or imaginary) which makes them feel welcome, safe and confident about themselves. Ask the children to explore their relationship with that place. What is it that makes them feel the way they do? Is it the place itself, or how it is cared for? Is it the atmosphere, the people and how they treat each other?

Remind the children of their work on good relationships with people. Can they treat a place in the same way as they would treat a friend who made them feel good?

Ask the children to pick out those places where they have felt unsure, not confident, not in charge of themselves, or where they have been asked to behave in ways which made them uneasy. Ask them to try to identify what made them feel this way. Was it the place, the atmosphere, how the people behaved, how they treated each other and the place itself?

Some places make us feel uneasy because:

They're dark you can't see what is happening.

I'm not sure what kind of people come here.

I'm not sure what people will ask me to do.

They're secret places.

Every one looks so grown up.

People push you about.

Its noisy, smoky, boozy, rough.

My mum wouldn't like me to go there.

I can't see anyone in charge.

There could be drugs and things.

it looks friendly but I don't know anyone.

How would we cope?

We'd think it over first.
We'd decide it was too risky.

We'd only go with friends.

We'd say 'Don't push me about please'.

We wouldn't go.

We'd try it and go home if it got rough.

We'd check up on who was in charge.

We'd take deep breath and relax.

We'd fall out about it. Some would want to stay. Some not.

We would stand back and watch first.

We'd look confident and copy the rest. Group 6

Hold brainstorming sessions with the children to help them explain why some places make them feel uncertain, ill at ease or unsafe, and to help them think of the kinds of strategies they might use to cope with these feelings. Ask them to write about these feelings and strategies.

There are opportunities here to revise and extend through role-play, the children's skills in resisting peer pressure, saying 'No', and avoiding potentially dangerous situations.

Activity 4 ● ***Special places for special people***

- Writing. Drawing.
- Pair or group activities.

Ask the children to work in pairs or small groups to try to build up a picture of places which would be friendly and welcoming to each of these categories of people:

— pre-school children.

— an infant school with a poor playground. (The organisation Inter Action might be helpful here.)

— 10 and 11 year olds and young teenagers (out of school).

— families (at the weekend).

— old people (in the winter time).

— people with special needs or disabilities (in the evenings).

Invite the pairs and groups to choose one category and begin to plan the kind of place which would make the people in that category feel confident and welcome.

Their plans could be expressed in illustrations and writing. Ask the children to focus on:

— the atmosphere they feel the place should have.

— the equipment they think would be needed.

— the activities they would encourage, discourage or ban.

— the rules they would introduce and methods of enforcement.

Ask the children to share their finished plans with other groups and to pinpoint similarities and differences.

Ask the children how the good relationship between the people and the place could be maintained. How would they encourage people to think that their place is special, and build a strong and caring relationship with it? What kinds of messages or notices would help to keep the place happy and healthy?

Activity 5 ● *What is a vandal?*

- Talking together. Writing. Drawing. Evaluating. Generalising. Empathy.
- Class or group activities.

Ask the children to recall times when, as young children, they made something at school, or at home, as a gift for someone, and it was put in a place of honour, or used daily. How did this make them feel?

Recall other occasions when in school, their work was praised, shared or displayed. How did they feel? How would the children have felt if the gift or the piece of work had been accidentally thrown away, ignored or spoiled? What might they have said, done, or not said? How would they have felt if someone had deliberately torn, scribbled on, thrown away or destroyed their work? What might they have done or said then? Invite the children to relate this to the things they make and the work they do in class at present.

Ask the children to contribute to two 'circles of feelings': one which shows how we feel when we make something and people value it, and one which shows how we feel when we make something and people spoil it deliberately.

Ask the children to suggest ways in which the school, and their class in particular, could ensure that everyone respects and values the work and belongings of others. This could be extended to look at ways of ensuring that people's feelings, relationships, ways of talking, appearance, bodies and the space immediately around them, are valued and respected.

Ask the children how they think they would feel if they came into their classroom to find it wrecked. How would they react? What would they say and do, or want to do? How would they feel about the classroom itself? Would they be able to build up their special relationship with the place again?

The children could look in local newspapers for reports about places spoiled by litter, vandals or pollution. Ask them to try to put themselves in the shoes of the people who suffered. What would they feel, say, do or want to do?

Ask the children, without prior discussion, to draw what they perceive a vandal might look like and to write down what the vandal is doing or planning to do, and why. Invite them to share their responses with others in the class and to pick out any common features. Encourage the children to identify and discuss any examples of stereotyping by race, sex, age or class.

Explore with the class what can be discovered about the original Vandals in the third and fourth centuries AD. How has their name become part of today's language? Ask the children to look at the ways in which today's vandals are similar to or different from the original Germanic armies.

Hold a brainstorming session with the children on destructive behaviour. As a starting point ask them if they think puppies and young children are vandals when they are destructive.

> Come and read our class brainstorm. Can you add to it?
>
> What makes puppies destructive? Is it vandalism? **NO**
> It's a game. its fun. they don't mean to ruin it. they're cutting teeth. they're just playing
>
> What makes little children destructive? Is it vandalism? **NO**
> they're learning about things. they don't know they shouldn't
>
> What makes vandals destructive?
> they enjoy spoiling things. they are jealous. They're bored. they think it's exciting, risky, dangerous. They can't think of anything else to do. they're stupid. they follow what other people do and don't think for themselves. they think it's clever

Emphasise the importance of setting a good example to other children. Ask the class to design some messages for younger children about:

— choosing safe places to play in.

— keeping places healthy and happy.

— litter and vandalism.

Cross-curricular links with environmental studies: this would be a good time to make use of the resources of the Environmental Health Officer and other national and local groups concerned for the care and conservation of the environment.

Family Worksheet Masters

The worksheet masters in the following pages are photocopiable so you can give them to the children to take home and work through with their families. The worksheets can also be used by the children with the teacher in a one-to-one session, or in group work. However, home use brings to your health education programme the important benefit of family involvement.

The worksheets vary in difficulty, and begin with worksheets for the younger children. They have not been age-graded as you will probably prefer to select them according to the needs of your class.

A photocopiable letter has also been provided which you can send home with the worksheets. This explains to the parent, or family, the purpose of the worksheets and suggests ways in which they could be used. You may wish to adapt this letter to your own needs.

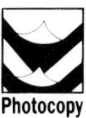

Dear

Family Worksheets

These worksheets are an important part of your child's health education. We would like you and your child to work on them together. They will show you some of the ways in which the children are finding out about themselves, their feelings, the feelings of the people who are part of their lives and about how they and their relationships grow and change.

The children are bringing these worksheets home so you can share in the work they have been doing at school. You can help them to get the most out of what they have learned. This is not the kind of homework which is taken back to school and marked, it is family work, everyone can share in it. We think you will learn a great deal from the way your child thinks about health and explains it all to you.

When you sit down with your child to start a worksheet, one way to start is to ask your child to explain what has been happening in health education sessions at school. The next step is to work together through the activities on the worksheet. Remember that there are no right and wrong answers. The important thing is to talk together. Don't worry if your child's drawings are not very clear, you can always ask her, or him, to tell you about them. Read the worksheet *with* your child or read it *to* your child, but don't make the reading a struggle. Write for your child if that is what she or he **would like you to do. Most importantly, feel free to contribute some** questions of your own, and think of other things to talk, draw and write about.

This school is working to promote health and your child is sharing that with you at home. This is your chance to help bring important health messages home to your child.

We hope you enjoy sharing these worksheets with your child.

Me and My Relationships

My name is ....

Special people

This is Sammy with his
special people

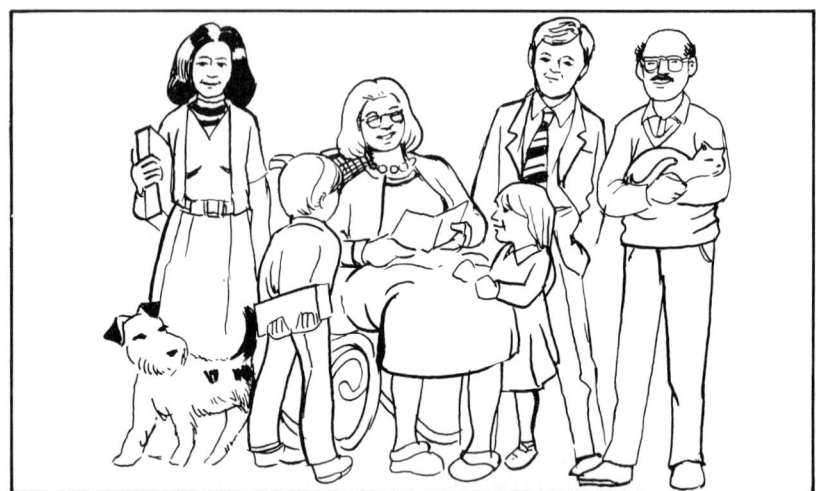

Talk about Sammy's special people.
Who are they?

_____

Talk about your special people.
Who are they?

_____

Can you draw yourself with your special people?

What are you all doing?

Me and My Relationships

 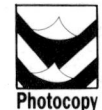
My name is ....

Feeling happy

Here are some happy people

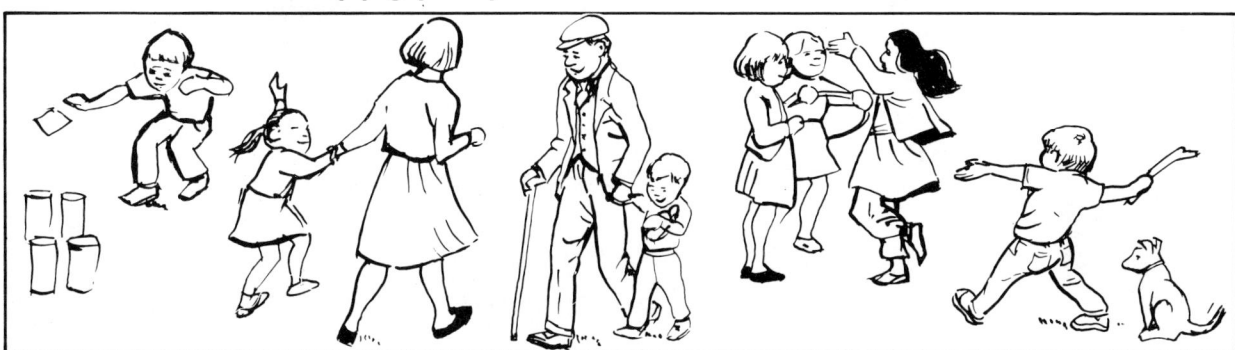

What are they doing?

_____

Why are they feeling happy?

_____

Draw yourself feeling happy?

What are you doing?

I am . . . .

. . . .

Talk about some of the things that make you feel happy.

Can you draw some of them?

Photocopy

Me and My Relationships

My name is ....

How do you feel?

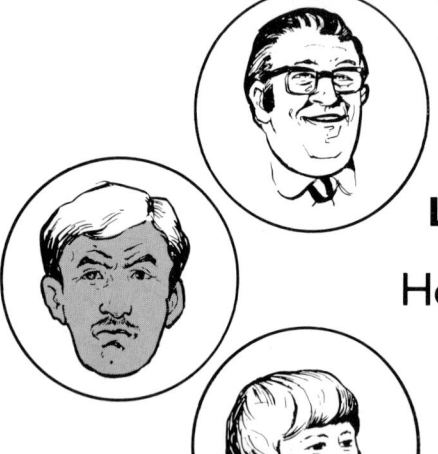

Look at these people

How are they feeling?
Are they happy?
Are they sad?
Are they cross?

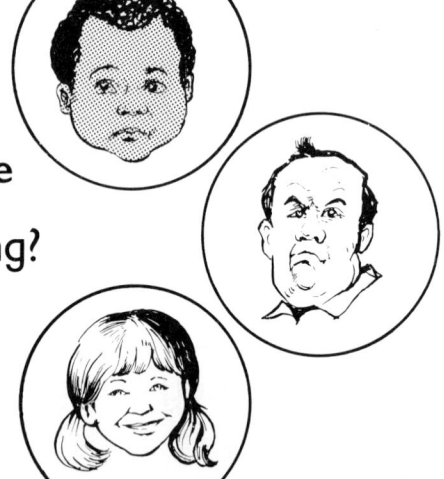

Draw yourself feeling cross.

Talk about the things that make you feel cross.
Can you draw some of them?

Talk about what makes you feel better.

Me and My Relationships

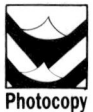

My name is ....

How do we make people happy? 1

Sammy is making his Granny feel happy.

What is he doing?

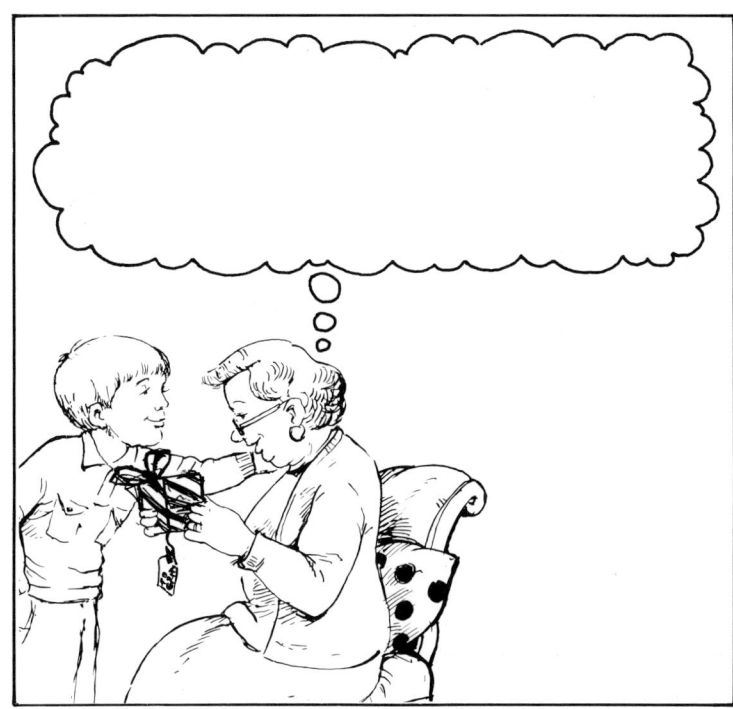

What is his Granny thinking?
Write in the thought bubble what she is thinking.

Talk about what you do to make your special people happy.

Tammy is making her friend happy.

What is she doing?

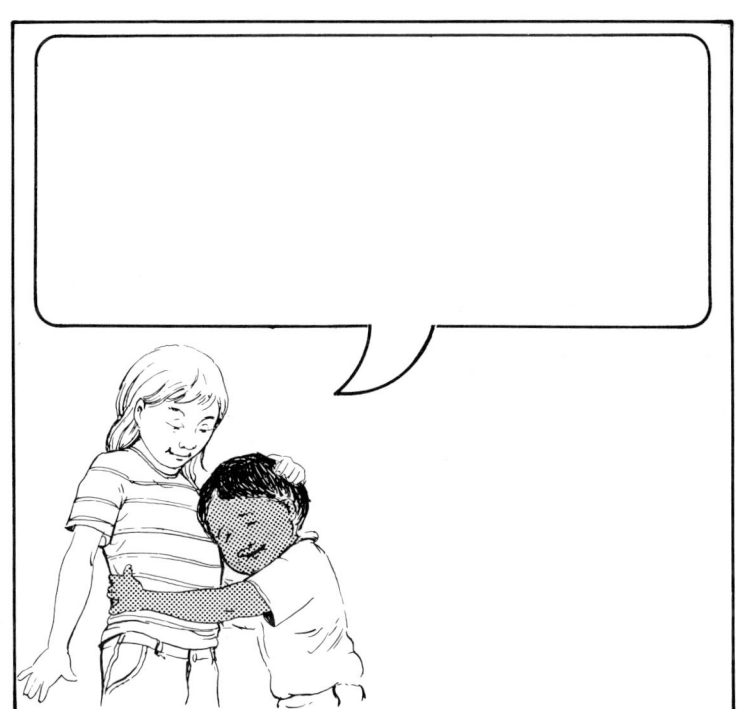

What is her friend saying?
Write in the speech bubble what you think he is saying.

Talk about what you do to make your friends happy?

Me and My Relationships

Family Worksheet

5

My name is ....

Why do people feel sad?

These people are making
Sammy feel sad.
What do you think they are doing?

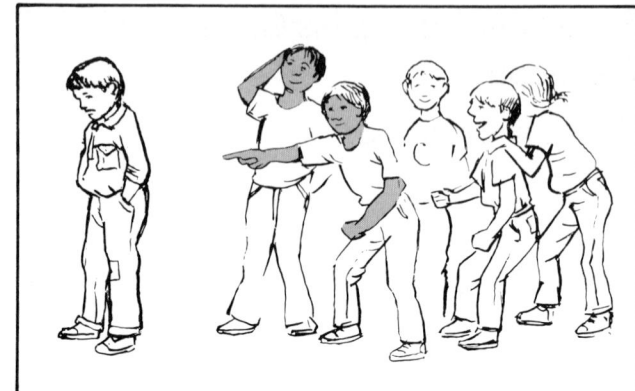

_____

What do you think Sammy will do?

_____

Draw someone making you feel sad.
What are they doing to make
you feel sad?

_____

What are you saying to them?

Me and My Relationships

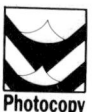

My name is ....

Why do we make people cross?

Sandy and Joey are making their family cross.

What are they doing?

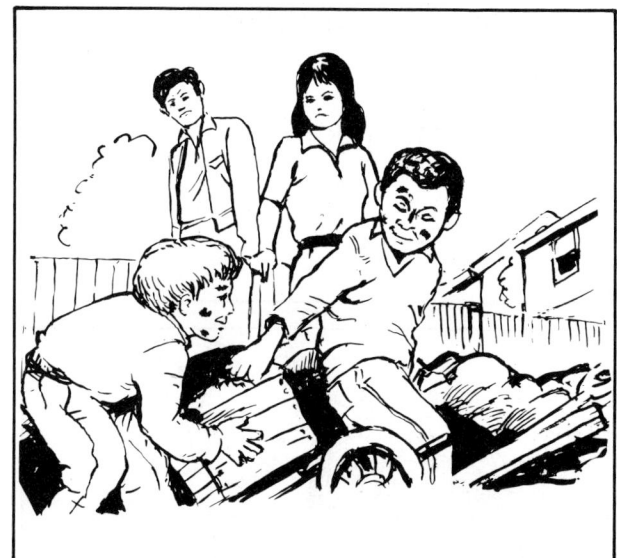

_____

What do you think will happen?

_____

_____

Draw yourself making someone cross.

What are you doing?

_____

_____

Why does it make them cross?

_____

What do you do to make them feel better?

_____

_____

What do they do to make you feel better?

_____

Photocopy

Me and My Relationships

My name is ....

How do we make people happy? 2

Linzi's friends are making her feel happy.

What are they doing?

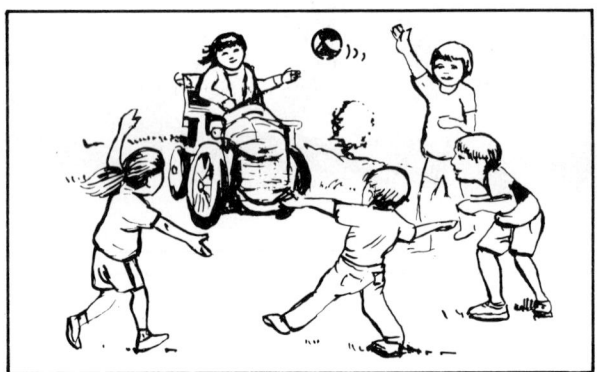

Why does she feel so happy?

Linzi is making her friend feel happy.

What is she doing?

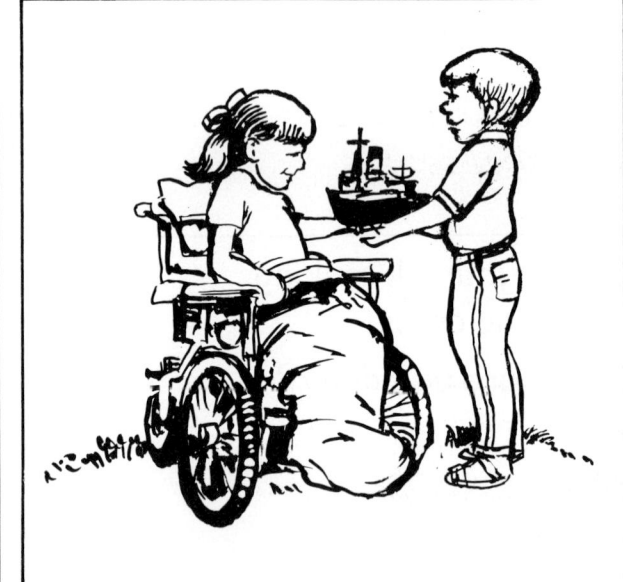

Draw your friends making you feel happy.

What are they doing?

What are you saying to them?

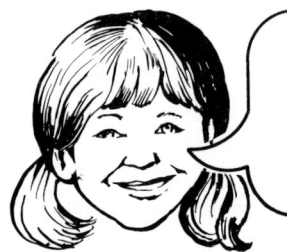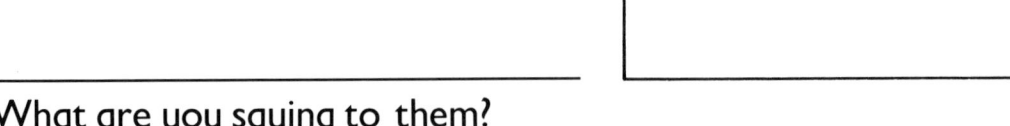

© Health Education Authority 1989

Me and My Relationships

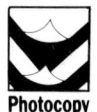

My name is ....

What makes us upset?

These children are upset.

What do you think has happened?

What are the children thinking?

Write what they are thinking in the thought bubble.

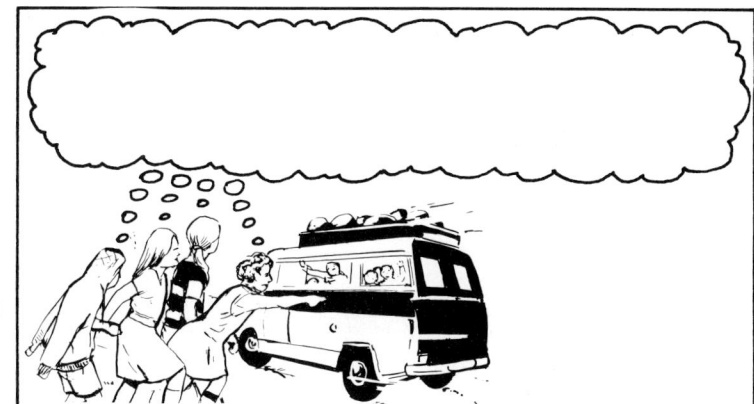

Talk about a time when you felt upset.
What happened?

Draw yourself feeling upset.

What made you feel better?

What did someone do?

What did someone say?

Me and My Relationships

My name is ....

Saying 'No'

This is Sandy saying 'No!' to a grown-up.

Why do you think Sandy is saying 'No!'.

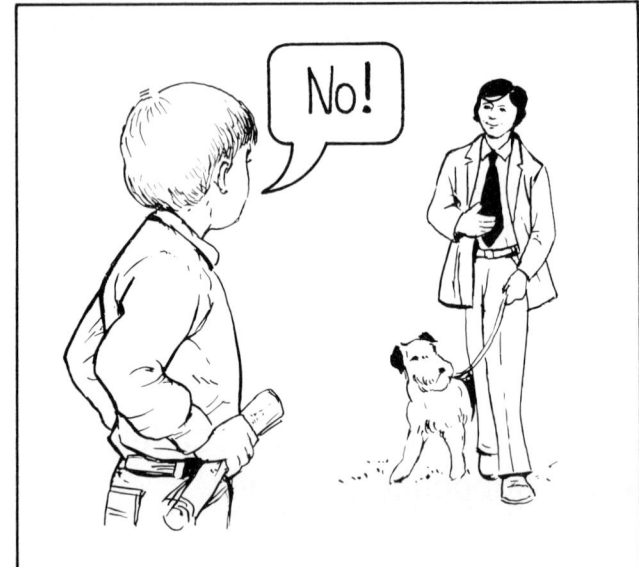

Draw yourself saying 'No!' to a grown-up.

Why are you saying 'No!'?

Talk about times when it is important to say 'No' to a grown up.

Me and My Relationships

 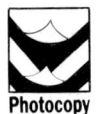
My name is ....

Making and breaking friends

Draw yourself with your best friend.
What are you doing?

_____

What other things do you do with your best friend?

_____

What do best friends do for each other?

_____

Sandy and Joey have stopped being friends.
What do you think has happened?

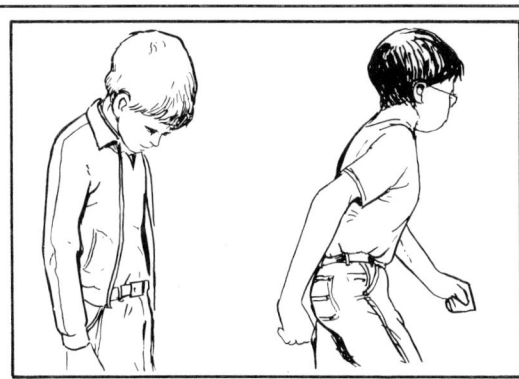

_____

How do you think they are feeling?

_____

Talk about how you feel when you stop being friends with someone.

Me and My Relationships

My name is ....

'Pretend' friends

Sammy has a pretend friend. He calls him Ben.
No one else can see Ben.

Why do you think he has a pretend friend?

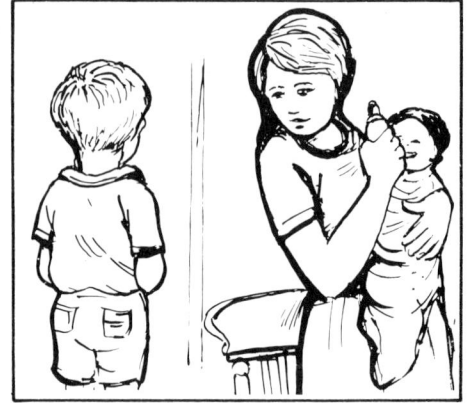

_____

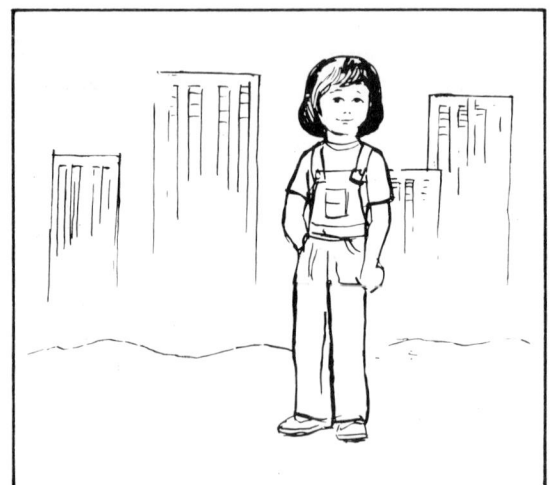

Tammy has a pretend friend.
It's a dog called Buster.
No one else can see Buster.

Why do you think she has a pretend dog?

_____

Do you know someone who has a pretend friend?

If you had a pretend friend
who would it be?

_____

Draw a picture of them.

Me and My Relationships

My name is ....

Why do we pretend? 1

Draw yourself pretending to cry.

Why are you pretending to cry?

Draw yourself pretending to go to sleep.

Why are you pretending to go to sleep?

Draw yourself pretending to be a grown-up.

What are you doing?

Is this pretending good?

Me and My Relationships

My name is ....

Why do grown-ups sometimes pretend?

This is a grown-up, pretending to be a tiger.

What is he doing?

_____

What is he saying?

_____

What are the children doing?

_____

Are they really frightened?

_____

Can you draw a grown-up
pretending to frighten you?

What is the grown-up doing?

_____

What are you doing?

_____

Are you really frightened?

_____

Talk about other kinds of pretending.

Me and My Relationships

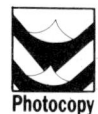

My name is ....

Playing safely

Sandra and Tom are playing with their friends.

What are they doing?

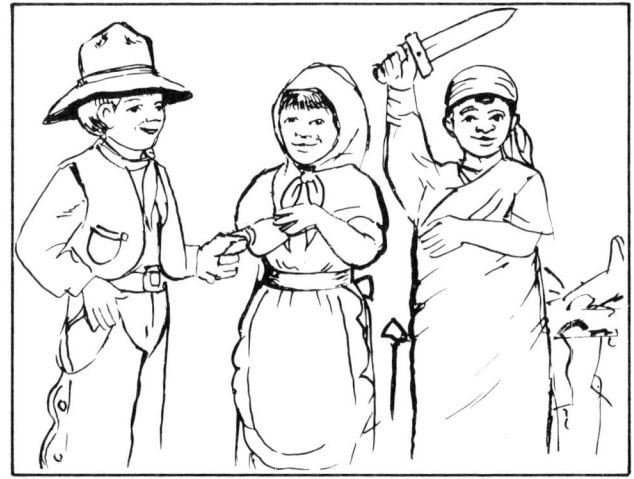

_____

Do you think they are safe here?

_____

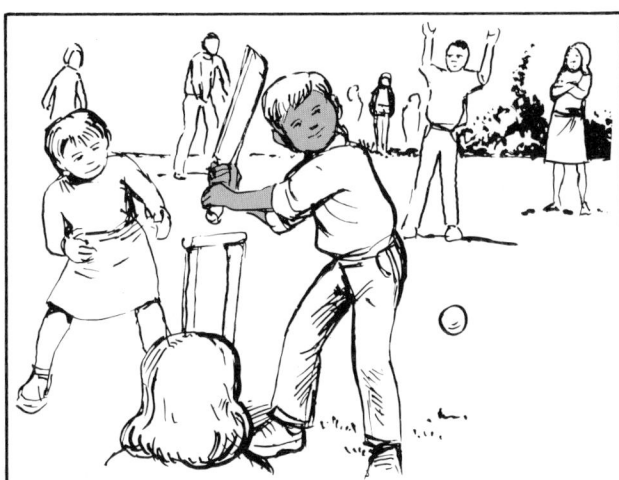

Sandra and Tom are playing with some grown-up friends.

What are they doing?

_____

Do you think they are safe here?

_____

This is someone pretending to be a friend to Sandra and Tom.

Do you think they are safe here?

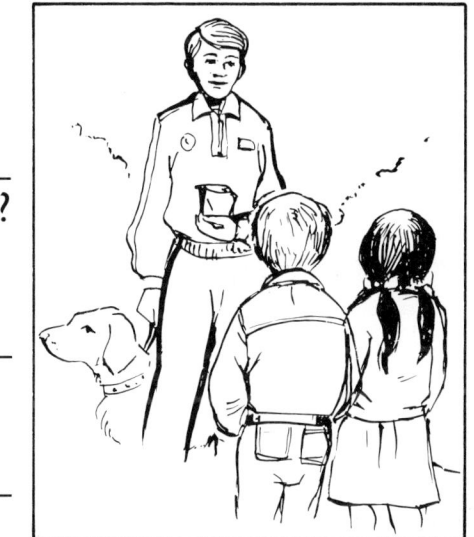

_____

What do you think Sandra and Tom should do?

_____

What should they say?

_____

Talk about what you would do.

Me and My Relationships

My name is ....

Special places

This is Tabby's special place by the fire.

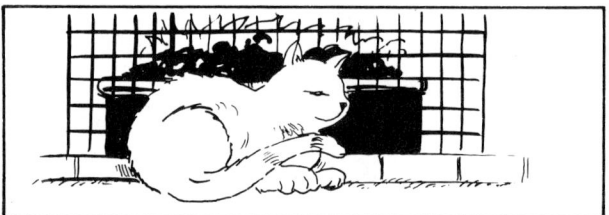

What makes it special for Tabby?

_____

What could spoil it?

_____

This is Jake's special place by the gate.

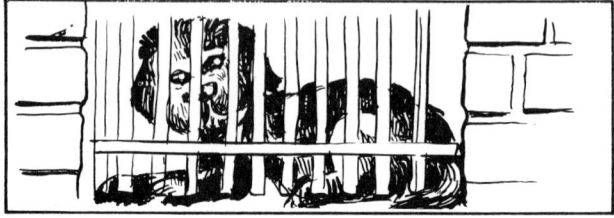

What makes it special for Jake?

_____

What could spoil it?

_____

Can you draw two of your special places?

Where are they?

_____

What makes your places special?

_____

What could spoil them?

_____

Talk about other people and their special places.

Me and My Relationships

My name is ....

Where are your special places?

Liza and Eric's special place is the children's adventure playground.

What do they do there?

_____

What makes it special?

_____

What could spoil it?

_____

Talk about some of your special places outdoors.

Draw a special place where you go with your family or grown-ups.
What makes it special?

_____

Would you go there alone?

_____

Draw a special place where you go with your friends.
What do you do there?

_____

What makes it special?

_____

Would you go there alone?

_____

Me and My Relationships

My name is ....

How can we keep our special places happy and healthy?

Liza and Eric are helping to keep the adventure playground happy, healthy and fun to be in.

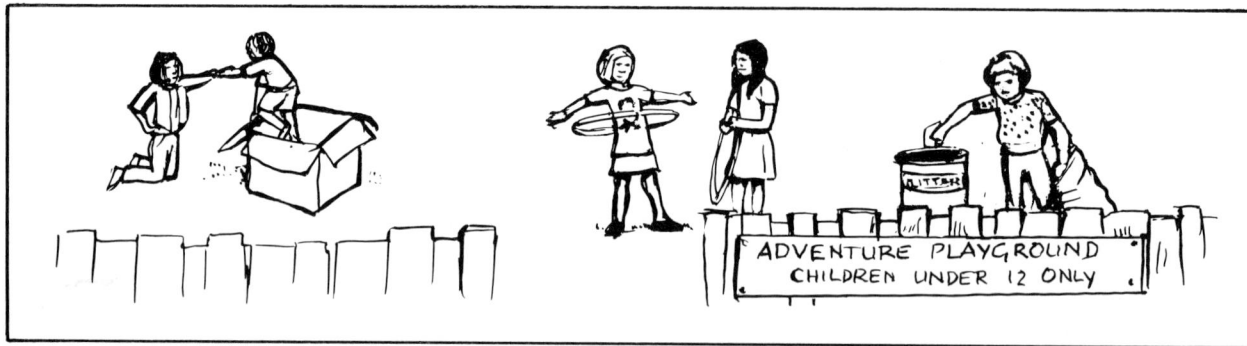

What are they doing?

Here are some things children do when they are in the adventure playground.

Can you ring the ones which help to keep the place happy, healthy and fun to be in?

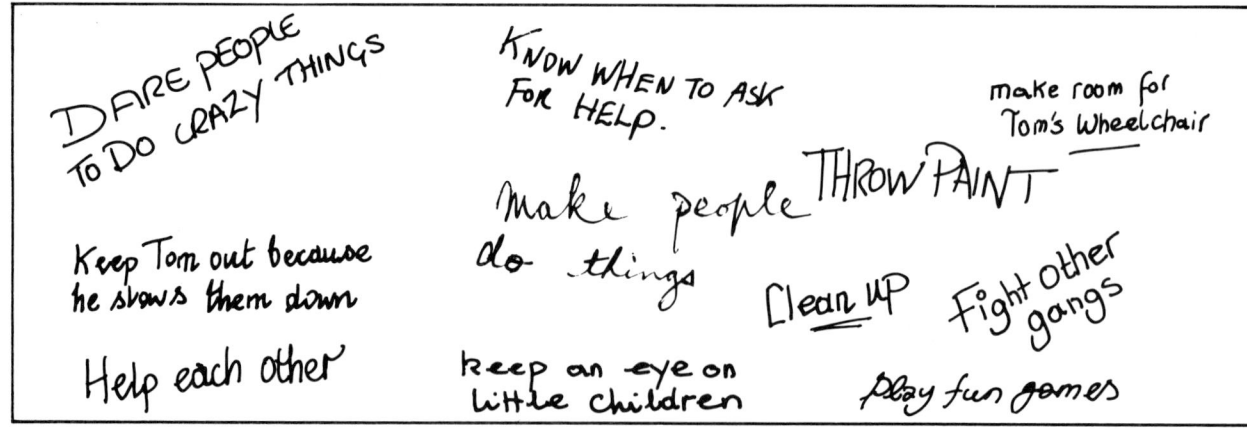

Can you think of any more?

Me and My Relationships

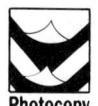
Photocopy

My name is ....

Why do we pretend? 2

You have hurt yourself.
Draw yourself being brave
and pretending it doesn't hurt.

Why are you pretending?

Draw yourself pretending
you like something someone
has given you.

Why are you pretending?

Draw yourself pretending
you want to do what your
friends are doing.
You don't really want to do it.
Why are you pretending?

Draw yourself saying, 'No,
I'm not going to pretend
about that'.

Why are you saying that?

Photocopy

Me and My Relationships

My name is ....

My family 1

Sandy has been drawing his family network

What does it tell you about him?

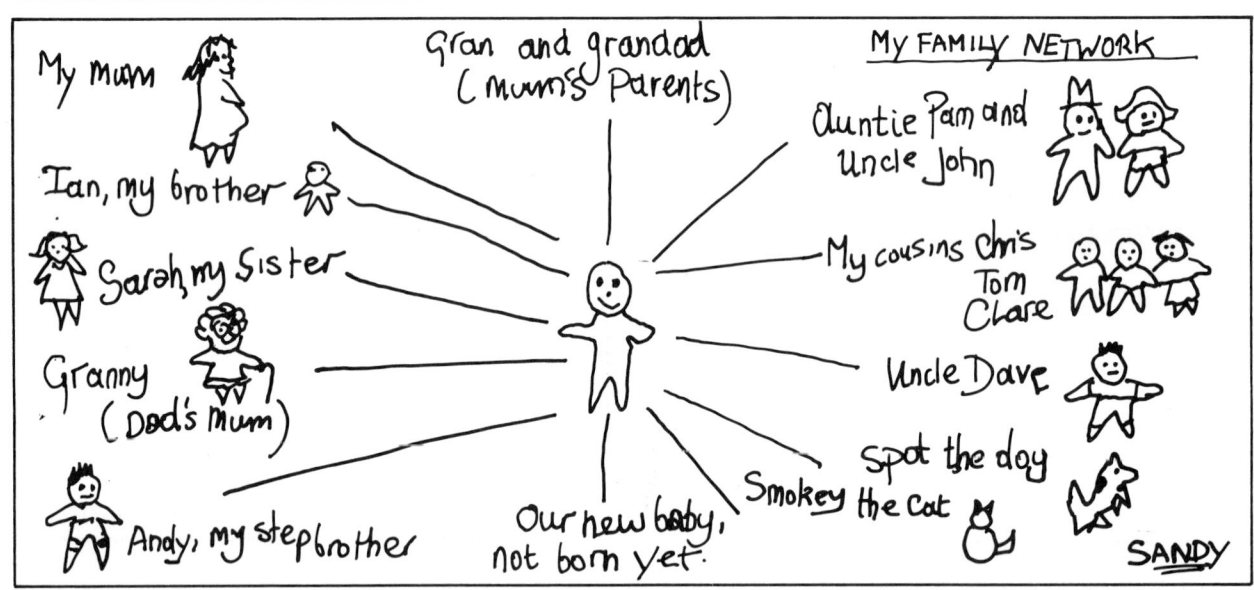

Talk about your own family network.

Can you draw it?

Talk about how it is different from Sandy's network.

Me and My Relationships

My name is ....

My family 2

Think about the people in your family network and
what you like most about each other.

Now try to finish these sentences:

What I like most about my family is:

What my family likes most about me is:

Talk about what you would like to change about your family.

Talk about what they would like to change about you.

How do you think you and your family could change things?

Photocopy

Me and My Relationships

My name is ....

What do me and my friends like about each other?

Think about the people in your network of friends and what you like most about each other.

Now try to finish these sentences:

What I like most about my friends is:

What my friends like most about me is:

Is there anything about them you would like to change?

Is there anything about you they would like to change?

How do you think you and your friends could change things?

Me and My Relationships

 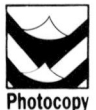
My name is ....

Quarrels

Draw yourself having a quarrel with a friend.

What are you quarrelling about?

_____

What are you saying?

_____

How do you feel?

_____

How do you think your friend feels?

_____

Talk about how you could make things better.

Draw yourself having a quarrel with someone in your family.

How did the quarrel start?

_____

How do you both feel?

_____

Talk about how you could make things better.

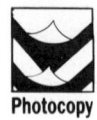
Photocopy

Me and My Relationships

My name is ....

Hurt feelings 1

Liza and Lennie are in trouble.
They were late home, but it
wasn't their fault. No one will listen
to them. Their feelings are hurt.

What could they do to feel better?

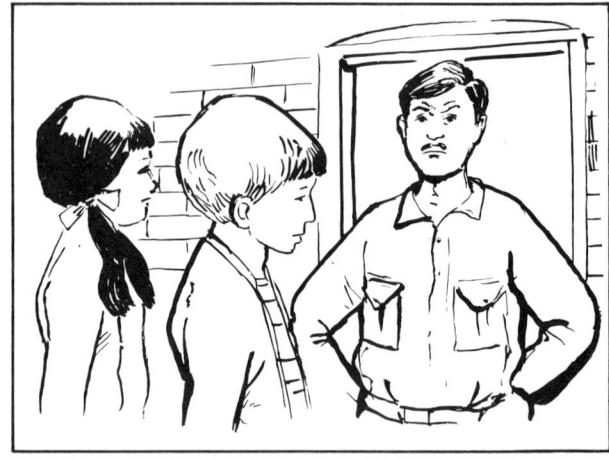

_____

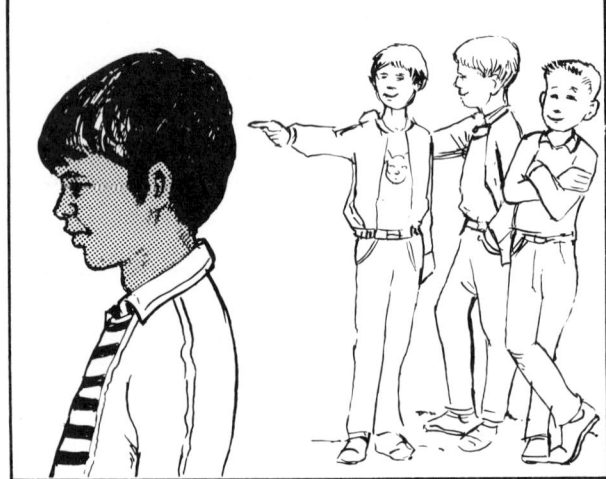

Ranjit's feelings are hurt. His friends
teased him about the way he looked.

What could he do to feel better?

_____

What would you have done?

_____

Karli's feelings are hurt.
Her best friend went off without her.

What could Karli do to feel better?

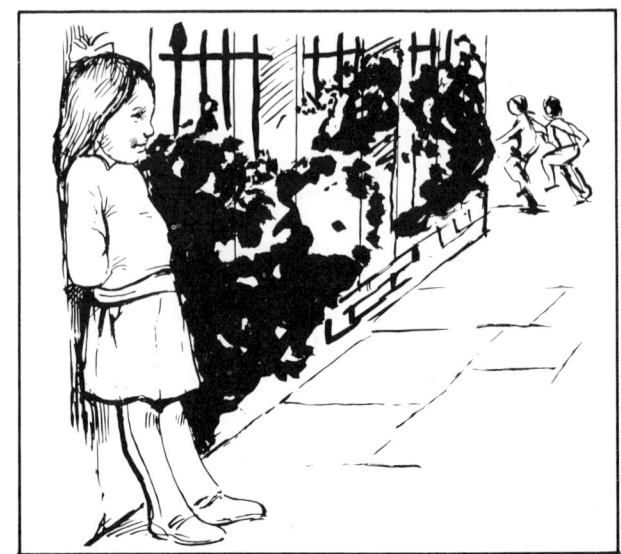

_____

What would you have done?

_____

Me and My Relationships

My name is ....

Good moods and bad moods

Tammy is in a bad mood and is sitting moaning about it.

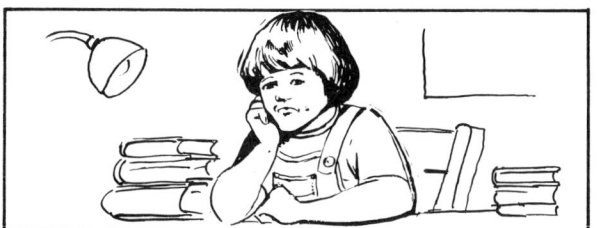

How could you help her to feel better?

Jo is in a bad mood and is sulking in his bedroom.

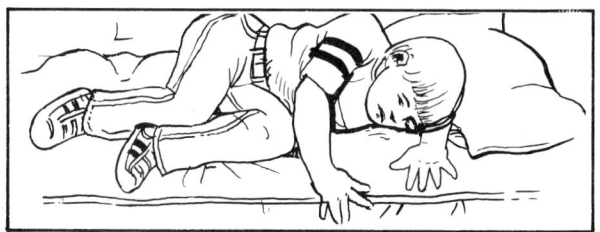

How could you help him to feel better?

Talk about the different moods you have.

Look at the mood-meter. Can you think of some more words to describe the moods you have? Write them on the mood meter

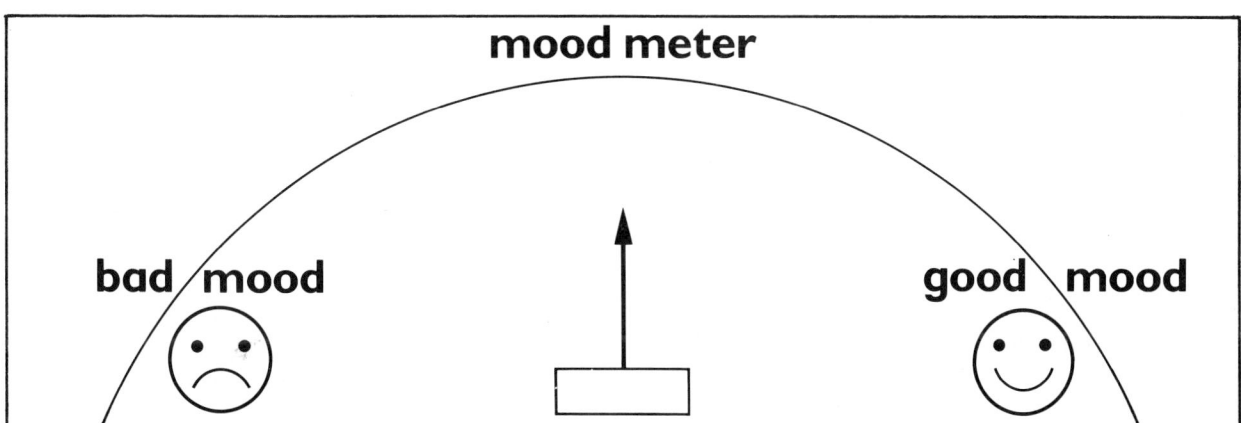

What puts you in a good mood?

What puts you in a bad mood?

What helps you get out of a bad mood?

Photocopy

Me and My Relationships

My name is ....

Hurt feelings 2

Can you remember a time when someone hurt your feelings?

Can you draw what happened?

What did you do to help yourself feel better?

_____

Can you remember a time when you hurt someone's feelings?

Can you draw what happened?

How do you think the person felt?

_____

How did you feel?

_____

What did you do to make things better?

_____

Talk about what else you could have done.

Me and My Relationships

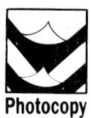
My name is ....

Memories

Smithy says she can remember being born.
Do you think she can really remember it?

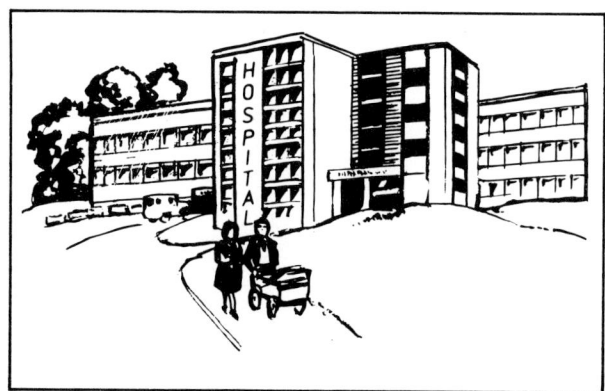

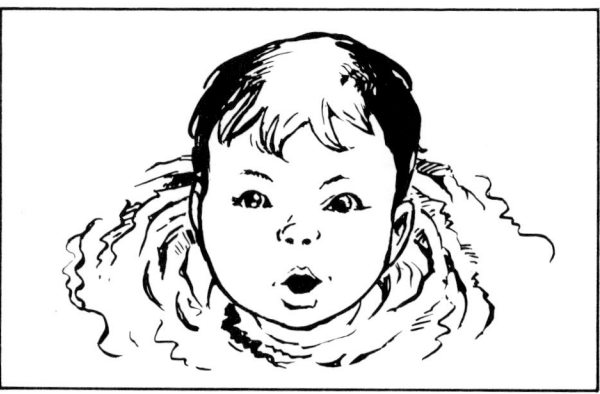

Martin says he can remember falling in the river. He was only 1 year old.
Why do you think he remembers it?

Sandy and Jo say they can remember their Gran coming to England for the very first time.
Why do you think they remember it?

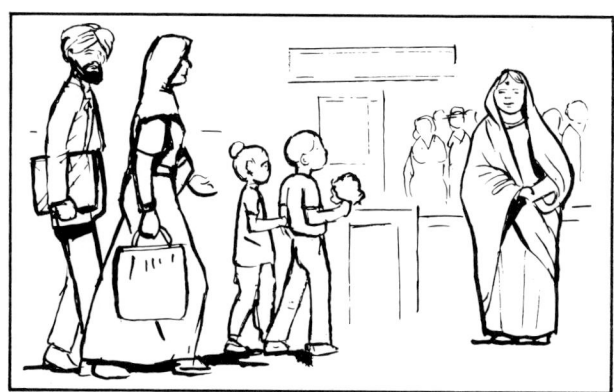

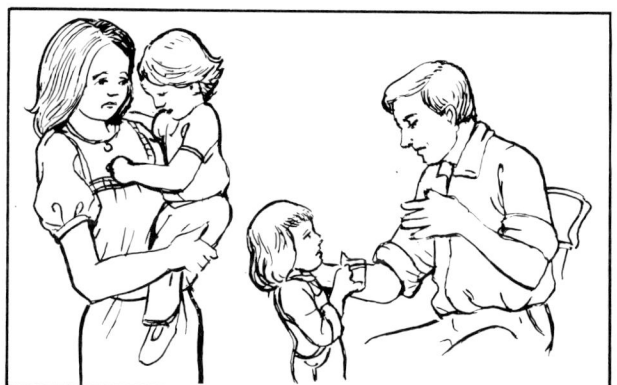

Liza and Lennie say they can remember their grandpa dying. They were only 2 years old.
Why do you think they remember it?

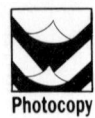
Photocopy

Me and My Relationships

My name is ....

Funny memories

Draw the funniest time you remember:

What made it so funny?

_____

Who else can remember it?

_____

Did they think it was funny?

_____

Why do you think you remember it so well?

_____

Talk with your family or your friends about the funniest
things they remember.
Do you remember any of them?

_____

Me and My Relationships

My name is ....

What are my happiest and saddest memories?

What is the happiest time you remember?

The happiest time I remember was

Draw a picture of it.

_____

When did it happen?

_____

Talk about what made it so happy.
Who else can remember it?

_____

Why do you think you remember it so well?

_____

What is the saddest time you remember?

The saddest time I remember was

Draw a picture of it.

_____

When did it happen?

_____

Talk about what made it so sad.
Who else can remember it?

_____

Why do you think you remember it so well?

_____

Photocopy

Me and My Relationships

My name is ....

Other people's quarrels

Draw yourself listening to some people you know having a quarrel.

Why are they quarrelling?

_____

How do you think they are feeling?

_____

Is there anything you can do?

_____

Talk about how you feel when you have a quarrel.
Draw yourself listening to some people you know quarrelling about you.

Why are they quarrelling?

_____

How do you think they are feeling?
How do you feel when people quarrel about you?

_____

Is there anything you can do?

_____

Talk about what you could say to them.

Me and My Relationships

My name is ....

Feeling sad

Sammy is feeling sad.
One of his special people has gone away and isn't coming back.

What could you say to Sammy to help him feel better?

_____

What could you do to help him feel better?

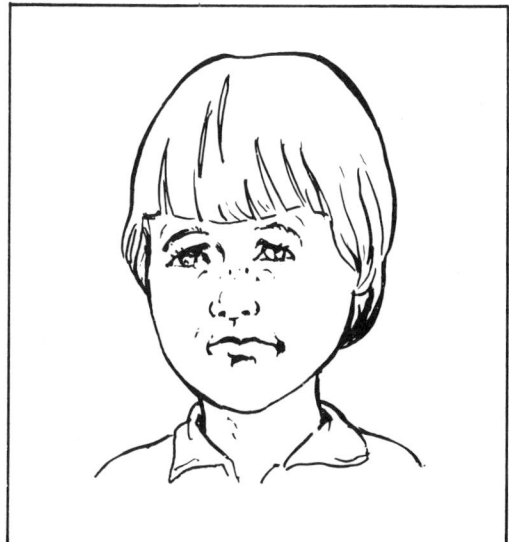

_____

Linzi is feeling sad.
One of her special people has died.

What could people say to Linzi to help her feel better?

_____

What would you have said or done?

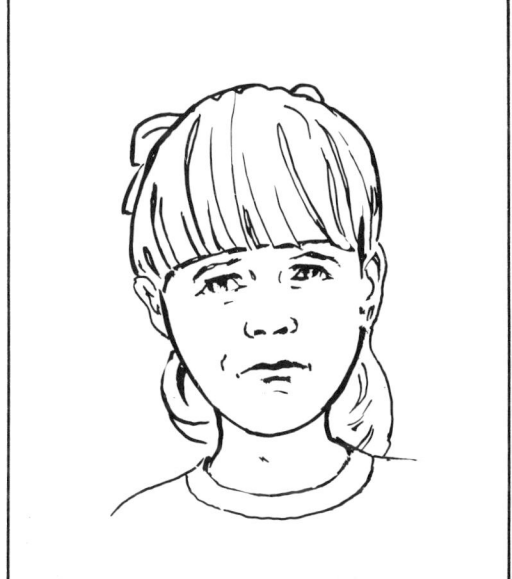

_____

Have you ever felt the way Sammy or Linzi felt?

_____

Appendices

Appendix 1
The Draw and Write Investigation Technique

This classroom technique was originally devised as part of the Health Education Authority's Primary School Project which investigated **The World of Drugs, Keeping Myself Safe** and **Me and My Relationships**. The investigation is described in *A Way in – Five Key Areas of Health Education* D T Williams, N M Wetton and A M H Moon (Health Education Authority, 1989). It is based on drawing and writing activities and can be adapted for use with children aged 4 and over. The children themselves can help in the analysis of the responses. It can be used not only to discover how far children's perceptions and explanations have developed but also as one way of monitoring changes in their perceptions as they work through the programme you have planned.

● *How to organise the draw and write activity for all three topics*

Introduction

Use the introduction given on the relevant instruction sheet. Remember not to discuss the topic with the children beforehand.

● Invite the children to draw and write (or dictate) in response to your instruction or questions. You will only be analysing the written statements (though you will find the pictures very illuminating) so it is important to tell the children that there must be some writing at the side of each picture.

● Remind the children who are dictating their captions or statements that it is important on this occasion to whisper to you, so that others cannot hear.

● Tell the children not to colour their pictures until the end of the activity.

Timing

The activity should be completed in one session. This can vary from 20–30 minutes depending on the age of the class.

Secrecy

To ensure the accuracy of the results, it is important that what the children produce is, as far as possible, their own unaided work. This is why you should prevent them from sharing their ideas. One way of explaining this is to tell them what they are doing is a secret activity, and if they need to ask you for help, they should whisper to you so no one else hears. You can tell older children they are taking part in a survey.

Spelling

If undue emphasis is placed on spelling this may detract from, or prolong, the activity in hand. It is recommended that the children do not use word books to check words they cannot spell; they could spell as they think words should be spelled, or you could write for them the words or phrases they need.

Labelling

It will be helpful when analysing the results if you label each child's paper with their sex and age.

Materials

One A4 sheet of plain paper per child. Pencils and crayons.

Instructions for explaining *The World of Drugs* investigation to the children

Spoken instructions	Permitted prompts and reminders	Beware
'Good morning/Hello. I am going to read you the beginning of a story and then I am going to ask you to draw and write some of your ideas about the people in the story and what they did.'	'Listen to the story carefully.'	Don't mention the word drugs before it appears in the story.
Introduce the activity. (See page 412.) Give suitable names to the children mentioned in the introduction.	Read the introduction twice if you think this is appropriate to your class.	Don't let the children comment out loud, or ask questions. Don't let them share their ideas with others. Don't give them any hints or clues.
Ask the questions on page 412 one at a time, asking the children to draw their answers, and to explain them in writing. Make your own decision about how many questions to ask the class. Ask the children to number their responses.	Remind the children that there are no wrong answers, that all their ideas are right. Remind them to draw and write every time, and to write as much as they like. (The written responses are the ones which are analysed.)	
Conclusion 'Now let's stop. I am going to read the questions through again. make sure you have numbered them.' 'Make sure you have some writing by every drawing.' Older children 'Put at the top of your paper your age and whether you are a boy or a girl, but do not put your name.' Younger children You will probably have to do this for them.	A two or five minute warning is useful. Some children may need your help to number their responses.	Look out for children who are still colouring and have not written anything.

The World of Drugs – the invitation and questions

1 Introduce the activity to the children:
'Cheryl (use any name) was walking home when she found a bag with drugs inside it. Draw what you think was in the bag. If you can, write at the side what it is you have drawn. If you can't write, whisper to me what it is you have drawn and I will write it for you.'

Next, ask the children to continue drawing and writing in response to the following questions and instructions. Not all of these will be appropriate for all the children. You know your children and will be able to make your own decision about where to stop.

2 'Who do you think lost the bag? Draw the person. If you can, write at the side who it is you have drawn. If not, whisper to me and I will write it for you. What kind of person is this?'

3 'Draw and write about what you think that person was going to do with the bag.'

4 'Draw and write about what Cheryl did with the bag.'

5 'What would you have done if you had found it? Write and draw what you would have done.

6 Can a drug be good for you? Can it help you? If so, when? Write and draw about it.

7 Can a drug be bad for you? Or hurt you? If so, when? Write and draw about it.

(The results of **The World of Drugs** investigation, and this technique, have been used by many schools under the name *Jugs and Herrings*. In the original research some 4 year olds interpreted 'drugs' as 'jugs', and many older children spelled 'heroin' as 'herring'.)

Instructions for explaining the Keeping Myself Safe investigation to the children

Spoken instructions	Permitted prompts and reminders	Beware
'Good morning/Hello. It's good to find you have all got here safely. Today I want you to think about all the things you have to keep safe from, and how you keep yourself safe indoors and outdoors. Don't tell me or anyone about them. Keep them in your head until we are ready to draw and write.'	'There are no right or wrong answers. All your ideas are right.' Think about keeping safe wherever you are, wherever you go, indoors and out.	Don't mention danger, dangerous people, places or things. Don't mention any recent accidents.
Invite the children to draw and write in response to the questions on page 414, and to work through them one at a time.	Tell the children they can draw as many pictures as they wish. Remind them that every drawing must have some writing alongside it. Remind them that they are thinking about *what* they are keeping safe from and *how* they are keeping safe.	Don't let the children comment out loud, or ask questions. Don't let them share their ideas with others. Don't give them any hints or clues.
Conclusion Remind the children that every drawing must have some writing alongside it. Ask the children to label their response sheets: *Indoors* on the front, and *Outdoors* on the back. You could write these two words on the blackboard.	Remind the children that there are no wrong answers, and that all their ideas are right. Remind them to draw and write every time and to write as much as they like. (The written responses are the ones which are analysed.) Make sure that each response sheet is marked with the child's age and sex.	Look out for children who spend too much time colouring their pictures and do not write. Suggest that colouring is left until the end of the activity.

Keeping Myself Safe – *the invitation and questions*

1 Ask the children to 'Draw yourself indoors keeping yourself safe'.

2 While they are drawing ask them the following questions:

a 'What are you keeping yourself safe from? Draw and write about all the things you are keeping safe from. If you need help with spellings or writing, whisper to me and I will help you.'

b 'How are you keeping yourself safe? Write down how you are keeping safe. If you need help with the writing, whisper to me and I will write for you.'

3 Tell the children: 'Now turn your paper over and draw yourself keeping safe outdoors.' Repeat questions 2a and 2b with the same offer of help.

4 Finally ask the children to draw and write in response to the question: 'Whose job is it to keep you safe wherever you are?'

Instructions for explaining the *Me and My Relationships* investigation.

Spoken instructions	Permitted prompts and reminders	Beware
'Good morning/Hello. Today I want you to think about the people who are very special to you. Don't tell me or anyone about them. Keep it in your head till we're ready to draw and write.'	'There are no right or wrong answers. All your ideas are right.' They can be people in your family or other people who are special to you.	Don't mention terms such as 'love', 'care for', 'care about', 'take care of', 'relationships' etc.
Invite the children to draw and write in response to the questions on page 415 working through them one at a time. Make your own decision about how many questions your class can cope with.	Remind them they are thinking about their special people.	Don't let the children comment out loud, or ask questions. Don't let them share their ideas with others. Don't give hints or clues.
Conclusion Remind the children that every drawing must have some writing alongside it. Ask the children to number their responses.	Remind the children that there are no wrong answers, that all their ideas are right. Remind them to draw and write every time, and to write as much as they like. (The written responses are the ones which are analysed.)	Look out for the children who spend too much time colouring their pictures and do not write. Suggest that colouring is left until the end of the activity.

Me and My Relationships – the invitation and questions

Ask the children to draw and write in response to these instructions:

1 'Draw the people who are special to you. If you can, write down who they are. If you can't write, whisper to me and I will write for you.'

2 'Draw what you do to make them happy. Write down how you make them happy. If you can't write, whisper to me and I will write for you.'

3 'Draw what you do to make them cross. Write down how you make them cross. If you can't write, whisper to me and I will write for you.'

The following questions will not be appropriate for all the children. You know your children and will be able to make your own decision about where to stop. Some children may prefer to draw first and add their written answers afterwards.

4 'What is the happiest thing you can remember? Write it down. If you can't, I will help you'.

5 'What is the saddest thing you can remember? Write it down. If you can't, I will help you.'

6 'Write down the things you like about your best friend.'

7 'Write down the things your best friend likes about you.'

8 'What do people do to make you happy?'

How to analyse the children's responses

You can use the following categories (used in the original research) to code and analyse each child's work. Alternatively you may wish to develop your own categories for analysing the responses your children make. On each child's paper make a note of, or code, the categories you think have been illustrated and written about.

The World of Drugs

Question 1   ***What was in the bag?***

- Tablets/powders/medicines.

- Cigarettes.

- Needles/syringes.

- Poison.

- Alcohol.

- Glue.

- Matches/foil.

- Straws/droppers.

- Specifically named drugs.

- Other objects.

Question 2   ***Who had lost the bag?***

- Legitimate owners (doctors, nurses, etc).

- Grown-ups.

- Teenagers.

- Relatives (my uncle, brother, sisters etc).

- Criminals ('robbers').

- Dealers/pushers.

- Addicts.

- Named people (including television characters).

Question 3   ***What was the person going to do with the drugs?***

- Eat it.

- Inject it.

- Keep it.

- Share or hand it on to others.

- Sell it.

- Dispose of it/destroy it.

Question 4 | **What did the child do with it?**

- Hand it to the authorities.

- Take it home to Mum/Dad.

- Eat/take/use/keep.

- Dispose of it, destroy it.

- Ignore it.

- Sell it.

- Find the owner.

Question 5 | **What would you have done?**

Categories as (4) above, including:

- Don't know.

Question 6 | **Can a drug be good for you or help you?**

- Yes.

- No.

- Yes and no.

- Don't know.

Question 7 | **Can a drug be bad for you or hurt you?**

Categories as (6) above.

Keeping Myself Safe

Question 2a | **What are you keeping safe from?**

- Imaginary dangers.
  For example, aliens, ghosts, monsters.

- Not quite so imaginary dangers.
  For example, the dark, outside, something creeping upstairs, frightening films and videos.

- People.
  For example, bullies, strangers, people who tell you off, glue sniffers, muggers and drunks.

- Places and situations.
  For example, dark places, rivers, traffic, dangerous buildings, getting lost, getting locked in or out, crowds, being attacked, getting involved in fighting, vandalism or taking drugs.

- Objects.
  For example, household or garden equipment, unknown liquids or powders, fireworks, alcohol, cigarettes and medicines.

Question 2b

How are you keeping safe?

(**From imaginary dangers**)

- Hide your eyes

- Hide under or inside beds, cupboards, bedcovers etc.

(**From people**)

- Stay with Mum.

- Run away.

- Shout and cry.

- Play close to home.

- Don't let them in.

- Keep away/ignore.

- Don't talk/take lifts.

- Tell someone.

(**From places and situations**)

- Don't go.

- Don't tease/boast/fool about.

- Don't get dragged in.

- Listen to instructions.

- Keep out of the way.

- Don't behave badly.

- Know the rules.

(**From objects**)

- Don't touch.

- Keep out of the way.

- Don't break things.

- Learn how to do things/ask a grown-up.

- Mind you don't . . .

- Watch out for little children's safety.

Question 4

Whose job is it to keep you safe?

- Parent/family member.

- Other adults.
  For example, police, crossing patrol person, teacher, doctor.

- Organisations.
  For example, church government, social services.

- Self.

Me and My Relationships

Question 1

Who are the people special to you?

- Parents.

- Nuclear family.

- Extended family.

- Friends.

- God.

- Teachers.

- Others.

Question 2

What do you do to make them happy?

- Help them.

- Be good/well-behaved.

- Love them.

- Give them things.

- Share things with others.

- Keep out of the way.

- Work hard at school.

Question 3

What do you do to make them cross?

- Misbehave.

- Tease/annoy.
- Hurt them.
- Damage things.
- Make mess or noise.
- Be unhelpful.
- Ask for money.

Question 4   *What is the happiest thing you remember?*

- Special occasions.
- Being given material things.
- Family life.
- Friendship.
- Personal achievements.
- Being young/being a baby.

Question 5   *What is the saddest thing you remember?*

- Death of grandparents/family member.
- Death of a pet.
- Personal injury/illness.
- Other people's illnesses.
- Missing special occasions.
- Family separation or break-up.
- People upsetting me.
- Being punished.
- Broken friendship.

Question 6   *What are the things you like about your best friend?*

- Playing with them.
- Personality.
- Getting their help.
- Their looks/the clothes they wear/the things they own.
- Sharing things.
- Gifts.

- Personality.
- Loyalty.

Question 7

What are the things your best friend likes about you?

- Playing with me.
- Because I give him/her things.
- My personality.
- My looks, my belongings.
- Sharing things.
- My qualities.
- My loyalty.

Question 8

What do people do to make you happy?

- Love me.
- Look after me.
- Give me things.
- Help me.
- Kiss and cuddle me.
- Listen to me.
- Respect me.
- Make me feel good.

Appendix 2

Resources

The books, videos and television programmes listed below are just a small selection from the many useful resources available. You will no doubt accumulate your own collection of materials, many children's books can be used in the context of work on 'health'.

As well as consulting teachers' centres and local libraries, you can contact your local Health Education Unit or 'Health Promotion Unit'. This may be listed under the name of your health authority in the phone book but if you cannot find it, contact the Liaison Section of the Health Education Authority or ask at your local Community Health Centre or local library. This service is normally run by Health Education Officers and generally includes advisory services, the loan of materials and the supply of Health Education Authority publications.

The Health Education Authority offers a subscription service to individuals and organisations concerned with Health Education. Subscribers receive a copy of the *Health Education Authority's Annual Report*, copies of the *Health Education News*, published bi-monthly, a copy of the *Library List and Journal Articles of Interest to Health Educators*, and a copy of each new leaflet and poster as published.

The Health Education Authority also supplies *Books for Children 5–8: an annotated bibliography with relevance to health education*, and *Teaching Aids for children 5–8: an annotated list with relevance to health education*. These lists are also available for ages 9–13. These are available free of charge from the Information Centre, Health Education Authority, Hamilton House, Mabledon Place, London WC1H 9TX.

The World of Drugs

Teacher's books and resources

What to do about glue-sniffing Health Education Authority (booklet)
Advice on the misuse of glue and other solvents.

Smoking and Pollution Family Smoking Project (Health Education Authority, 1988)
Pupils' booklet, parents' leaflet, teachers' guide. Promotes discussion about the effects of smoking on health, other people, the atmosphere and developing countries.

Health Education – Drugs and the Primary School Child TACADE (Teachers' Advisory Council for Alcohol and Drug Education, 1986)
A curriculum package for use with 9–11 year-olds consisting of an introductory unit, modules for teachers, parents and pupils, plus 61 slides. The pack aims to create awareness amongst pupils, teachers and parents of drugs, and their use and abuse.

My Body A Health Education Council Project (Heinemann Educational Books 1983)
Workcards, games pack, teacher's book. A curriculum project for 10–12 year olds, designed to help pupils learn about their bodies and explore various aspects of human biology and health care. Contains a strong anti-smoking element.

The Good Health Project Trefor Williams, Noreen Wetton and Alysoun Moon (Forbes Publications Ltd, 1986)
A series of booklets containing teaching notes and photocopiable worksheets designed to accompany the Central TV Series.

Television programmes

Good Health – Drugs (Channel 4)
For 8–12 year olds. The aim of this series is to promote health education within the primary and middle school and to encourage children to take increasing responsibility for looking after themselves and each other.

Useful addresses

ISDD (Institute for the Study of Drug Dependence) 1–4 Hatton Place, Hatton Place, London, EC1N 8ND. 01–439–1991.

TACADE (Teachers' Advisory Council on Alcohol and Drug Education) 3rd Floor, Furness House, Trafford Road, Salford, M5 2XJ. 061–848–0351.

Health Matters, 7 Wetherburn Court, Brunell Centre, Bletchley, MK2 2OH. 0908–270426.

Health Information Service, Lister Hospital, Corey's Mill Lane, Stevenage, SG1 4AB. 0438–314333, ext 520 or 431.

Help for Health, Health Information Centre, Grant Building, Southampton General Hospital, Southampton, SO9 4XY, 0703–779091.

Facts Centre, Frenchay Hospital, Frenchay, Bristol, BS16 ILE, 0272–701212, ext 2033.

Asthma Society and Friends of the Asthma Research Council, 300 Upper Street, London, N1 2XX. 01–226–2260.

British Diabetic Association, 10 Queen Anne Street, London, W1M OBD. 01–323–1531.

British Epilepsy Association, Anstey House, 40 Hanover Square, Leeds, LS3 1BE, 0532–439393.

National Eczema Society, Tavistock House East, Tavistock Square, London, WC1H 9SR, 01–388–4097.

Keeping Myself Safe

Teacher's books and resources

Preventing Child Sexual Assault Michele Elliott (Bedford Square Press/NVCO, 1985)
A helpful starter and 'confidence booster' for anyone wishing to tackle this crucial subject in school or at home. Michele Elliott gives practical advice on teaching children about their right to be safe. She also suggests what to do if abuse is suspected or occurs, and gives a list of organisations to turn to for further support.

Child Abuse: an educational perspective ed. Peter Maher (Blackwell, 1987)

Play safe Understanding Electricity Education Service. Three A3 posters and one A5 leaflet. Free. The leaflet illustrates accidents involving children and electricity to warn them of the dangers, while the posters can be used to back up the film/video 'Play Safe', or as an independent teaching aid conveying the same message.

Safety at Home and School Chris North for Science Horizons: West Sussex Science 5–14 Scheme (Macmillan Education, 1984)
A 46-page, A4 book consisting of loose-leaf sheets in a slide binder, with information for the teacher followed by 'activity sheets' which can be photocopied. *Safety at Home and School* is from Level 2a of the Science Horizons Scheme and is designed for use with 7–11 year olds. The aims of the unit are to make pupils safety-conscious at home and school, to highlight dangers and help children avoid accidents, and to teach the safe use of tools and apparatus.

Children and Traffic (Macmillan)
A pack of books and cards

Play it Safe (Health Education Authority, 1987)
How to prevent accidents to babies, toddlers and young school-age children.
Includes what to do in an emergency and basic first-aid.

A Curriculum for Road Safety Education (RoSPA, 1983) 6-page A4 booklet,
illustrated in colour. Copies available free from the Safety Education Department,
RoSPA.
A basic curriculum guide looking at the early and middle years of schooling, and
suggesting a rationale, goals and possible content of road safety education for both
age ranges, as well as briefly listing suitable RoSPA materials. A handy starting
point for any teacher planning work on this topic.

Books for children

No More Secrets For Me Oralee Wachter (Puffin, 1986)
Four stories with a multi-cultural background, about preventing child abuse.

First Aid R. Thomson (Orbis)

Not Now, Bernard D McKee (Anderson Press)

Television programmes and videos

Kids Can Say No! Rolf Harris video (Rolf Harris Video Ltd., 1985)
Also available from CFL Vision/Concord Films Council Ltd. for hire and purchase).
A 20-minute video for 5–11 year olds aimed at preventing child sexual abuse. Four
abusive incidents are enacted, ranging from approaches by strangers to sexual
advances by the father. The children talk about what to do – say 'No', get away fast
and tell someone you trust. The video comes with teaching notes and two books –
Preventing Child Sexual Assault by Michele Elliott, and *Sexual Abuse within the
Family* by the CIBA Foundation. Asterisks appear at the bottom of the screen
when suitable points to break for discussion occur.

Feeling Yes, Feeling No Video by the National Film Board of Canada (Educational
Media International/Concord Films Council Ltd., 1984) A video in four sections,
three for children and one for adults. Total running time 71 mins. Aimed at any
educator concerned about the prevention of sexual abuse of children.

Good Health – Keeping safe (Channel 4) See page 423 for a description of the
series.

Watch Out! (Central TV. Guild, Sound and Vision Ltd.)
Zab, the robot from outer space, finds out about safety on the road and in the
home.

How to have an Accident at Home (Walt Disney Productions, 1956)
An animated cartoon in which Donald Duck suffers every imaginable accident in his home through carelessness. Still amusing and instructive despite its age.

Rolf Harris Water Safety (Rolf Harris Video Ltd, 1982, purchase only. CFL Vision/Concord Films Council Ltd, hire and purchase)
A video in three parts: 'Spot the Danger' (14 mins) 'Boating and Falling into Cold Water' (17 mins), and 'Reach, throw, wade, row' (23 mins). The presentation is sometimes verbose, but Rolf's advice is friendly and informal and twice reinforced with catch songs. Four young swimmers help him to give practical demonstrations of most of the safety messages.

One Step Ahead (Devon Educational Television Service, 1981)
9 minute video, purchase only. A film which covers aspects of road safety that are particularly relevant to children living in rural areas. Situations featured include getting off the school bus in a country lane, crossing the road safely, and how to walk along a country road with no pavement. The children are encouraged to follow the example of the fox shown in the film by being alert to possible dangers and always thinking ahead.

Say No to Strangers (COI for the Home Office, 1981, CFL Vision)
15 minute video, for hire (free) or purchase. A film to alert 8–10 year olds to the dangers of accepting lifts, sweets etc from strangers. Support from parents and teachers is vital if the film is to succeed in warning rather than frightening the children. (The Home Office advise that a police officer be present at the screening.)

All Year Round – Keeping safe (Channel 4)
A series to encourage the development of science and health education with top infants and first year juniors.

Whirligig (Channel 4)
For lower juniors. A unit in the summer term entitled 'Looking after Me' may contain programmes of relevance. Topics covered include health and hygiene; safety in the home, park, playground and streets; coping with the loss of a relative or friend; and saying 'No'.

Useful addresses

Understanding Electricity Education Service, Electricity Council, 30 Millbank, London, SW1P 4RD.

RoSPA (Royal Society for the Prevention of Accidents) Cannon House, The Priory, Queensway, Birmingham, B4 6BS.

Child Accident Prevention Trust, 28 Portland Place, London W1N 4DE.

Home Surveillance, Department of Trade and Industry, Millbank Tower, Millbank, London SW1P 4QU.
(A source of statistics on accidents in the home.)

Me and My Relationships

Teacher's books and resources

Startline Schools Council Moral Education 8–13 Project (Longman Group, 1978).
The aim of the pack is to encourage children to develop greater social awareness,
to appreciate the needs and feelings of others and to acquire basic social skills. The
pack is made up of many separate items, including stories, posters, workcards and a
handbook entitled 'Moral Education in the Middle Years'.

Personal and Social Skills Nigel Leech and Arthur D. Wooster (Religious and Moral
Education Press, 1986)
A book of activities for children.

Sex Education: Some Guidelines for Teachers D. J. Went (Bell and Hyman, 1985)

What Shall We Tell the Children? Peter Moyle (W. H. Allen, 1979)
About divorce.

Roles, Relationships, Responsibilities. Chris Abuk for the Lambeth Health
Education Project, 1982. (ILEA Learning Resources Branch.)
Pack of 48 black and white A4 drawings on stiff card with notes for teachers. The
drawings are of a wide range of open-ended and multi-ethnic situations relevant to
young people. Teachers of health and personal and social education should find one
or more cards useful in many of their classes to trigger small-group discussion or
stimulate role-play. No written information or questions are attached to any of
the drawings in order to encourage a variety of interpretations.

Books for children

A Baby in the Family Althea Braithwaite (Dinosaur, 1981)
For parents to read to children about the arrival of a new baby.

Jane is Adopted Althea Braithwaite (Souvenir Press, Brightstart Series, 1980)
A straightforward book about adoption that will help families discuss the topic
openly.

George and the Baby Althea Braithwaite (Dinosaur, 1973)
A dog feels rejected, thereby expressing the feelings other children have when a
new baby arrives.

My New Family Althea Braithwaite (Dinosaur, 1984)
The transfer from a home to being fostered reveals for the first time to a primary
school girl that families can have rows without splitting up.

Peter Pig Althea Braithwaite (Dinosaur, 1973)
Peter finds that people who look different can still be friends.

Smith, the Lonely Hedgehog Althea Braithwaite (Dinosaur, 1977)
Smith is shy and lonely, but eventually finds a friend.

It's Your Turn, Roger Susanna Gretz (Armada, 1986)
A humorous book about a little pig learning about taking turns.

Moving Molly Shirley Hughes (Armada, 1981)
A little girl moves house, but soon finds new friends.

Badger on the Barge Janni Howker (Heinemann Educational Books New Windmills Series, 1987)
Five stories which focus on encounters between young and old.

The Young Puffin Book of Verse compiled by Barbara Ireson (Puffin, 1970)
Contains 'Cats Sleep Anywhere' by Eleanor Farjeon and many more enjoyable verses for the youngest children.

My Naughty Little Sister Dorothy Edwards (Magnet, 1982)
A mother's stories, told to her children about the little sister of her childhood.

Trouble with Jack Shirley Hughes (Corgi, 1986)
Picture Lion series. The trouble with Nancy's brother Jack was that he was not a tidy person at all, but she had to learn to put up with him whatever he was like.

Titch Pat Hutchins (Picture Puffin, 1974)
Titch was the smallest in the family. He had a big sister and an even bigger brother, and everything they had seemed bigger and better, until Titch planted a seed that grew, and grew.

We are Best Friends Aliki (Bodley Head)

Feelings Aliki (Bodley Head)

He is your Brother R Parker (Hodder & Stoughton)

David and his Grandfather P Rogers (Young Puffin)

Comfort Herself Geraldine Kaye (Heinemann Educational Books New Windmill Series, 1987)
The story of a black child moving between two countries: England and Ghana.

Television programmes and videos

Watch BBC2
A series of five programmes for 5–7 year olds which aims to widen the experiences of young children and to stimulate project work.

Sex Education (BBC Enterprises, 1983)
(Film Hire and Purchase.) Three programmes: 'Growing', 'Someone New', 'Life Begins' (each 20 minutes)

Who – me? (BBC)

For the upper primary level. A series exploring some of the personal and social issues affecting children's lives. Each programme is a fictional drama based on children's experiences or a dramatic reconstruction of real events. Topics include moving home, family responsibilities and peer group pressures.

Problem Page (Central TV Guild, Sound and Vision Ltd.)

A group of schoolchildren investigate bullying. Some children are bullied because they are fat, or because of their skin colour. Some are called names, others teased, and some are physically abused. What can be done about the problem?

Good Health – Summer Story (Channel 4)

A programme about relationships in which Alan and Kim have different ideas about their responsibilities towards their younger sister when they set out to explore a lake near their holiday caravan.

Useful addresses

Family Planning Association, Education Unit, 27–35 Mortimer Street, London,
W1N 7RJ.

InterAction, HMS President, Victoria Embankment, London EC4Y 0HJ.